THE RISE AND FALL OF NATIONAL WOMEN'S HOSPITAL

THE RISE AND FALL OF NATIONAL WOMEN'S HOSPITAL

A HISTORY

LINDA BRYDER

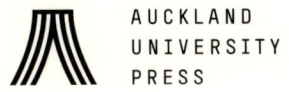

AUCKLAND UNIVERSITY PRESS

First published 2014

Auckland University Press
University of Auckland
Private Bag 92019
Auckland 1142
New Zealand
www.press.auckland.ac.nz

© Linda Bryder, 2014

ISBN 978 1 86940 809 1

National Library of New Zealand Cataloguing-in-Publication Data
Bryder, Linda.
The rise and fall of National Women's Hospital : a history /
Linda Bryder.
Includes bibliographical references and index.
ISBN 978-1-86940-809-1
1. National Women's Hospital (Auckland, N.Z.)—History.
2. Women's health services—Auckland—New Zealand—History
—20th century. I. Title.
362.11099324—dc 23

This book is copyright. Apart from fair dealing for the purpose of private study, research, criticism or review, as permitted under the Copyright Act, no part may be reproduced by any process without prior permission of the publisher.

Cover design: Duncan Munro
Front cover: National Women's Hospital staff, early 1960s.
Photograph courtesy of Glenda Stimpson
Back cover: 'National Women's Hospital: Perspective View from Green Lane', c. 1960.
Archives New Zealand, Auckland

Printed in China through Asia Pacific Offset Limited

CONTENTS

Acknowledgements		vii
Abbreviations		ix
Introduction		1
1	Childbirth Services in New Zealand, 1900–1939	9
2	National Women's Hospital and the Postgraduate School of Obstetrics and Gynaecology	26
3	A Tripod: Patient Care, Research and Teaching, the 1950s to 1963	46
4	A Woman's World: Mothers, Nurses and Midwives at National Women's, the 1950s to 1963	70
5	From Premature Nursery to Paediatric Department, 1950s to 1963	88
6	A Bright New Age: Advances in Reproductive Medicine, 1964–1980s	103
7	The New Patient and Perinatal Medicine	117
8	Contraception, Sterilisation and Abortion	142
9	Obstetrics and the Winds of Change, 1964–1980s	166
10	Feminists, Midwives and National Women's Hospital	190
11	A Hospital in Trouble, 1990–2004	210
Conclusion		234
Notes		243
Bibliography		294
Index		314

ACKNOWLEDGEMENTS

Since it opened in 1946, National Women's Hospital has been a special place for many Auckland women and the host to a very important event in their lives: childbirth. This includes my mother, my sister and me. My sister was born at the hospital and I paid a brief visit to the 'premature ward' as a one-day-old. My sister's children and my children were subsequently born there, although my first (in 1992) had been planned as a home birth, following the social trends of the day. This generational story can no doubt be repeated by many Auckland women. However, this personal connection was not the motivating factor in writing this history. My academic career has always been in the field of medical and social history, and my interest in the hospital was sparked whilst working on the history of the Royal New Zealand Plunket Society (*A Voice for Mothers*, AUP, 2003). It was not difficult to see that the absence of an academic history of National Women's Hospital was a major gap in Auckland and New Zealand's medical and social history. In 2003 I successfully applied to the Royal Society Marsden Fund to research the history of women's health with a special emphasis on National Women's Hospital. During the course of my general research into the hospital I was diverted into investigating one aspect of the hospital's history, the 1987–88 Cartwright Inquiry. I felt it important to understand this important event in the hospital's history, and my research led me to some surprising conclusions (*A History of the 'Unfortunate Experiment' at National Women's Hospital*, AUP, 2009). Now my original, more encompassing, history has finally reached fruition.

Overseas trips to speak to specialist groups and to participate in international conferences are an important part of the research process, enabling constructive feedback and ensuring an eye to international trends. I wish to thank the Marsden Fund for facilitating these opportunities, as well as my colleagues overseas who so willingly listened to me and commented on my work. The Marsden Grant also funded related graduate research projects, completed with distinction by Claire Gooder (PhD thesis) and Gabrielle Bourke and Christina Jeffery (MA theses).

I wish to thank Dr Jenny Carlyon for conducting the interviews for the project, which she undertook with flair and sensitivity. I also wish to thank the people who so generously gave their time and memories of the hospital to enhance the project, and Barbara Batt for typing the transcripts. Thanks too to Glenda Stimpson for facilitating the placement of the Joan Donley papers at the University of Auckland Special Collections, ensuring that this valuable archive is in a secure location for future historical research, and to Stephen Innes, Manager of the Collections, for his speedy and efficient cataloguing of the material. I also appreciated the helpful and friendly staff at the other archives I visited, including the libraries of Parents' Centre, Wellington, and the Royal College of Obstetricians and Gynaecologists, London. The team at AUP have my deep appreciation and in particular AUP director Dr Sam Elworthy for his unstinting support and enthusiasm for history. I am very grateful to Dr Ginny Sullivan for once again bringing an astute eye to the manuscript as copy editor, and for her unerring commitment to the task despite nursing a broken foot. I wish to thank my sons, not only for giving me the experience of childbirth but for being there, and finally my partner Derek for his eternal support and patience. I dedicate this book to my mother, Else Bryder, and to my sister, Janne Saunders.

ABBREVIATIONS

AJHR	*Appendices to the Journals of the House of Representatives*
AMA	Auckland Museum Archives
ANZA	Archives New Zealand, Auckland
ANZW	Archives New Zealand, Wellington
BMJ	*British Medical Journal*
CPAP	continuous positive airways pressure
FNZPC	Federation of New Zealand Parents' Centres
FRCS	Fellow of the Royal College of Surgeons
HMC	Hospital Medical Committee
IUD	intrauterine device
IVF	*in vitro* fertilisation
MRCNZ	Medical Research Council of New Zealand
MRCOG	Member of the Royal College of Obstetricians and Gynaecologists
NCW	National Council of Women
NICU	Neonatal Intensive Care Unit
NMRB	Nurses and Midwives Registration Board
NZBMA	New Zealand Branch of the British Medical Association
NZCOM	New Zealand College of Midwives
NZFPA	New Zealand Family Planning Association
NZFUW	New Zealand Federation of University Women
NZH	*New Zealand Herald*
NZMA	New Zealand Medical Association
NZMJ	*New Zealand Medical Journal*
NZNJ	*New Zealand Nursing Journal: Kai Tiaki*
NZOS	New Zealand Obstetrical Society
NZOGS	New Zealand Obstetrical and Gynaecological Society
NZPD	*New Zealand Parliamentary Debates*
NZSPWC	New Zealand Society for the Protection of Women and Children
NZWW	*New Zealand Woman's Weekly*
PSA	Plunket Society Archives

RCOG	Royal College of Obstetricians and Gynaecologists
RDS	respiratory distress syndrome
SCBU	Special Care Babies Unit
SPUC	Society for the Protection of the Unborn Child
UOAA	Archives, Office of the Vice-Chancellor, University of Auckland
UOASC	University of Auckland Library, Special Collections
WHO	World Health Organization

INTRODUCTION

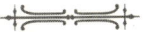

AT THE OPENING OF NEW ZEALAND'S NEW PURPOSE-BUILT NATIONAL Women's Hospital in 1964 Sir Douglas Robb, Chancellor of the University of Auckland, recounted his feelings upon returning from overseas and hearing the news of the first-ever successful antenatal blood transfusion, performed at the hospital. He said, 'No longer do we necessarily turn our back on intellectual and scientific progress when we leave Europe and America for "down-under". Here we were heading towards the news and not away from it. It was a grand feeling for a native New Zealander.'[1] Almost fifty years later an expatriate professor of haematology at the University of Cambridge wrote, 'The incorporation of advances in medical science into clinical practice is led by the great teaching hospitals of the world. Not only are these found in the predictable clusters of Boston, London and Paris but they are also dotted in unexpected places throughout the globe. New Zealand has one such centre of excellence, the National Women's Hospital in Auckland.' He proceeded to explain that National Women's was an acknowledged international leader in the medical care of mothers and the newborn, through the specialties known as obstetrics and gynaecology, and that its reputation was built on the quality of its teaching and patient care together with the constant research and questioning that was the mark of a teaching hospital.[2] This view was not uncommon. On her appointment as professor of obstetrics and gynaecology to the hospital's postgraduate school in 1992, British doctor Gillian Turner declared that most obstetricians in Britain had been brought up knowing about National Women's Hospital: 'it was a household name in Britain'.[3] Profiled in the *New Zealand Herald* later that year, she recounted how, when she undertook obstetrical and gynaecological training at London's Hammersmith Hospital in the 1960s, everyone knew of National Women's. She said it had 'an enormously high international profile'.[4]

By the time of Turner's appointment, however, the hospital's research programme was in tatters, its leaders in disgrace and its public image at an all-time low. When her predecessor as professor, Dennis Bonham, died in 2005 the *New Zealand Herald* declared that he would be best remembered for the role he played in the 'Unfortunate Experiment', and ignored his long and distinguished career, both nationally and internationally, which had spanned three decades.[5] The so-called 'Unfortunate Experiment' led to the 1987–88 Inquiry into Cervical Cancer at National Women's Hospital, also known as the 'Cartwright Inquiry' after its chair, Silvia Cartwright. In the popular consciousness, this drama continues to overshadow other aspects of the hospital's history. It was for this reason, during my research into the history of the hospital, that I decided to publish separately on that episode.[6] It is now time to try to restore some balance to the history of what was clearly an important institution in New Zealand's medical history.

Yet this is no celebratory history of the achievements of the hospital and the medical advances it introduced. While it is important to explain how New Zealand, a small and remote South Pacific country, came to contribute so significantly at an international level, this is not my sole intention. Rather, I argue that other aspects of the hospital's history are equally important. Specifically, through exploring the hospital's social history and the interaction of its staff with patients, consumer and professional groups, and the government, this study will contribute to our understanding of the broader development of services relating to reproductive health during the second half of the twentieth century. A *New Zealand Listener* article, which appeared in the mid-1980s before the publicity surrounding the Cartwright Inquiry hit the headlines, declared: 'National Women's is news; always has been. Over the last two decades, women's health has become a hot topic and women's bodies have been the focus for some ferocious power struggles, and some of the messiest battles going – abortion, the politics of birth, the status of women's bodies in a teaching hospital, contraceptive crises like the Dalkon shield debacle.'[7] This history sets out to investigate some of these 'messy' social and ethical issues through the lens of National Women's Hospital.

My previous book, on the Cartwright Inquiry, focused on the history of gynaecological cancer and pre-cancer at National Women's Hospital. This history briefly revisits the Inquiry and the issues surrounding it in order to explain its impact on the hospital and as one aspect of the hospital's history. However, the predominant focus of this volume is reproductive health: childbirth, fertility and perinatal medicine. Since the 1970s there have been many studies internationally on the history of childbirth, prompted by the new discipline of the social history of medicine and the emerging women's movement. In the introduction to her ground-breaking 1986 history of childbirth, *Brought to Bed: Childbearing in America, 1750–1950*, Judith Walzer Leavitt explained, 'This book focuses on the phenomenon of birth precisely because of its centrality to women's lives. By understanding childbirth we can understand significant parts of the female experience.'[8] Leavitt's study included an analysis of diaries, letters and autobiographies, from which she concluded that women were active agents of change in American childbirth history, until, she said, childbirth moved to the hospital when they lost control over the birthing experience to the medical profession, 'and began their quest, continuing today, to recover some of that control'.[9]

The history of twentieth-century childbirth by some feminist historians has been a story of women's disempowerment as they were forced by a male medical profession into hospital and into accepting ever-increasing technological interventions, often through scare tactics. In her 1998 study of the history of childbirth in Ireland, Jo Murphy-Lawless described the historiography since the 1970s: 'writers have converged around the convincing thesis that male medical control of childbirth has disempowered women as mothers and as care-givers, principally through its argument that childbirth is full of risks and danger, that it is pathological and thus requires the medical expert to oversee the event'.[10]

Obstetricians have been given a particularly bad press in these histories. Barbara Ehrenreich and Deirdre English's 1973 study, *Witches, Nurses and Midwives*, portrayed American obstetricians as 'self-serving individuals who "had no real commitment to improved obstetrical care", and who systematically sought to outlaw midwifery in order to gain a monopoly over this potentially lucrative field of practice'.[11] In Britain an influential history by medical sociologist Ann Oakley, *The Captured Womb* (1984), sought to explain the evolution of antenatal care and obstetrical intervention as a 'strategy for the social control of women'.[12] Whilst she acknowledged that 'in the battle to prevent every fatality that is conceivably preventable, medical antenatal care must be counted as an essential ally',[13] she nevertheless labelled obstetricians and the state as 'misogynist', and explained how 'womanhood and motherhood have become a battlefield for not only patriarchal but professional supremacy'.[14] A decade later a 'critical history of maternity care' in Britain, written by Marjorie Tew, argued that women were indoctrinated by doctors, through an 'unremitting campaign of propaganda', to go to hospital to give birth rather than stay home.[15] She explained, 'The policy of the increasing hospitalisation of birth advocated by doctors, allegedly to improve the welfare of mothers and babies, was in fact a very effective means of gaining competitive advantage by reducing the power and status of midwives and confirming the doctors' ascendancy over their professional rivals'; she also claimed it was a 'promising gateway to assuring their [doctors'] social importance'.[16] Nor, in her view, did this change once women were in hospital, where the obstetrician 'reasserts his superiority most emphatically when he cuts open the womb and extracts the baby without any co-operation from the mother, an intervention apparently so deeply satisfying to the operator that, now that its danger to life is relatively small, is imposed on ever slighter pretexts'.[17]

New Zealand had its own local variants of this mode of history writing in books by Joan Donley (1986), and Elaine Papps and Mark Olssen (1997).[18] Donley's book, *Save the Midwife*, spanned the period from the start of colonisation and included a chapter on National Women's Hospital. During the 1988 Inquiry, she sent a copy to Judge Cartwright, who thanked her for her assistance in 'putting into perspective certain historical matters'.[19] In her obituary of Joan Donley in the *New Zealand Herald*, Phoebe Falconer wrote of *Save the Midwife* that Donley 'charted the history of the profession'.[20] Yet Donley's was a very particular perspective, for she approached the subject as a midwife and feminist activist, providing a view of the history of childbirth in which doctors were depicted as self-interested whilst midwives acted in the interests of their clients, the mothers. She explained her views on women's lack of agency in the past when she wrote in the introduction to the 1998 reprint of *Save the Midwife* that, 'After 50 years of being "under the doctor" it is difficult for women to overcome their fear-based medical dependence and opt to regain control of their bodies and their births.'²¹ She set out her perspective on National Women's Hospital in her comparison of the logo used by the National Women's Postgraduate School of Obstetrics and Gynaecology (the women's earth sign, surrounding a map of New Zealand) with those of organisations that were led by women and/or midwives such as 'La Leche League, Plunket, Parents' Centre, NZ Homebirth Association, Midwives Section NZNA, and Save the Midwives'. She wrote that while the latter organisations used logos that 'reflect their concern with mothers, babies and families, the Postgraduate School of O & G indicates their desire to encompass and control all the women of New Zealand!'²²

Internationally, some recent histories have questioned this victimisation/oppression model of the history of childbirth. A recent historian of childbirth in Canada, Wendy Mitchinson, reminded her readers that doctors were not a monolith, and different groups within the profession disagreed with one another and at times expressed concern about the direction their colleagues and medicine itself were taking.²³ She also noted that much of the historical literature had romanticised traditional home birth.²⁴ A recent volume I jointly edited with Scottish historian Janet Greenlees on the history of Western maternity included chapters that questioned a romanticised view of traditional childbirth and women's lack of agency in determining the form childbirth services took over the twentieth century.²⁵

This book will contribute to that international literature by challenging some popular assumptions about the history of childbirth, activist women's groups, and the medical, midwifery and nursing professions in New Zealand. Chapter 1 investigates the background to the founding of National Women's Hospital in 1946 by surveying childbirth services from the beginning of the twentieth century and the lobbying for changes to those services. Specifically, it explores the pressures that doctors and women's organisations together exerted on the government to create the maternity services which eventually included National Women's Hospital. Chapter 2 traces the debates about the form the new hospital would take, such as combining obstetrics and gynaecology into one institution, and including the functions of medical training and research as well as childbirth and clinical services. This can be understood only in the context of international developments, and chapter 2 also explores the interaction between British medical professionals and local doctors, and particularly the activities of one influential local doctor, Doris Gordon.

Chapter 3 outlines the work of the hospital under Harvey Carey, who was professor of obstetrics and gynaecology there from 1955 to 1962, a time when the hospital began to establish its international reputation. This chapter questions any automatic correlation between hospitalisation and medicalisation. While National Women's was a major medically controlled teaching hospital, this did not mean an unbridled enthusiasm for medical technology; on the contrary the chapter explores how and why senior staff embraced 'natural' childbirth. Chapter 4 moves the attention to the nurses and midwives of National Women's during this period, arguing for their centrality in hospital developments as well as the way in which they became a primary target for patients' complaints. In exploring consumer attitudes to conditions at National Women's, the chapter engages with a new important consumer group in childbirth that emerged in the 1950s, the Federation of New Zealand Parents' Centres. Chapter 5, which also deals with the 1950s to 1963, considers the increased emphasis on treatment of the newborn which was a feature of that time, with the premature nursery evolving into a paediatric ward. The chapter describes how National Women's made a dramatic contribution to the new discipline of perinatal medicine (with 'perinatal' defined as the period from 28 weeks' gestation to the end of the first week of life). Research at this hospital placed New Zealand on the world map in medical research, primarily through the work of Bill (later Sir William) Liley, who has been dubbed the 'founder of fetal medicine'.[26]

Chapters 6 to 10 address the period from 1964 to the 1980s, one of dramatic social change, which could also be described as the 'Bonham era' of the hospital's history. This is no hagiographic reference to Dennis Bonham, the professor from 1964 to 1989, but it does indicate his centrality to events during this time. Chapter 6 explores the glamour of fertility services with which the hospital was crucially involved, bringing into the limelight the rights and status of the embryo and the fetus, and showing how those working in this discipline were becoming involved in broader ethical and social debates, offering differing perspectives but also subject to rising patient expectations. The next chapter develops this further by focusing on work relating to perinatal medicine, with a particular emphasis on respiratory distress syndrome, identified as a major risk factor for newborn babies. This chapter explores mechanical respirators, the drama of the discovery of the effects of corticosteroids, and the introduction of ultrasound and other prenatal diagnostic tests. Again, it looks at rising public expectations and new ethical issues that were coming to the fore. Mont (later Sir Graham) Liggins' work on corticosteroids propelled the hospital into world fame, whilst he saw his major contribution to obstetrics not so much in terms of a therapeutic advance, vitally important as it was, but rather a new conceptualisation of the fetus as a 'hitch-hiker in the womb'.[27]

Chapter 8 moves the discussion to contraception, sterilisation and abortion, areas with which the hospital became involved through its clinical services, research and teaching. While it shows how the new women's health movement saw these areas as integral to its feminist agenda of women reclaiming control of their bodies, it also reveals that there was no clear-cut division between a predominantly male medical profession and its female patients. The views held by clinical staff were as diffuse as those of the women they served, spanning the full spectrum from Liley's involvement in the Society for the Protection of the Unborn Child (SPUC), to Bonham's commendation in the feminist magazine *Broadsheet* for his views on abortion.[28] Staff contributed in manifold and diverse ways to the national debates on these socially sensitive issues, but ultimately had a service to provide.

Chapter 9 concentrates more directly on the relationship between women's groups and the clinical staff at the hospital. Given their conviction that hospitals were the safest places for women to give birth, those working at National Women's became involved in public debates and were cognisant of the need to make the experience for birthing women as attractive as possible. The changing hospital environment was the result of negotiations between health professionals and those they served, and this chapter addresses issues such as the role of husbands in childbirth and feminising the profession. The following chapter turns attention to those who rejected hospital births altogether in favour of home births. It examines the new alliance between midwives and feminists that was emerging in the 1980s, and the role of feminist activist and independent midwife Joan Donley in particular. Hospital staff did not shy away from engaging in these debates. However, as the 1980s progressed, feminists gained more political power and public support, and the 1987–88 Inquiry into Cervical Cancer was a major blow to the hospital's public image. Chapter 10 also examines the effects of the Inquiry on the hospital and on childbirth services more broadly, specifically leading up to the 1990 Nurses Amendment Act that gave midwives autonomy in childbirth services. Finally, chapter 11 looks at the aftermath of the Cartwright Inquiry, and the struggles of the hospital to regain its public support and staff morale, in the face of staff shortages, new management structures and legislative changes to maternity services in the 1990s, until the time the hospital itself was relocated in 2004. Again, this chapter engages with national debates around childbirth services and the contributions by National Women's staff.

The history of National Women's Hospital cannot be divorced from the broader trends within maternity services, and focusing on this hospital illuminates those trends and the politics of maternity nationally and internationally. This volume is more than a history of one institution. It utilises the experiences of those associated with the hospital as a window into wider social issues during the second half of the twentieth century in New Zealand, and shows how doctors, nurses, midwives and consumer groups interacted to create health services for women during this period. All had a role to play, as did the government. The narrative is a complex and engaging one about the interface between science, medicine and society. The story also has a transnational component, for events in Auckland can only be understood in the context of what was happening overseas, and what happened in Auckland also contributed to that international environment.

CHAPTER 1

CHILDBIRTH SERVICES IN NEW ZEALAND, 1900–1939

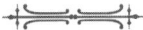

National Women's Hospital was opened in 1946, at a time when most New Zealand babies were born in hospital. This had not always been the case. The twentieth century opened with New Zealand's Liberal government firmly committed to developing childbirth services managed by midwives and not necessarily located in hospital. Yet just over three decades later, a Labour government passed legislation giving all women the right to give birth in hospital free of charge and with a doctor in attendance. The views expressed in a government inquiry into maternity services, set up by the Labour government in 1937 under Labour MP and general practitioner Dr David McMillan, were crucial to this development.[1] This chapter investigates those views, and in particular the role of doctors and consumers in persuading the government to go down the path of hospitalised childbirth, and to found a new maternity hospital in Auckland, which became National Women's Hospital.

A State Midwifery Service and the New Zealand Obstetrical Society
Under the Liberals who governed New Zealand from 1891 to 1912, New Zealand gained an international reputation as a 'social laboratory', as a consequence of its extensive social legislation.[2] Reforms that New Zealand proudly

boasted as world firsts included granting women the vote in 1893, setting up a Department of Public Health in 1900 and passing a Nurses Registration Act in 1901. In 1904 the government passed the Midwives Registration Act with the aim of improving maternity services in New Zealand. The Act provided for the registration of midwives and for setting up maternity hospitals where they would be trained and where the wives of working men would be catered for. Seven public maternity hospitals, called St Helens after the birthplace in Lancashire of New Zealand's Premier (Prime Minister), Richard Seddon, were established by 1921.

The Liberal government's interest in maternity services arose directly from its preoccupation with the future strength of the nation, an anxiety that New Zealand shared with other Western nations and as part of the British Empire.[3] A popular slogan of the early twentieth century, which New Zealand borrowed from Australia, was 'Babies are our best immigrants'. Introducing the midwives' Bill into the Legislative Council, Attorney-General Albert Pitt explained that the aim of registering and training midwives was to reduce infant deaths.[4] The government considered a growing population a national asset. Discussing the Infant Life Protection Bill a few years later, one member of New Zealand's Legislative Council declared, 'The real reason for our solicitude . . . is that population, which is decreasing, is indispensable to national safety and national progress. We must have soldiers and workers, or our prosperity will be imperilled and our industry will decay.'[5]

In the early twentieth century the government assumed that midwives would play an important role in future maternity services in New Zealand, which is why it wished to upgrade their training. Conjuring the image of Charles Dickens' fictional character Sarah Gamp, Seddon declared that some midwives 'indulge[d] a little too freely, and . . . the sooner we have legislation which will ensure competent midwives – sober and especially clean midwives – the sooner you will prevent loss of life'.[6] Dr Duncan MacGregor, Inspector-General of Hospitals and Charitable Institutions, predicted that, 'With the passing of the Midwives Registration Act the day of the dirty, ignorant, careless woman, who has brought death or ill health to many mothers and infants, will soon end.'[7] While this was not a true reflection of the competency of many midwives, 761 of whom were registered under the Act as midwives 'of good character', it was part of the professionalising trend of midwifery. The future midwife was to be a young, single, professional woman, just like the new nurse mandated by the 1901 Nurses Registration Act.[8]

The St Helens hospitals, set up following the 1904 Act and under the jurisdiction of the Department of Public Health, accommodated married women whose husbands earned less than £4 a week and who would contribute towards the cost of confinement to avoid the stigma of receiving charity.[9] The hospitals also provided a district maternity service for women who chose to have their babies at home. Midwives ran these hospitals, and there were no resident doctors; the latter were called only to deal with complications. Medical superintendents were appointed to the hospitals but they did not live on site and were summoned at the matron's discretion.[10]

The Health Department continued to view the St Helens hospitals and a midwifery service as central to maternity care in New Zealand well into the 1930s. The 1937 Committee of Inquiry into Maternity Services noted that in a number of countries, 'the trend is towards a service in which the bulk of the normal midwifery is conducted by highly trained midwives' and that 'in such a scheme the general practitioner is excluded from all normal midwifery practice'. This was specifically the case in Holland and Scandinavia 'where the maternity services are recognized to be of a very high order'. The report referred to a British committee representing the Ministry of Health, the British Medical Association (BMA), and the British College of Obstetricians and Gynaecologists, which recommended a national midwifery service for England and Wales, 'based on the principle of midwife attendance in normal labour' and which had been introduced there in 1936.[11] The report cited the evidence of Dr Henry Jellett, formerly master of the Rotunda Hospital, Dublin, who had immigrated to New Zealand in 1920 and was consultant obstetrician to the Department of Health from 1924 to 1931. In Jellett's view, for normal births, 'it is a mistake to bring in the complication of the medical man who has to attend all kinds of disease, statistics and history having proved over a period of years in other countries, and also at Home, that these cases can be attended more satisfactorily by midwives'.[12]

Generally, however, the 1937 committee did not favour the British model of a midwifery-based service. While two of its six members, Dr Sylvia Chapman, medical superintendent of Wellington's St Helens Hospital, and Dr Tom Paget, the Health Department's inspector of hospitals, advocated a midwifery service, the report endorsed doctor attendance for all births in hospital.[13]

Doctors had lobbied against a midwifery system for a decade prior to this inquiry. In 1927 a group of doctors formed the New Zealand Obstetrical Society (NZOS) to represent the interests of doctors who practised obstetrics.

At its 1929 meeting, members resolved to draft a maternity services plan since 'Dr Jellett had recently published his proposals for the future midwifery service of this Dominion, which proposals eliminate the doctors from attending cases of normal confinement.'[14]

In the midst of the economic depression in 1933, the Obstetrical Society noted that Paget had recently ordered the various hospital boards which ran New Zealand's public hospitals to make provision for indigent maternity cases within their areas, based on a scheme that was 'an exact parallel of the English midwife service'. The society was concerned that this policy, perhaps introduced as an emergency measure, might become the 'thin edge of a permanent wedge'. It resolved to reaffirm the principle that 'the ideal obstetrical service for every confinement in this Dominion is a doctor and a midwife or a doctor and a maternity nurse attending'.[15] The following year the society repeated this resolution in the light of a perceived trend for more women to be confined by midwives alone, declaring their belief that 'for reasons of safety to mother and infant, reasonable pain relief, and elimination of future pelvic weaknesses', a doctor and a trained nurse should be present at every delivery.[16]

Dr Bernard Dawson, professor of obstetrics and gynaecology at the Otago Medical School, warned his colleagues that 'a small cloud can herald a thunderstorm'. With an eye to Britain, where he said the percentage of midwife deliveries had increased from 58 to 75 over the previous decade, he averred, 'It is usual for methods adopted by England to be advocated sooner or later in her Dominions', adding that the midwife system of maternity service already had advocates in New Zealand. He advised the medical profession to devise a scheme that included midwives 'rather than be left inarticulate and bereft when some Bill for Maternity Services detrimental to our interests becomes an enactment'.[17] Dawson clearly saw midwives as competitors.

Dr Thomas Corkill, at that time president of the NZOS, not surprisingly was also outspoken about doctors' involvement in births. Graduating in medicine at Edinburgh in 1915 (where he also completed his MD in 1920), Corkill practised obstetrics in Wellington from 1921. He became a member of the (British) College of Obstetricians and Gynaecologists in 1934, and a fellow in 1937. In a 1933 article in the *New Zealand Medical Journal (NZMJ)* he addressed the argument put forward by Jellett, among others, that maternal mortality was much lower for midwife-conducted births than doctor-attended cases.[18] He noted that textbooks often warned against a doctor's presence during labour, as this was 'more likely than anything else to promote weariness and tempt interference' which were detrimental to the woman's welfare. Yet he argued that one advantage of the doctor's presence at the time of delivery was 'much more satisfactory anaesthesia'. His main argument in favour of doctors attending normal births, however, was that only by such experience could they gain a sense of the abnormal.[19] In his view, doctors should be involved in normal births to enhance their knowledge of obstetrics for the greater good of all. Corkill was one of the members of the 1937 Committee of Inquiry into Maternity Services.

The 1937 inquiry was not swayed by medical argument alone, however. Three members of the committee of seven represented women's organisations, Mrs Amy Hutchinson, Mrs Agnes Kent-Johnston and Mrs Janet Fraser.[20] Whilst the latter was the wife of the Minister of Health and later Prime Minister Peter Fraser, she was also active in women's issues in her own right. All three were explicit about their preference for hospital births, as were some of the women who came before the committee as witnesses. For instance, when Dr Paget asked Mrs McGuire of the Onehunga Labour Party whether she preferred a maternity hospital or a nurse service in the home, she replied, 'We think a hospital is the better.'[21]

Hospital Births and Pain Relief: Women's Demands

In the early twentieth century most women delivered their babies at home. In 1920 fewer than 35 per cent of births occurred in hospital (defined as an institution with two or more beds).[22] At that time the Health Department's Director of Nursing, Hester Maclean, supported home births, believing that the 'large majority' of births could take place at home provided conditions were 'reasonably comfortable'.[23] Yet a decade later 57 per cent of New Zealand births occurred in hospital.[24] In 1936 Dawson maintained that the fact that over 60 per cent of New Zealand women gave birth in hospital proved that the majority preferred hospitals, 'even in perfectly normal confinements'.[25] The 1937 Committee of Inquiry contrasted New Zealand with England and Wales, where only 15 to 25 per cent of births took place in hospital compared to 81.75 in New Zealand.[26] This was the case despite the fact that in New Zealand most women had to pay for the privilege.

New Zealand's health system prior to the 1930s was a mixture of private and public hospitals. Public hospitals, run by elected hospital boards, were funded by a combination of government subsidies, voluntary donations and patients' fees, with those patients who could pay being required to do so.

In 1930, with a population of under 1.5 million and about 27,000 births per annum, New Zealand had well over 1500 maternity beds available in institutions. This included 76 public hospitals containing maternity wards or maternity annexes, providing 506 maternity beds. New Zealand also had 274 private maternity hospitals; most of these were small, with an average of fewer than four beds per institution (and 873 beds in total). There were also unregistered private one-bed institutions run by midwives; Auckland alone had at least 25 of these in the 1930s. Finally, the St Helens hospitals, with their heavily subsidised fees, accounted for an additional 121 beds.[27] Still it was not enough. By the 1930s New Zealand women almost took it for granted that the best services for childbirth were hospital-based. New Zealand's National Council of Women (NCW), which had been set up in 1896, had long kept a watching brief over women's affairs.[28] When the Auckland branch of the NCW set up a sub-committee to look into maternity services in 1936, they called it 'The Committee on Maternity *Hospital* Services in New Zealand'.[29]

This was partly a reflection of the changing public image of hospitals generally. In the nineteenth century, hospitals had been regarded as places of last resort, where someone would go when they could not be cared for at home. The advances in scientific medicine changed the public image of hospitals; gradually the public came to accept them as respectable places of curative medicine. Women in childbirth wanted all the advantages that modern science could give them. Historian Judith Leavitt noted of America that 'women in alliance with obstetrical specialists decided to move childbirth to the hospital', and explained that 'they made this decision because they believed in medical science'.[30] Canadian historian Wendy Mitchinson also argued that Canadians had developed faith in science, and that, 'Much in a hospital setting gave the patient the feeling that everything that modern medical science could offer was available to her.'[31] Jane Lewis concluded from her research into the history of maternity in Britain that women went into hospital because of fear of the pain and the health consequences of childbirth.[32]

In New Zealand too childbirth was feared in the early twentieth century. In her history of childbirth in nineteenth-century New Zealand, Alison Clarke explained that women were very aware of their vulnerability as they prepared to give birth. She noted that letters frequently included expressions of relief and gratitude following childbirth, reflecting the very real dangers women had faced.[33] These fears were common knowledge. Premier Richard Seddon was not alone when he spoke of 'the dark hour of maternity', and nor was another MP who referred to 'that great dread which is felt as the time of maternity approaches'.[34] This apprehension was heightened after the First World War when it was announced that New Zealand had the second-highest maternal mortality rate in the Western world.[35] Women were not reassured by a pronouncement of a Board of Health committee set up in 1921 to look into this situation that, 'Childbirth is a normal physiological process, and to the healthy woman in healthy surroundings is attended with very small risk.'[36]

There were reasons other than health concerns for women to prefer hospitals for childbirth. Lewis wrote of Britain, 'A ten-day rest in hospital made sense in the context of the hard household labour performed by working-class women.'[37] In the American context, Leavitt considered the physical and psychological isolation of many women to be important in their decision to enter hospital; they could not find the help they needed in their own homes.[38] With its perennial shortage of domestic servants and the frequent absence of extended family, New Zealand shared these characteristics. Dr Emily Siedeberg McKinnon, medical superintendent of Dunedin's St Helens Hospital, mentioned a factor counterbalancing the attraction of hospital births, however, when she told the 1937 Committee of Inquiry, 'I do not know whether it is difficult to get [domestic] help or not, but I do know that a fair number of mothers are afraid of the infidelity of their husbands. That is a definite difficulty in persuading a woman to go into hospital, and even when they do go to hospital they are always anxious to get home again on that account. As a member of the Society for the Protection of Women and Children I have encountered many such cases.'[39]

One of the clearly recognised drawcards of hospital births (and probably outweighing any concerns about their husbands' infidelity) was that pain relief was more readily available in hospital than at home. Pain relief dates back to the mid-nineteenth century. First administered in 1846 by an American, Dr William T. G. Morton, it quickly spread to Europe and began to be used in childbirth as well as surgery. In 1847 Professor James Young Simpson of Edinburgh gave a birthing woman ether inhalation anaesthesia, and later tried another inhalational anaesthetic, chloroform. Shortly after, an American dentist, Horace Wells, published his work on nitrous oxide. Very soon these three general anaesthetics became widely known and were all used in childbirth. Some opposition persisted, based on the biblical injunction that 'in sorrow thou shalt bring forth children' and the related belief that women were meant to suffer in childbirth. Opponents of pain relief, sometimes including husbands, also argued that anaesthesia gave doctors unchecked powers over their patients. Opposition faltered, however, after Queen Victoria had chloroform for her eighth delivery in 1853. Wealthy women, in particular, began to pressure doctors for chloroform. With regard to America, Leavitt described nineteenth-century women as more eager than their physicians to invest in pain-relieving agents such as chloroform and ether.[40] The same was true in nineteenth-century New Zealand. In her history Alison Clarke related the story of Amy Barkas who demanded chloroform: 'Amy was a determined woman, wealthy enough and assertive enough to find a doctor willing to do what she wanted.'[41]

In the early twentieth century another form of pain relief was introduced in an attempt to avoid the risks related to total anaesthesia. A narcotic analgesic consisting of injections of scopolamine and morphine, dubbed 'twilight sleep', caused a state of semi-consciousness in the woman; it did not abolish pain but the memory of it. In America a group of women, mostly suffragettes, set up the National Twilight Sleep Association in 1914 to pressure doctors to provide this alternative to painful childbirth. They argued that the availability of analgesia was a fundamental right.[42] As historian Donald Caton commented, 'In articles and editorials alike American physicians were accused of rejecting Twilight Sleep because of its promotion by patients rather than medical colleagues, because of procrastination in learning about the subject, or a callous indifference to the pain of women in labor.'[43]

Twilight sleep had major drawbacks. In America the campaign in its favour suffered a setback in 1915 when one of its leading advocates died in hospital whilst undergoing a twilight sleep delivery.[44] British historian Irvine Loudon explained that twilight sleep often produced a disorientated and restless mother, unable to cooperate and extremely difficult to manage, who needed constant attention throughout labour. He noted that it was virtually abandoned in America and Britain in the 1920s, the whole affair being regarded as the 'twilight sleep fiasco'.[45] In New Zealand Dr Doris Gordon, whose activism in obstetrics will be discussed in the next chapter, pioneered the use of twilight sleep in childbirth, and continued to favour this method of pain relief long after it had fallen from favour in Britain. In 1937 she claimed that her private hospital in Stratford had been a 'twilight sleep' hospital for 20 years.[46] She reported that the stillbirth rate was much lower than at the St Helens hospitals, a point she stressed because during 1925–30, she said, the Health Department had strongly opposed its use and had convinced the public of its dangers. She claimed that many women who had been afraid of giving birth were more willing to have children once they had experienced twilight sleep in her hospital, but she added, 'Twilight Sleep can only be given by people who are really enthusiastic about it, and I usually spend the night in hospital when there is a case here.'[47] She also championed chloroform, which continued to be the predominant form of obstetric pain relief in Britain up to the Second World War, particularly for women in private hospitals.[48]

Many women seemed to favour doctors' involvement in childbirth because of the latter's ability to dispense pain relief. In 1933 the Auckland branch of the NCW sent a remit to the national conference that resident medical officers should be appointed to all St Helens hospitals in the Dominion. Two months later they clarified that they meant 'medical officers in the capacity of anaesthetists'.[49] The secretary was instructed to find out whether St Helens' matrons and nurses were qualified and authorised to administer chloroform, and whether they gave it 'only in cases of extreme difficulty; *also may the patients have it if they wish*'.[50] They viewed pain relief as a woman's right. Mrs Amy Hutchinson spoke in support of the remit and read a lengthy letter from Mrs Stanley Baldwin, wife of the British Prime Minister, giving details of the management of maternity hospitals 'at Home'.[51]

Mrs Stanley (Lucy) Baldwin had helped set up and was vice-president of a British voluntary organisation, the National Birthday Trust Fund, founded in 1928 to improve maternity services. The organisation focused on three issues: increasing the availability of health services for poor women, improving nutrition for young children and relieving the pain of childbirth. Mrs Baldwin assumed responsibility for the fund's efforts to increase the availability of obstetric anaesthesia. She later formed the Anaesthetic Appeal Fund, an organisation separate from, but affiliated with, the National Birthday Trust Fund.

Baldwin believed passionately that all women should be offered pain relief in labour as a fundamental right, regardless of their social status or income. She admired Finland, 'that little progressive nation which was the first in Europe to give the franchise to women', where she said anaesthesia in childbirth was always given. The novelist Virginia Woolf also suggested that one advantage of the political empowerment of women would be a government that provided every mother with chloroform in childbirth.[52]

Modern women, like their male counterparts, believed in the efficacy of modern science. The National Birthday Trust Fund allied itself with the

British College of Obstetricians and Gynaecologists, and underwrote college research projects such as that by R. J. Minnitt, a part-time obstetrician at Liverpool Maternity Hospital, who was developing a nitrous-oxide-and-air apparatus for obstetric use. The college conducted trials in 1936, concluding that nitrous oxide was safer than chloroform, and the National Birthday Trust Fund began distributing gas-and-air machines, free or at a discount, to hospitals.[53]

Women in New Zealand shared a similar objective to their British counterparts. To Vera Crowther, a British-born nurse and feminist who had immigrated to New Zealand in 1924 and subsequently joined the Communist Party, it was a class-based issue. She believed it unfair that women who were ill-nourished, overworked and mentally distraught with domestic and financial worries should 'suffer depletion and exhaustion of all their human powers in childbirth'. She compared the movement to provide universal pain relief with the suffragettes' fight to gain the vote. She wrote in 1937, 'to gain the confidence of working mothers is to know without doubt that disinclination for children is caused [first] from fear of the actual confinement'. Accused by certain doctors of exacerbating this fear herself, she responded that those who were most frightened were the ones who had already had the experience (she herself only had one child).[54]

Crowther's was not a lone voice. The New Zealand Society for the Protection of Women and Children (NZSPWC), like the NCW, had been set up in 1893 and also kept a watching brief over women's affairs.[55] In 1936 the Auckland branch summed up what appeared to be a widespread consensus among women when it sent a set of recommendations to Health Minister Peter Fraser for improved state maternity services:

> This Society is anxious that every woman, married or single, rich or poor, giving birth to a child shall be provided with the utmost attention and relief from pain which science can provide. As this can only be obtained by the services of both a Doctor and a nurse, the Society urges: 'That hospital accommodation for all classes of maternity work be extended, and that in such hospitals, resident medical officers specialised in obstetrics and gynaecology, be appointed, one of whom shall be present at every delivery.'[56]

The report stated that the existing practice at the St Helens hospitals resulted in 'prolonged and unnecessary suffering for the patient'.[57]

A 1937 report of a government inquiry into abortion that led to the subsequent inquiry into maternity services stated that several witnesses had suggested that fear of pain relief being withheld in labour was a factor in women seeking illegal abortions. The report declared, 'an erroneous idea seems to be prevalent among certain sections of the laity that the total abolition of pain during labour is possible for every patient'.[58]

The NZSPWC was particularly critical of the practices at the St Helens hospitals. Its representatives reported having interviewed seven women who had given birth at Auckland's St Helens Hospital. 'Without exception', they said, these women stated that only financial reasons prevented them from having a doctor present.[59] One of the society's representatives, Mrs Nellie Molesworth, explained in 1937 that she had been an inspector for the society for nine years, and had interviewed many of these women 'of the poorer class'. She claimed to have heard 'very distressing stories of unnecessary suffering', because unless the case was 'abnormal' they had received inadequate pain relief. Most were given a 'Murphy Inhaler', which could be administered by midwives and consisted of a teaspoon of chloroform, but, she said, they found it 'almost useless', and moreover, 'very often it is taken from the patient and they are told to do more to help themselves'. She also heard of stitches being inserted by the matron or a sister without anaesthetic. She reported that many women who had to go to St Helens because of their financial circumstances 'dread a confinement so much that they have told me that they would rather die than face it again'.[60] Janet Fraser was equally outspoken about pain relief. She reported that she had heard that mothers who went to St Helens were afraid because no anaesthetic was given there, and she was clearly not persuaded by Dr Paget's retort that this was an impression deliberately conveyed by the medical profession.[61]

The NZSPWC told the 1937 Committee of Inquiry into Maternity Services that it believed that adequate relief should be given in all cases and research carried out to improve methods, declaring that, 'painless maternity is every woman's right'.[62] Most women's groups that addressed the inquiry agreed with the Auckland Women's Branch of the New Zealand Labour Party, which demanded 'complete relief from pain by the most modern methods providing there is no danger to either the mother or infant'.[63]

The campaign for pain relief in New Zealand differed to some extent from that in Britain. The latter focused primarily on providing safe analgesia that midwives could administer without supervision.[64] By contrast New Zealand women appeared to favour doctor attendance. Mrs Kent-Johnston explained that from a psychological point of view, a 'woman prefers to have a doctor'. The seven women interviewed at St Helens 'expressed the feeling that it would give confidence to know a doctor would attend them'. One of the women went so far as to declare that 'she had known a young woman who lost her baby "because she lost confidence"'.[65] Doctors were the arbiters of medical science and therefore the best service included their involvement. Nurses agreed: the Obstetrical Branch of the New Zealand Registered Nurses Association stated that the 'highest ideal' was to have a doctor present and regretted that such services were not currently available.[66]

Women drew on professional authority to support their case. In a letter to the Minister of Health in 1936, the NZSPWC cited a 1934 report of the New Zealand Obstetrical Society which, it claimed, 'definitely supports our resolution' of having a doctor present at every delivery to ensure the health and safety of mother and infant and for 'reasonable' pain relief.[67]

The 1938 Social Security Act

In November 1935 the first Labour government swept into power in New Zealand, promising social security from the cradle to the grave. The commitment of the new government to social justice, and the importance it attached to building a strong population base, ensured that maternity services were high on its agenda. Founded in 1916, the New Zealand Labour Party had included 'nationalisation of the medical services and free medical and maternity attention' as one of its election platforms from the 1920s.[68] In 1938 the government passed the Social Security Act; among its provisions was a free maternity service under which all women could give birth in hospital with a doctor in attendance.

The political goal of 'national efficiency' that had led to reform of childbirth services in the early twentieth century was heightened by the imminent threat of another war. The Obstetrical Society (from 1935 the New Zealand Obstetrical and Gynaecological Society, NZOGS) marshalled this argument. It had established contact with the English Population Investigation Committee in the late 1930s, and, claiming a 'definite responsibility for arousing public opinion to heed the immediate dangers of race suicide', it offered to assist the government to investigate the reasons for falling birth rates.[69] At the close of the Second World War the society again pointed to the importance of increasing birth rates, and declared that the welfare of mothers and infants was a 'matter of Dominion defence'.[70]

Women likewise took advantage of this national concern to push for the kind of maternity services they wanted. For example, Mrs Cassey, representing the Women's Auxiliary of the Unemployed Workers' Union, and Mrs Stewart of the Devonport Housewives' Union, told the 1937 Committee of Inquiry into Maternity Services that, 'If you want population then you must cater for them in the proper way' through a state maternity service. Mrs Cassey added that as the government considered the child to be an 'asset to the country', it should 'be prepared to maintain that asset and bring it into the world free'.[71]

The recommendations of the 1937 Committee of Inquiry led to the inclusion of a maternity benefit in the 1938 Social Security Act, effective from 1939. This benefit allowed women to give birth in hospital and stay there for fourteen days free of charge, or to access the services of maternity nurses and midwives for a home birth and for fourteen days thereafter. An 'obstetric nurse' could claim a benefit as a midwife (practising without a doctor in attendance) or a lower benefit as a maternity nurse (assisting a doctor), and a total of 290 obstetric nurses signed contracts to provide maternity services. Women thus had the choice of home or hospital, doctor or midwife. Over the next ten months, 22,652 women gave birth in hospital and 1854 (or 7.5 per cent of all births) at home.[72] So, according to Joan Donley, the maternity benefit completed the medicalisation of childbirth.[73] Or, as Doris Gordon put it, New Zealand was the first country in the British Empire to allow women in childbirth to be the 'financial guests of the Government'.[74]

The argument for improving facilities to train doctors in maternity care was strengthened once the government had endorsed doctor-led maternity services and it became clear that women were taking up this option. As the NZOGS pointed out in 1945, without providing postgraduate training for doctors, the government could not purchase what the public wanted, that is, 'a most efficient State obstetrical Service'. It argued that paying inexperienced doctors would court disaster, and that the Maternity Benefits Scheme should incorporate within its framework the establishment of an up-to-date women's hospital located in Auckland, the most populous area of New Zealand. That hospital would train house surgeons who wished to specialise in obstetrics, provide courses for young doctors proposing to work in the Maternity Benefits Scheme and refresher courses, and assist in the training of sixth-year medical students.[75]

A New Maternity Hospital for Auckland

In 1936 the NZSPWC sent a deputation to the chairman of the Auckland Hospital Board, the Reverend W. L. Wood, regarding hospital facilities for childbirth in Auckland. Wood replied that he was fully aware of the poor maternity facilities for Auckland with its rapidly growing population, and told them the matter had been drawn to the government's attention for some time. He said that the board frequently paid for private hospital treatment or provided a nurse in the home for those who could not be accommodated at St Helens. Wood assured them that the board would be willing to shoulder the responsibility of a new maternity hospital for Auckland with the cooperation of the Health Department. He advised that newly published plans for Auckland Hospital did not include a maternity block because the board envisaged the time when a new, separate and modern maternity hospital would be built. Following this meeting, the deputation concluded, 'The women of Auckland, as those most interested, should do all in their power to gain the sympathetic interest of the Minister [of Health], Hon P Fraser', and recommended sending a deputation to him.[76]

The 1937 Committee of Inquiry reviewed the status of maternity services in Auckland. As the NCW noted following the inquiry, their representative on the committee, Amy Hutchinson, 'travelled throughout New Zealand . . ., and reported that Auckland sadly lags behind other parts of New Zealand in its maternity facilities'.[77] Auckland's St Helens Hospital had 32 beds; in 1936 there were 635 deliveries there.[78] There was no separate accommodation for maternity cases at Auckland Hospital, although 90 women had given birth there in 1936. Dr Joseph Craven, the hospital's medical superintendent, told the inquiry that 62 of those women should have gone to St Helens as they were 'uncomplicated cases', but no accommodation had been available.[79] There were two church homes for single women giving birth in Auckland, who were still refused admission to St Helens: the Salvation Army's Bethany Home with twelve beds (and about a hundred births per annum), and the Church of England's St Mary's Home in Otahuhu with six beds (about 50 births per annum).[80] Bethany opened to private paying cases in the mid-1930s, owing to increasing demand, and by 1937, 20 out of the hundred births per annum were private. There were also private maternity homes, usually run by midwives; as noted earlier, Auckland had at least 25 unregistered one-bed institutions run by midwives.[81] Anne Nightingale, who trained as a midwife at Auckland's St Helens Hospital in the 1950s, recalled that there were 'dozens' of little private maternity homes in Auckland run by midwives.[82] Other wards were attached to general surgeries; one witness told the 1937 inquiry that on Auckland's North Shore, there were some local private hospitals that accommodated maternity along with medical and surgical cases. However, these hospitals were short-staffed, and if a couple of 'operation cases' came in, they required the complete attention of the nursing staff, and the mothers and babies were 'just left to get along as best they could under the care of girls who were not qualified'.[83] This witness believed the service at St Helens to be far superior. In November 1939 the NZSPWC reported that St Helens was booked up for two months ahead and Bethany Hospital was booked up for six months ahead, concluding, 'Accommodation in Auckland for confinements is absolutely at a premium.'[84]

The NCW was delighted when the Minister of Health promised a new and larger St Helens Hospital for Auckland.[85] However, an enlarged and refurbished St Helens Hospital would not provide the doctor-run modern services many women wanted. When the NZSPWC sent a deputation to the Minister of Health in 1937, they found that his advisers, Drs Paget and Michael Watt, insisted that it was neither necessary nor desirable to appoint resident doctors to St Helens, believing that this hospital should continue to function primarily as a midwives' training school.[86]

Neither would an enlarged St Helens solve the problem of medical education in obstetrics. The training of medical students was a longstanding issue. In 1904 Premier Richard Seddon and Assistant Inspector of Hospitals Grace Neill, responsible for setting up the St Helens hospitals, had insisted that these institutions should be for the use of midwives and mothers and not for the 'convenience of embryo doctors'.[87] By 1918, at the request of the Medical Faculty of the University of Otago, the Health Department agreed to admit medical students into Dunedin's St Helens Hospital. In 1921 the St Helens hospitals in Auckland, Wellington and Christchurch were also opened to medical students along with trainee midwives.[88] However, midwives had priority in training in these hospitals during the following decades. In 1941 Dr Michael Watt, the Director-General of Health, explained to Doris Gordon in relation to the St Helens hospitals, 'Until I'm forced to acknowledge the rightness of your agitation I'll always train midwives to the exclusion of doctor graduates.'[89]

Professor Charles Hercus, Dean of the Otago Medical Faculty, told the 1937 Committee of Inquiry that his faculty believed that it was 'most essential that the future doctor be regarded as the most fundamental unit in our national maternity service', and that being the case the doctor must take precedence over the midwife in training. He thundered that 'all the recognised medical authorities on the subject' supported him. He drew the committee's attention to the 'extraordinary anomaly' that he believed to be 'unique in the world':

> [that] a State hospital, set up to do the whole of the maternity work of the country, where obviously one would expect medical education as well as nursing education to be catered for, should set up a barrier by making it necessary for women to sign a form stating that they are willing to allow the student to attend. I submit that this is a gross anomaly and that there is nothing whatever to support that extraordinary regulation. A good many cases are lost to us on account of that regulation.[90]

There was clearly a shortage of 'clinical material' in Auckland. Dr Selwyn Kenrick, medical superintendent of Auckland's St Helens Hospital, explained to the inquiry that the University of Otago had a branch faculty in Auckland, comprising seven doctors, whose duty it was to train sixth-year medical students coming to Auckland. They felt they could not provide adequate training unless more cases were made available. The problem was that midwives and nurses had first claim on the cases at St Helens, requiring for their training about 612 out of the 650 cases admitted each year. Kenrick pointed out that he trained both midwives and medical students, and declared, 'I cannot help being struck by the excellent facilities provided for the training of midwives in practical obstetrics compared with the poor facilities provided for the training of [medical] students.' He said that about 20 medical students had come to Auckland the previous year and, as they had on average done about six deliveries in Dunedin, they still needed to attend fourteen each to meet the Medical Council minimum requirements.[91] The poor facilities for medical students meant they were not as well trained as the nurses and midwives. In Kenrick's recent experience, the medical students had performed less well than the nurses when required to sit the same examination paper. Committee member Mrs Kent-Johnston agreed: 'The main point is that for the future mothers of New Zealand it is essential that the [medical] students should have every facility given in their training.'[92]

In 1926 Dr Henry Jellett had also stressed the importance of postgraduate courses for medical practitioners, if only to guard against unnecessary intervention. He believed that doctors performed caesarean sections too often to compensate for inadequate obstetric experience. He cited an American professor who believed that the operation was 'frequently employed unnecessarily; and . . . that even when strictly indicated, it was not always performed at the time of election, with the result that its mortality becomes needlessly high'.[93] Jellett reminded his readers that he was referring to America, but said he wished to avoid such a situation arising in New Zealand. Neighbouring Australia shared this concern to improve medical education in order to avoid unnecessary interference by doctors in childbirth.[94]

In 1939 when the Auckland branch of the NCW again appealed to the Minister of Health for better maternity facilities in Auckland, it met with a favourable response. Fraser assured it the matter was receiving attention.[95] The NCW had worked hard to improve maternity facilities, which it firmly believed ought to be hospital-based and should include doctors. The introduction of the maternity benefit under the first Labour government in 1939 could be seen as a triumph for the medical profession in monopolising childbirth services for their own professional and financial interests. Yet it was an outcome aided and abetted by women. Through their organisational networks such as the NCW, the NZSPWC and the women's branches of the New Zealand Labour Party, women had played a key role in lobbying the government for this generous welfare provision. These women clearly believed this would benefit themselves, their families and the nation, and managed to persuade the government to fund it. Their submissions reveal much about public attitudes around the middle of the twentieth century to science, medicine and medical professionals, as well as to community responsibilities and individual rights. Their sense of achievement was summed up in the memoirs of a member of the 1937 Committee of Inquiry into Maternity Services, Mrs Amy Hutchinson, when she wrote, 'After so many years of interest in these matters it was a thrill for me to have my name on the [National Women's] Hospital's Foundation stone.'[96]

CHAPTER 2

NATIONAL WOMEN'S HOSPITAL AND THE POSTGRADUATE SCHOOL OF OBSTETRICS AND GYNAECOLOGY

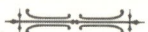

CHAPTER ONE SHOWED HOW THE AUCKLAND HOSPITAL BOARD WAS committed to providing a new maternity hospital in Auckland by 1939, owing to considerable public pressure particularly from women's groups. This ultimately resulted in the founding of National Women's Hospital, which also housed a Postgraduate School of Obstetrics and Gynaecology. This chapter traces the origin of the idea of combining obstetrics and gynaecology within one institution that would be a centre for medical training and research as well as birthing and treatment. In particular it considers the influence of Dr Doris Gordon in bringing about and shaping this new maternity facility.

Dr Doris Gordon and the Obstetrical Society

Australian-born Doris Gordon (née Jolly) had immigrated to New Zealand with her family at the age of four in 1894. As a teenager she wanted to become a medical missionary amongst the 'purdah-bound women of India', an evangelical zeal that she did not lose despite spending her life in New Zealand. She graduated MB ChB from Otago Medical School in 1916, having topped the lists in both the medical and surgical examinations in 1915. The year after graduation she married a fellow medical graduate, William (Bill) Gordon, in Palmerston North. Following the First World War when Bill served overseas, they took over from Dr Tom Paget a general practice in Stratford with a small private hospital attached. This was their base for the rest of their working lives, and Gordon was probably accurate in her assessment that the two of them became as much a part of the Stratford landscape as Mt Taranaki. 'Dr Doris', as she was known locally, later described 'back-block' practice as 'bog, bush and candle-light' medicine. She specialised in the treatment of women and children.[1]

Gordon set the course of her career while she was still a medical student. She decided to devote herself to midwifery, and specifically the quest for 'a safe, universally applicable method of pain relief' in childbirth. She helped found the New Zealand Obstetrical Society in 1927, of which she became joint honorary secretary and treasurer with her husband. Bill Gordon described the aims of the new society as 'the scientific study of obstetrical work in New Zealand and an endeavour to give the art of obstetric practice the dignity and status it rightly deserved but, at present, lacked'.[2] Gordon herself gave a more graphic description when she later explained that it had been 'first conceived as a banding together of doctors to refute allegations that obstetricians were a forceps-interfering pest-bearing coterie'.[3] This was in response to the Health Department's 'safe maternity campaign' and its officials who argued that medical interference was the main source of infection during childbirth.[4] One of the first initiatives of the new society was to found an obstetrical scholarship in 1928 for New Zealand medical graduates to gain experience as residents for six months at Melbourne's Royal Women's Hospital.[5]

Gordon saw the interests of the profession and women as one and the same; of the Obstetrical Society she said, 'Our aim was *the genuine welfare of every mother*, irrespective of colour or complexion, and her inviolable right to be treated with the same consideration as would be extended to a Prime Minister's daughter.'[6] Although she was no socialist in that she was highly suspicious of state control, her espousal of social justice was to fit well with the ideology of the first Labour government (1935–49). She took on the post of director of Maternal and Infant Welfare under that government to further her goal of improving obstetrical services for women. In 1945 she confided to Dr Helen Deem, medical adviser to an infant welfare organisation, the Plunket Society, 'Frankly I am only tempted to leave a comfy home and my beautiful province because a strict sense of duty tells me that by so doing, for a few years, I might finalise all developments for the Women's Hospital, Auckland, and possibly persuade the male mind political to BUILD requisite new St Helens in Christchurch and Wellington.'[7]

The 1930 Obstetrical Endowment Appeal and the Professor of Obstetrics

The University of Sydney appointed its first professor of obstetrics (Dr John Windeyer) in 1925, following a public campaign. As Dr Henry Jellett, consultant obstetrician to the New Zealand Health Department, noted the following year, 'The University of Sydney has, I understand, been compelled by the pressure of public opinion to create such a Chair [of Obstetrics].'[8] This had followed a meeting of women's organisations in 1924 at the Feminist Club that discussed maternal mortality and resolved that the university establish a chair immediately.[9] Jellett thought New Zealand should follow suit, arguing that midwives were better trained in New Zealand than were doctors.[10]

Jellett found a ready ally in Doris Gordon, who set out to stir up women's groups in New Zealand. In 1929, the same year that the University of Melbourne established such a chair, the New Zealand Obstetrical Society, under Gordon's stewardship, sent an official appeal to women's organisations, urging them to support their campaign.[11] Women responded with enthusiasm. The Auckland branch of the NCW considered that the 1930 Obstetrical Endowment Appeal would contribute to 'a noteworthy advance in maternal welfare long advocated by the National Council of Women'.[12] The NCW passed a resolution urging the creation of such a chair, 'in view of the high rate of maternal mortality in New Zealand . . . to control more efficiently this most important branch of the medical profession'.[13]

In February 1930 the Obstetrical Society recorded that the campaign was well organised, with 'multiple women's committees' working around the country.[14] Within a short time they had raised over £30,000. Gordon noted that most of the support came in the form of 'silver' subscriptions, which showed the wide public interest in maternal welfare, and was particularly impressive in light of the deepening economic depression. Gordon also reported the important role played by women doctors in the campaign, naming more than a dozen practising women doctors. She pointed out that Helen Deem had 'nearly doubled the quota asked of her district' (Wanganui); and added that many other medical women who were married and had retired from professional work also joined in, bringing their considerable experience to the campaign.[15] The involvement of women doctors suggests that they believed this was an area in which they had a special responsibility or interest.

The appeal achieved its goal, and acknowledging the role played by Gordon, an early historian of the Otago Medical School noted, 'It was felt that Dr. Gordon was by no means over-decorated in 1935 with the M.B.E.'[16] On the retirement in 1931 of Dr Frederick Riley, professor of obstetrics and gynaecology since 1929, Dr Bernard Dawson became the first full-time incumbent. English-born and trained, Dawson had immigrated to Australia where he set up antenatal and postnatal clinics.[17] The Obstetrical Society suggested that he tour Europe and America before taking up the post at Otago, so as to be aware of the latest trends in obstetrics. The appeal had been so successful that it accrued surplus funds. The Obstetrical Society placed these into its travelling scholarship fund; scholars would now spend six months in Australia and eighteen months in Britain.[18] By 1937 nine doctors had been awarded the scholarship but only one of them had returned to practise obstetrics in New Zealand.[19] In 1938 when Gordon was planning a trip to Britain, Dawson suggested that she contact the scholars to find out why they had not returned home.[20]

Dr Doris and the Empire Congress: Combining Obstetrics and Gynaecology
Doris Gordon's trip to Britain in 1939 proved to be an important step in the establishment of the Postgraduate School of Obstetrics and Gynaecology in Auckland. She represented the Obstetrical Society (renamed the New Zealand Obstetrical and Gynaecological Society in 1935) at the Empire Congress of Obstetricians and Gynaecologists in Edinburgh. At that conference she met another New Zealander, obstetrician John Stallworthy. She explained how, following her contribution to a session on pain relief in labour:

> Within an hour of my impromptu defence of Simpson's chloroform, a triangular friendship started between Professor William Fletcher Shaw, Stallworthy, and the woman doctor from New Zealand, that was eventually to result in the beginnings of a Post-Graduate School of Obstetrics and Gynaecology in New Zealand.[21]

John (later Sir John) Stallworthy, son of Arthur Stallworthy, New Zealand's Minister of Health from 1928 to 1931, had been awarded an obstetrical scholarship to go to Melbourne and then to Britain in 1933.[22] In 1939 he was clinical assistant to Professor Chassar Moir in the Nuffield Unit of Obstetrics and Gynaecology in Oxford. Earlier that year Stallworthy had been listed first for a chair in Canada but, according to Gordon, Sir Farquhar Buzzard and others in Oxford started a counter-move to keep him in Oxford, giving him the right to private practice and postgraduate teaching. Gordon claimed that a New Zealand professor in Oxford started a 'secret-second-counter-move' to procure Stallworthy's services for New Zealand.[23] This was undoubtedly Robert (later Sir Robert) Macintosh, another obstetrical scholar who was appointed Nuffield Professor of Anaesthetics in 1937.[24] According to Gordon, 'Jack' (as she called Stallworthy) 'was deeply interested in the project'.[25]

In Britain, Gordon pursued Dawson's suggestions of tracing the obstetrical scholars. She spoke with William Fletcher Shaw, president of the Royal College of Obstetricians and Gynaecologists (RCOG), chairman of the Dominions' Committee, and professor of obstetrics and gynaecology at the University of Manchester. Shaw convened a meeting of the scholars in London, to which almost all of them came, to find out why they did not return to New Zealand.[26] Gordon later reported that the reason was clear. If the scholars stayed in Britain, with their membership of the RCOG and the Royal College of Surgeons, they could get consultant provincial appointments at a retaining fee of £750 per annum and the right of private practice. In New Zealand they would have to rely on private practice alone.[27] New Zealand's hospital boards did not offer such posts, she said, because of the influence of general surgeons who were reluctant to see gynaecology elevated to a specialty. Shaw had explained to her that the British college had been established a decade earlier, in 1929, precisely because he and his colleagues had been fighting for recognition of gynaecology as a specialty apart from general surgery.[28]

The British College of Obstetricians and Gynaecologists became a Royal College in 1938. Combining the two branches of gynaecology and obstetrics had been some time in the making, presaged by their merger into a single section of the Royal Society of Medicine in 1907.[29] Shaw, as one of the RCOG's founders, explained that its primary object was 'to prevent gynaecology from becoming a mere subdivision of surgery while obstetrics is left to those who have nothing better to do'. He and his colleagues hoped that having control over standards of training and of entry into the combined profession of obstetrics and gynaecology would undermine the surgeon's dominance of gynaecology. The college would also 'speak as a representative body of all obstetricians and enhance their status and public visibility'.[30]

One outcome of this new alliance of obstetrics and gynaecology was that obstetricians were encouraged to be more surgically minded. Victor Bonney, a leading London obstetrician who was invited to New Zealand in 1928 to address the first Annual General Meeting of the New Zealand Obstetrical Society, declared that midwifery was a 'purely surgical art'. He likened the baby to a 'neoplasm' and regarded labour as a process accompanied by self-inflicted wounds, and the puerperium as a period of surgical healing.[31] It was at this AGM that a resolution was passed urging the Council of Otago University to establish a chair of obstetrics and gynaecology. The society appointed Bonney to the recommendation committee set up in Britain to search for candidates for the chair.[32]

The renaming of the New Zealand Obstetrical Society as the New Zealand Obstetrical and Gynaecological Society (NZOGS) in 1935 reflected this modern trend.[33] At the time Christchurch obstetrician and gynaecologist Dr Leslie Averill, who was medical superintendent of the local St Helens Hospital from 1929 to 1962, explained the reasons for the name change. He contrasted the 'tendency in New Zealand . . . to separate Gynaecological and Obstetrical interests' with the policy in 'all other civilised countries'. He explained that obstetricians must be 'gynaecologically minded'. Otherwise, he said, 'not only might a woman's happiness be wrecked by such disturbances as a septic cervix, relaxed uterine supports, parametritis etc., but a husband's success in life might be retarded and children cheated of their rights to a happy childhood, as no patient with the above gynaecological disorders could give her best to husband and home'. Similarly, it was essential that gynaecologists be 'obstetrically minded', since only by the possession of such knowledge could they decide what operative procedures were suitable for a particular case; he argued that gynaecologists could perform their work successfully only by taking into consideration the effect on future childbearing of the operative procedure they proposed. Following his formal paper, Averill spoke about the specialists who had influenced him during his recent visit to the USA; a single certification board for the two fields had been established there in 1930.[34]

In 1937 the Dean of the Otago Medical Faculty, Dr Charles Hercus, also referred to the modern trend combining obstetrics with gynaecology, regretting that in New Zealand gynaecology was still the terrain of general surgeons.[35] Similarly, Dr Louis Levy, president of the NZOGS, in discussions on the shape of the new maternity hospital in Auckland in 1940, argued that the sciences of obstetrics and gynaecology overlapped, and 'for this reason all progressive countries always group Obstetrics and Gynaecology together in one special women's department'.[36]

The linking of obstetrics and gynaecology ruled out developing the local St Helens hospital. In 1945 the NZOGS declared, 'In view of Dr Paget's recent statement that Gynaecological work would never be incorporated in St Helen's services, the Committee feel that no enlargement, etc, will make St Helen's a suitable Medical Centre.'[37]

The 1940 Dominion Conference

The decision to set up a Postgraduate School of Obstetrics and Gynaecology was made at a national conference of interested parties in Wellington in 1940, and once again, Doris Gordon was a central figure. On her return from Britain earlier that year, Gordon set out to lobby for the new school. She presented her 'confidential report' on the scholars' conference and discussions with Shaw at an NZOGS meeting. In the light of the obstetrical scholars' failure to return to New Zealand, she proposed that New Zealand set up its own training school for membership of the RCOG. Even training two candidates per annum, she argued, would meet New Zealand's needs and ensure that the scholarship money would be spent in New Zealand. This, she said, would please the Minister of Finance more 'than the present export of both brains and capital'.[38]

The NZOGS meeting endorsed her proposal. The society had also received a letter of support from the RCOG president, Fletcher Shaw, who thought the new hospital should serve as a training school for membership of the RCOG. The NZOGS resolved to approach the New Zealand Branch of the British Medical Association (NZBMA) seeking its approval for a campaign to establish a postgraduate obstetrical and gynaecological unit in Auckland. To this end it proposed a joint deputation to the Department of Health asking for a round-table conference to explore the project, with wide representation of medical and women's interests.[39]

The NZOGS again commissioned Gordon to address women's groups.[40] She did not need much coaxing, and while she certainly courted women's groups, it was a two-way process. She was frequently invited to speak to such bodies. For instance, a month before the national meeting in Wellington to discuss the proposed hospital, she was invited to address the Auckland branch of the NCW.[41]

Gordon marshalled considerable arguments to advance her cause. She argued that the government spent more on cows and their hormones than on women, referring to the well-paid scientists attached to the Dairy Board. In her view:

New Zealand thinks of women's health solely in terms of a creditably low infantile and maternal death rate (women are assessed by their breeding values, and poorly assessed at that, for today NZ has not one special clinic for the diagnosis and cure of sterility). This Dominion does not yet realise that women have a right to POSITIVE good health, and that modern discoveries correctly taught at a Post-Graduate centre would soon cure 75% of the troubles hitherto passively accepted as 'women's lot'.[42]

She stressed that her cause was non-political. She wrote at length about it to her friend Nina Barrer, then vice-president of the Women's Division of the New Zealand Farmers' Union.[43] She believed that the onus rested on women leaders, telling Barrer, 'We want all the publicity we can, but still hope to avoid flinging brickettes like the old rampant suffragettes.' She feared that as long as she alone pushed for the new hospital, politicians would ignore the request, but that 'If hundreds of women appear to want it they will suddenly find it's their hearts' desire.'[44]

According to Gordon, the context of the Second World War made the matter urgent. She pointed out that, owing to war restrictions, doctors could not go abroad to study and yet there were no facilities in New Zealand for postgraduate training in obstetrics. This meant that future doctors would be forced to treat complicated obstetrical cases with no higher experience than they had at the time they graduated. She explained that the Queen Mary Hospital in Dunedin, which had opened in 1938, was unable to provide postgraduate courses as the number of undergraduate students had increased.[45] There were no obstetrical hospitals in New Zealand big enough to employ house surgeons, and it had been decided that St Helens hospitals were not suited to carry house surgeons, owing to their size, architecture and 'principles of running'. The new hospital she was proposing would concentrate on 'abnormal' obstetrical cases and so would complement rather than rival St Helens, and would only train nurses and not midwives.

Again referring to the war, she argued that returning doctors would need refresher courses in women's and infant health to offset the four or five years of military and masculine work. Gordon concluded with a flourish that the home front was no less important than overseas, and that final victory would come to the country 'who paid attention to the health and happiness of its mothers and children'.[46]

Following Gordon's address to them, the Auckland branch of the NCW passed a motion that it strongly supported the proposal to establish a modern obstetrical hospital in Auckland, which, while providing services for the women of the city and suburbs, would function as a postgraduate teaching centre for the advancement of knowledge of diseases of women.[47] In September 1940 a sub-committee of the NCW waited upon the NZBMA Council and pointed to the 'dangerous state of affairs now that war isolated the Dominion from all overseas' experience'. More than willing to come to the party, the NZBMA agreed that its president, Dr Alexander Wilson, and NZOGS president, Dr Louis Levy, should call a 'Dominion conference' to discuss the maternity situation.[48]

This conference, held on 11 December 1940, saw the coming together of various interest groups, specifically those who believed there was a need for better maternity services for women in Auckland, and those who wished to set up a new training school for obstetrics and gynaecology to improve medical education and promote the specialty. It was attended by various women's organisations, as well as delegates from the NZOGS, hospital boards, the NZBMA, the University of New Zealand and the Department of Health. Gordon was appointed secretary.

Women's organisations were well represented. Delegates included Mrs Agnes McIntosh, Dominion president of the NCW; Miss Amy Kane, then Dominion president of the Country Women's Institute and a former president of the NCW; Mrs Adams, Dominion president of the Women's Division of the Farmers' Union; Mrs Isabel Averill, representing the Canterbury branch of the NCW and herself a doctor; Mrs Charles White, vice-president of the New Zealand League of Mothers; Miss Kirk, JP, Dominion secretary of the Women's Christian Temperance Union; Mrs Amy Hutchinson, chairwoman of the Auckland Women's Committee for Better Maternity Services; Mrs Rhoda Bloodworth, representing the Auckland branch of the NZSPWC and formerly Dominion secretary of the NCW; Mrs David Smith, Wellington branch of the New Zealand University Women's Association; and finally Dr Hilda Northcroft, representing the Auckland branch of the NZOGS and former president of the Auckland branch of the NCW and Dominion secretary.

The chairman of the Auckland Hospital Board, Allan Moody, put forward the motion which was carried unanimously, 'That the time has arisen for the establishment in New Zealand of a Postgraduate Centre for Obstetrics and Gynaecology.' A motion by Levy to locate the hospital in Auckland was also carried unanimously. Levy linked the occasion with the 1930 endowment appeal, which he said had opened the first chapter in the history of 'New Zealand Obstetrical Science'. This conference, he said, heralded the second.[49]

Control: Health Department or University, Dunedin or Auckland?

Doris Gordon did not simply campaign for the establishment of a women's hospital in Auckland; she also had a clear idea of how this hospital should be controlled and run: 'There might be an all-in-war abroad, but within me there was one driving obsession: the midwifery of NZ might be paid for by the state, but if it was controlled by the state it would be over my dead body!'[50]

Gordon disapproved of government interference in professional practice. She later explained her misgivings about state control by referring to the events of 1924 when the Health Department had apparently threatened to shut down her private hospital if she persisted in using twilight sleep drugs.[51] Like many of her medical contemporaries she was convinced that state control would undermine medical practice as she knew it, and create a new generation of indifferent salaried doctors. She asked:

> Would mothers count as individuals in a State Service? . . . . Dawson had stated dogmatically, 'Your Auckland project will be state controlled.' And we, who had battled so long for it, wanted university control, plus affiliation with the Royal College of Obstetricians and Gynaecologists – as the best insurance, for all time, that the service would be humane, that the feelings of individuals would count, that modern treatment would be given and accurate reports released![52]

The alliance between women's groups and medical professionals continued following the December 1940 conference. The NZOGS set up a coordinating committee to prepare the scheme, including Levy, Dawson, Gordon and Northcroft, along with Mrs McIntosh, Miss Kane and Mrs Hutchinson. Sir Thomas Hunter, professor of mental and moral philosophy at Victoria University College 1907–48 and Vice-Chancellor of the University of New Zealand from 1929 to 1947, was also a member. This committee delegated most of the practical work to two sub-committees: one for finance and site building (convened by Northcroft), and the other for staffing, control and salaries (convened by Dawson).

The coordinating committee was soon joined by another influential person. Gordon explained, 'while I was laboriously writing up the minutes and drafting letters to the inquiring women (again, God bless them)', a letter arrived from a local thoracic surgeon Douglas (later Sir Douglas) Robb. Robb had a deep interest in medical politics; in 1940 he had published *Medicine and Health in New Zealand: A Retrospect and a Prospect*. In this publication, among other things, he criticised the quality of postgraduate medical education, and the inadequacies of the New Zealand hospital system, including the lack of specialist consultants. He expressed his concern that such deficiencies were driving talented doctors overseas. In 1943 he helped set up, and became secretary of, the Auckland Postgraduate Medical Committee, and from the mid-1940s he worked towards obtaining a second medical school based in Auckland.[53] He told Gordon in 1941, 'I am advised that your Obstetrical Society contemplates a unit at Auckland for the advancement of higher teaching and research in obstetrics and gynaecology.' He asked to become a member of the society in order to help the campaign.[54] As Gordon wrote flamboyantly, 'So began a history-making correspondence between Professor William Fletcher Shaw at Manchester, Stallworthy at Oxford, Robb at Auckland, and a menopausal woman at Stratford . . . . I concentrated on the "inquiring women" knowing that, through their massed opinion, lay the road to political approval.'[55]

Among those 'inquiring women' was her friend Helen Deem, to whom Gordon appealed to help ensure the hospital be placed under university control.[56] On the same day she wrote to Mrs Daisy Begg, the Dunedin-based president of the Plunket Society, imploring her along with Deem and Lady Fergusson (the wife of the Governor-General) to 'bring to Conference the experienced academic perspective specially on the all important matter of University control'. She added that she had written to Deem 'who will doubtless discuss my letter with you'.[57] The correspondence gives a sense of Gordon's lobbying and networking, and the importance she attached to marshalling influential women. Deem assured her that she would do all in her power to support the proposal and stress the importance of university control.[58]

Gordon had women's groups behind her all the way. The NCW, through its Maternity Services Sub-committee, kept a watching brief over the proposal for the new hospital. In 1941 and 1942 it sent resolutions to the Auckland Hospital Board and the Minister of Health, making clear that the scheme should benefit the whole of New Zealand and not just Auckland.[59] As Gordon had predicted, Health Minister Arnold Nordmeyer announced as a pre-election promise in 1943 that Auckland was to have a large new obstetrical hospital modelled on the lines of the teaching hospital in Dunedin.

Fundraising was a strategy to keep control of the new postgraduate school out of government hands. Gordon suggested to the NCW that they should thank the government for their promise of a costly hospital, and undertake to endow the professor's salary 'in order to ensure that it should be an institution worthy of the city and the Dominion'.[60] She used the same strategy when she lobbied the business community. She addressed the Rotary Club in Auckland, reminding them that the Minister of Health had recently promised that a large obstetric hospital would be built in Auckland. She asked them 'to decide whether this would be a mediocre state-controlled institution or one enjoying university status and therefore open to affiliation with the Nuffield chain of post-graduate hospitals [in Britain]'. As a result, a group of Auckland businessmen wrote to the Minister of Health, asking to be permitted to endow the teaching work, so that the director could have full status under the University of New Zealand.[61]

The appeal, organised by businessman Percy Shaw and largely run by women, attracted a huge voluntary effort. Shaw told Gordon enthusiastically in 1945, 'The wharf labourers raised £52 in a collection without notice', adding that he had 'just been tapped for £5 by a lady with one of our collecting books'.[62] Three years later the NCW congratulated Shaw on the success of the appeal, which had raised £100,000.[63] When the appeal closed in September 1948, it had raised £104,595.[64]

While the public endowment ensured university control of the new school, the next question was whether this control would be vested in the only medical school in the country, located at the other end of the country, Dunedin, or in Auckland University College which had no medical school. The advisory committee for the chair, set up by Nordmeyer in 1943, could not agree on this point. While Hunter, Gordon and Robb all favoured Auckland University College control, Dawson disagreed. Hunter suggested that the new school should focus on postgraduate teaching and research only, as he thought the proposed inclusion of undergraduate teaching was the source of the opposition.[65] However, not all Aucklanders supported local control; Gordon told Robb that she had heard that 'the Auckland financiers would prefer to see money for medical purposes handled by Otago [rather] than administered by the AUC [Auckland University College] as that body was too reformatory and employed too many pacifists, leftists etc on its staff for their liking'.[66]

As part of their strategy to get the school up and running, Robb, Gordon and Auckland obstetricians Geoff Fisher and Tom Plunkett decided to invite

Fletcher Shaw to New Zealand to advise on the new venture; each contributed £100 towards his fare.[67] However, they also recognised the 'need to be tactful towards Dunedin. The RCOG won't fancy sending their president out here if there's going to be a border war about this new unit in Auckland.'[68]

A University of New Zealand senate meeting in 1946 discussed the new postgraduate chair of obstetrics and gynaecology to be located in the school. William Cocker, president of Auckland University College from 1938 (and later Chancellor), proposed that it be attached to Auckland University College.[69] An amendment was put to the meeting that the professor should be appointed to the Faculty of Medicine of the University of Otago. Robert Bell, professor of mathematics at Otago from 1920 to 1948, spoke against the amendment. He believed that those opposing Auckland control did so because they believed it contained the embryo of a second medical school, 'with Auckland playing the part of Ahab in the biblical story of Naboth's vineyard'.[70] Bell made a strong case against remote control of the chair, pointing to problems such as attending meetings and carrying out administrative duties. Senate approved the Auckland proposal; in a subsequent summary of the setting up of the school, Auckland gynaecologist Herb Green referred to Bell and 'just how much Auckland and the School owe to this far-sighted Scot'.[71]

With Auckland control secured, the visit by Fletcher Shaw proceeded. It is not known how they met the rest of Shaw's fare, as Shaw himself discovered that the journey cost £780 and wryly commented, 'I wonder whether, from their point of view, any of us is worth the money.' He also told Eardley Holland (who had replaced Shaw as president of the RCOG in 1943) that he had learned from British Airways that the journey involved 'three continuous days and nights travelling, going down on the various aerodromes for only an hour. The chairs are reasonably comfortable and tip up, but there are no beds and no undressing.' He added, 'The idea of such a long period of sitting in one chair in the same clothes is rather appalling.'[72] Nevertheless, he made the journey in late 1946, staying nearly four months, followed by two months in Australia.[73]

Dr Cecil Lewis, later the first Dean of Auckland's Medical School which was eventually established in 1968, commented that Shaw's report of his visit, presented to the University Council, read 'rather like a regal tour of Italy in the last century'. He dined with the Governor-General and the Archbishop of New Zealand; the mayors of Wellington, Auckland and Christchurch welcomed him with a reception, one attended by the Prime Minister. The government gave him a free pass for railway and bus services and allowed him the use of their motor cars in the four principal cities. Lewis commented that his report was sixteen pages long but the part dealing with the postgraduate hospital covered fewer than three pages, despite his acknowledgement that this was 'the primary object of my visit to New Zealand'.[74] Yet the visit achieved its goal: the Auckland unit became a recognised training school for membership of the RCOG.[75]

The Hospital and the New Professor

At the conclusion of the Second World War, the Auckland Hospital Board acquired a military hospital that had been built in 1943 by the United States Army to accommodate two thousand Pacific battle casualties.[76] It was a light wooden construction, typical of army hospitals, with a corridor 800 yards long and side branches leading off at intervals; it was rumoured that the American orderlies cycled down the corridors and one later employee remembered seeing a 'No cycling' sign at one end of the long corridor.[77] The board decided to use half the building to accommodate geriatric patients and the other half for obstetrics and gynaecology. The NZOGS regarded this as a temporary measure. Its 1945 pamphlet, written 'on behalf of women's groups', stressed that this arrangement was no excuse for forgetting the 'full objective' of a new building, adequately equipped and staffed, 'to assist in the future improvement of New Zealand's obstetrical and gynaecological services'.[78]

The first baby was born at the makeshift hospital on 9 June 1946, and the following day a fourteen-bed ward was opened with part-time staff Drs Geoff Fisher, Tom Plunkett, Jefcoate Harbutt and Alastair Macfarlane (a former obstetrical scholar), with Lilian Knights as sister in charge.[79] On 18 August 1946 a gynaecological ward opened. Until 1955 the unit was known as 'The Obstetrical and Gynaecological Unit, Cornwall Hospital, Green Lane West'.

At the same time the Auckland University College began to plan the new school, setting up an advisory committee for that purpose, chaired by Cocker. It laid out certain principles. Obstetrics and gynaecology would be taught in the one institution, both in the interests of the institution itself and in order to obtain recognition from the RCOG. The professor would be required to devote his entire time to the duties of the chair and would have no right of private practice. His annual salary was fixed at £2,250 with living quarters, or £250 in lieu. He was to be responsible for the development and maintenance of postgraduate education and research in obstetrics and gynaecology, but might also be called upon to help train undergraduates in Auckland. He was to be appointed director of the obstetric and gynaecological unit, the appointment being for five years. These conditions were formalised in section 7 of the Hospitals and Charitable Institutions Amendment Act 1947.

The committee spelt out other details for the functioning of the new institution. The hospital was to include a self-contained laboratory for clinical needs, teaching and research. The committee affirmed that the school would train maternity nurses and not midwives, so as not to interfere with the local St Helens and so that resources would be concentrated on medical students. Medical staff would be divided into four teams, one led by the professor and the other three by senior consultants. Each team would have 25 obstetrical and 25 gynaecological beds. A paediatrician and a radiologist would be appointed on a part-time basis. Other consulting staff would include a surgeon and physician, ophthalmologist, psychiatrist, ENT surgeon and skin specialist.[80]

The committee looked primarily to Britain for applicants to the chair. Robb wrote to his friend Robert Aitken, then Regius Professor of Medicine at Aberdeen, Scotland, asking for suggestions. Aitken had graduated in medicine from Otago in 1923, the year after Robb, and had gone to Britain on a Rhodes Scholarship. (He returned to be Vice-Chancellor of Otago University, from 1948 to 1953, and was knighted in 1960.) Aitken showed Robb's letter to Dugald Baird, professor of obstetrics and gynaecology at Aberdeen, who told him that there was 'an appalling dearth of obstetricians whose interest and training are academic'. Aitken referred to the low salary: 'One trouble is that the good man, with drive, in obstetrics, as in surgery, can make four or five thousands in consulting practice, and is not attracted by a chair carrying £1500–£2500.'[81]

John Stallworthy, as a New Zealander in Oxford, was pinpointed as a possible candidate. Baird, however, did not think it likely Stallworthy would be attracted to apply. He told Aitken that he had seen Stallworthy recently, and 'got the impression he had developed along the Charles Read lines – profitable practice and the grand manner'. Read was another New Zealand obstetrical scholar who prospered in Britain (subsequently elected president of the RCOG in 1955 and knighted in 1957).[82] Nevertheless, Gordon thought Stallworthy might be persuaded. She told Robb in 1947 that she had received a long letter from Stallworthy, in which he expressed interest provided he would be able to continue some private practice. She also said he made a 'good point' explaining why the salary for a professor of obstetrics and gynaecology should be double that of a professor of English, as 'the [former] works well nigh the year round while the [latter] works little more than half the year. Also the O. and G. Professor has broken nights and week end work.'[83] Gordon added, 'The rigors of English life are acting in N.Z. favour', and commented earlier that 'he wants to see his son in the surf on a western beach'.[84]

However, Stallworthy did not pursue the offer but remained in Oxford where he became Nuffield Professor of Obstetrics and Gynaecology in 1967 and was knighted in 1972.[85] Gordon came up with a second suggestion, Dr William Hawksworth, another obstetrical scholar who, she said, was possibly a more tactful administrator than Stallworthy.[86] Hawksworth had gone overseas as a scholar in 1936. He had first met Gordon at medical school and, delivering the first Doris Gordon Memorial Oration in 1962, admitted that he thought her 'a bit of a dragon'. She invited him to her home at Stratford, he thought to vet him as a possible scholar. In 1939 he attended the scholars' meeting in London, and he and Gordon kept in touch.[87]

The academic advisory committee approached Hawksworth in 1949. He replied that he was interested in the post provided that his salary was £2,600 per annum, and that he was entitled to private practice within the unit. The committee gained the government's approval of the salary, and suggested that Hawksworth visit New Zealand, which he did in November 1949.[88] However, the Minister of Health did not agree to his request to have private beds and fee-paying patients, and so Hawksworth declined the offer.[89]

Hawksworth returned to Oxford where he lived and worked until his death in 1966, although, according to Stallworthy who wrote his obituary, he 'remained very much a New Zealander with a love of sunshine, hot sandy beaches, warm seas, and the freedom of an open air life'.[90] From his position in Oxford he continued to flourish and mentor New Zealanders who worked in obstetrics and gynaecology. As Dr J. E. (Ed) Giesen wrote on Hawksworth's death, 'No person had done more to assist young New Zealanders and also more senior members of the College in their postgraduate training. His hospitality, advice and help to all was almost a legend.'[91]

With no appointment to the chair in Auckland pending, the NCW kept up the pressure. Its Auckland branch recorded in 1950: 'The NCW which raised funds expressly for the appointment of a Gynaecologist in Auckland, note with dismay the discussions, and subsequent breakdown of plans, in appointing a specialist for Auckland. They hope a settlement will be reached.'[92]

In April 1951 Dr Gerald Spence Smyth from Johannesburg, South Africa, was appointed to the Auckland chair. Born in the Transvaal in 1903 of Irish parentage, Spence Smyth had taken his medical degree at Trinity College, Dublin, graduating MD in 1932 and was elected a fellow of the Royal College of Physicians, Ireland (1931) and of the RCOG (1947). Before coming to Auckland he had been a senior lecturer in obstetrics and gynaecology at the University of Witwatersrand.[93] He took up his appointment in Auckland in November 1951, after spending three months touring Britain, Sweden, Holland and the USA studying modern developments in hospital planning and equipment. A year after taking office he complained that he was 'still without any academic staff'.[94] He wryly told the university, 'I would take a great pleasure in directing an academic unit if one existed. Instead, I find myself spending a great deal of time performing the duties of a Hospital Superintendent.' He added, 'highly important though it is, hospital administration per se does not interest me in the least, and I shall be glad when the time comes for me to be relieved of this time-consuming and unacademic part of my work'. He also referred to public criticism that he was not practising obstetrics, but said that 'having no staff of my own – not even a house surgeon – it would be quite impractical for me to do justice to any obstetrical patients'. However, he added peevishly, 'it is clearly for me to decide what clinical work I do and when I do it'.[95] The job was not what he had expected and seemed to leave him exasperated and defensive.

Despite being on a five-year contract, Spence Smyth resigned in March 1954.[96] Subsequent assessments of his contribution to the hospital were generally negative, though it was acknowledged that he worked under disadvantages. In his history of the postgraduate school, Green noted the lack of facilities for Smyth.[97] Others commented on his lack of research and teaching experience, and that he was confronted with a well-established group of senior obstetricians and gynaecologists. Nor did his wife and children adapt well to their new home; they left before Christmas 1953. Spence Smyth returned to South Africa, and when Green contacted him ten years later he was working at Montebello Mission Hospital in Zululand. He died in 1975.[98]

Irwin Bruce (Bill) Faris, an obstetrical scholar (awarded in 1942, although interrupted by war service with the RNZAF 1943–45) who gained his MRCOG in 1949 and FRCS in 1950 before returning to New Zealand, held the position of temporary assistant to the professor and medical director from 1952 to January 1954.[99] The post of 'Assistant to the Medical Director' was advertised in Britain, and one of the applicants was Harvey Carey, who was appointed from January 1954.[100] Carey accepted this post on information he received in London that there was the prospect of very rapid promotion to professor.[101] Indeed, when Spence Smyth left two months later, Carey became temporary professor and medical director until December 1954, when he was confirmed as the new professor and director from 1 January 1955.[102] Bernard (Bernie) Kyle, another obstetrical scholar, arrived back from England in May 1954 to fill the position of assistant director. Faris continued on the part-time consultant staff.

In 1955, the year before she died, Gordon wrote a long letter to Barrer about the 'misuse of Trust money'.[103] She explained how for seven years the advisory committee of Auckland University 'had set its face against a top drawer salary, presumably not to raise jealousy amid other University Professors'. She stated that, 'The Auckland Endowment, like the Otago one, was raised on the public slogan of World parity for a teacher of world standing.' Once the money was handed to the Auckland University College and its advisory committee, however, they 'hesitated and baulked at a salary calculated to attract the best clinical Professor'. She referred to the original goal of the fund, 'to bring home one of our own most outstanding scholars', and claimed that at least three of these scholars, apart from Stallworthy, were very interested but were deterred by the inadequate salary and the refusal to grant private practice. She claimed that if the professor were allowed to see just 30 private patients per annum he would earn the difference over which they haggled and that had wrecked the project.

Gordon told Barrer that she was the only one of the committee who strongly opposed the appointment of Smyth, 'which was another of their bad bargain purchases obtained by the policy of hunting in bargain basements, when all the time they hold an open cheque to go up and find the best'. She added that in the end they could not get rid of the South African quickly enough.

She also told Barrer that she had dissented at the 1954 university meeting to 'the present unsuitable appointment' of Harvey Carey.[104] She held that research had not been mentioned as a major duty of the professor in the original endowment drive; rather, he was to have an able bedside manner. But, she said, Auckland, 'determined not to pay an unusual salary, pushed in a pure scientist. Clever no doubt. But the type who would never succeed in routine private practice.' How then, she asked, could he teach doctors the proper bedside manner or how to win the patient's confidence so she would reveal her domestic stresses or sorrows? Gordon concluded crossly, 'This is not a confidential letter. It's just the truth . . . . The University of New Zealand at least ought to know that a big public trust is being mismanaged under the caption of equal salaries for all.'[105]

Doris Gordon and Her Obstetrical Dream

Auckland got its new hospital, postgraduate school of obstetrics and gynaecology, and professor. Doris Gordon was a key figure in bringing this about. She was determined and politically astute; she never lost her missionary zeal. In a tribute after she died in 1956, Douglas Robb aptly described her as a 'crusader with a sword'. Robb said:

> No one who knew Dr Doris Gordon, or at least no one who was being used by her for her high purposes would remain long in doubt about her tenacities and inflexibilities in pursuit of her ends. A mere male, the ordinary decent peace-loving type might even be a little afraid of her energy and of the services she required. Fear was even on occasions known to develop into alarm as the pressure was put on and as the chariot wheels revolved faster and faster. To be of any use to Dr Doris you had to be ready to write letters, ring people up, try to put pressure on them, write newspaper articles, and generally leave your bed at any hour of the day or night . . . . Some mere males have even been so peevish as to characterise her communications as unparliamentary or even unscrupulous but these persons take no account of Doris Gordon as a creative woman.[106]

Gordon made both friends and enemies by her stance. Professionally she was highly regarded. She was awarded MBE in 1935. In 1925 she had been the first woman in Australasia to gain a fellowship of the Royal College of Surgeons of Edinburgh. She was elected a foundation member of the British (later Royal) College of Obstetricians and Gynaecologists, was elected to a fellowship in 1937 and, unusually, was appointed an honorary fellow in 1954. At the time this honour had been bestowed on only 20 leading obstetricians in the world. She was the sole woman outside royalty to be so honoured, and the only recipient in the southern hemisphere.[107]

Gordon was extremely energetic and driven. Mrs Norma Jenkin, who worked in Gordon's surgery at Stratford, later remembered how, when she was working on her autobiography, she would 'dash in about 5 a.m., write a chapter for me to type and then start work'. Pointing out that Gordon had four children, Jenkin wrote, 'she would work right up to her own confinement.

I remember that she once delivered a baby and then had her own only a few hours later.'[108]

Gordon could be described as a 'maternalist', working for the welfare of women and children in a political way.[109] In 1955 she wrote that a committee of inquiry into maternity should be appointed every five years or so, as a non-party committee and including women MPs and mothers. She thought that 'leading women sociologists [should] report to the Government of the day upon their <u>own</u> Maternity Affairs. The alternative would be to give every detail of Maternity affairs and buildings into Women's hands.'[110] Further, she claimed, 'If you relax your watching care of what is a feminine aspect of living, the males will let your services slide or drift or be regimentalized so mothers are just cogs in an inhuman State machine.'[111] Gender roles were very clear to Gordon; she believed women held responsibilities and she had boundless confidence in the ability of women to win the day.

Gordon did not entirely realise her dream; she was not happy with the appointment of Harvey Carey and the emphasis on scientific research. However, the appointment committee for the chair had envisaged research as coming within the professor's remit. Moreover, there is no reason to assume that Stallworthy or Hawksworth would have taken the hospital in a different direction. The 1950s was a decade of great excitement about the future potential of scientific medicine, with widespread and unquestioning faith in the powers of science and technology. Nor did women necessarily become disempowered by, or disapprove of, these new developments; the NCW, together with other women's organisations, continued to monitor developments within the field of maternity closely, as will be seen.

CHAPTER 3

A TRIPOD: PATIENT CARE, RESEARCH AND TEACHING, THE 1950s TO 1963

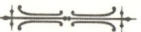

In his foreword to the first clinical report of the Obstetrical and Gynaecological Unit, Cornwall Hospital (1948–49), Auckland Hospital Board chairman John Grierson declared that it fulfilled a vital role in the life of the community. That year almost 1500 women had given birth there, over 1300 had been admitted with gynaecological problems and many more had attended as outpatients. The compilers of the report, Drs Frederick Clark and Herb Green, considered it important to mention in their introduction that the hospital aimed not only to serve the public, but also to improve the educational facilities in obstetrics and gynaecology for the whole country.[1] As a teaching hospital National Women's was similar to the Obstetric Unit at University College Hospital, London, whose director from 1946 to 1966 was William Nixon. Nixon likened the work of his unit to a tripod whose three legs represented clinical work, research and teaching, and declared that the failure of any one would cause the tripod to fall.[2] A direct link with this unit was established in 1964 when Nixon's assistant Dennis Bonham was appointed postgraduate professor in Auckland. However, even under Bonham's predecessor, the parallels were strong; Harvey Carey too emphasised the importance of the hospital as a teaching and research unit alongside its role as a women's hospital.

Harvey Carey: Teaching and Research

Harvey Carey was appointed postgraduate professor and head of the 'O & G Unit' in January 1955. From that time on, the hospital became known as National Women's Hospital, in recognition of its role as a national training and research centre. Carey revealed his views on medical research a few years later when the NCW asked him why he thought New Zealand had fallen from having the lowest infant death rate in the world in the early twentieth century to seventh place by the 1950s. He believed there was in New Zealand a 'reluctance to experiment' and a tendency to 'wait for new and modern techniques to be thoroughly tested overseas before they were practiced here' and this, in his view, led to 'frustration and stagnation'.[3] Given charge of New Zealand's largest women's hospital, Carey was determined that it would be at the forefront of innovative research at a time when there was great optimism attached to the possibilities of medical science.

Harvey Carey was born in Whangarei on 21 April 1917. His father, Mark Warren Carey, was an Australian and his mother a New Zealander. After three years in Whangarei they moved to Sydney and then, two years later, to South Africa, where Carey remained until he returned to Australia as a medical student. Carey's father was a Seventh-day Adventist (and later a Methodist) and Carey was, like his father, deeply religious; as an undergraduate he was president of the Evangelical Union of Sydney University and after graduation was a lifelong member of the Christian Medical Fellowship. He graduated in medicine at the University of Sydney in 1941. He also gained a BSc (Med) Hons in physiology (1939), and subsequently an MSc (1946) and a Diploma in Obstetrics and Gynaecology (1948). From 1943 to 1945 he did war service in the Royal Australian Air Force. During the war he met Grace Pinkerton, who was also studying medicine, and they married in Adelaide in 1948.[4] Achieving his MRCOG (London) and FRCS (Edinburgh) in 1950, he took up a post as senior registrar in obstetrics and gynaecology at the Royal Postgraduate School at Hammersmith Hospital, London. There he worked with Ian Donald, subsequently Regius Professor of Midwifery at the University of Glasgow from 1954 to 1976 where he pioneered the use of diagnostic ultrasound in medicine. Whilst Carey was at Hammersmith in 1951 he was awarded a University of London travelling fellowship to spend a year in America, where he worked at Johns Hopkins Hospital, Baltimore.[5]

Carey began his teaching career early; he supported himself through medical school by providing concise notes for other students.[6] In 1955 he contributed a chapter to Ian Donald's textbook, *Practical Obstetric Problems*. Two commentators later said of Donald and his textbook: 'He questioned every accepted obstetric procedure and his provocative and never to be forgotten book *Practical Obstetric Problems* . . . spread his teaching all over the world.'[7] Donald noted in the preface, 'The toxaemias of pregnancy are not easy to deal with in a modern way without becoming "woolly", and I am therefore very glad of Harvey Carey's chapter thereon with his uncompromising clarity.' In the third edition Donald commented on Carey's 'intellectual stamina which I learned to appreciate in him when we were together at Hammersmith Hospital'.[8] In 1951 Carey received a standing ovation for his presentation of a research paper, on pregnancy-induced hypertension, at the Royal Society of London.[9]

Carey brought a sense of mission to the new hospital when he was appointed in 1955. His wife Grace said he was married to his work, leaving her to bring up their four children, all of whom were born in Auckland. One of the secretaries at the hospital, Betty Port, agreed. Many was the time, she said, when he did not go home to his wife at the appointed hour: 'His work was his hobby because he was always working', she explained.[10]

In 1946 those running the hospital allowed private medical practitioners to deliver their patients there, owing to the shortage of childbirth facilities in Auckland. However, they regarded this as a temporary concession, stating that private practitioners would eventually be banned, 'in order that the wards could fulfil their true purpose of providing post-graduate training for the doctors'.[11] Bernard Dawson, professor of obstetrics and gynaecology at Otago, thought it was better from an academic point of view if there were no private beds (also called 'open beds') at the hospital.[12] As part of his negotiations to take up the chair in 1949, William Hawksworth asked for the right to treat private fee-paying patients in hospital, as he said he wished to treat 'all classes of patients'. William Cocker, chair of the academic advisory committee for the post, told him, 'There is not in this country the social prejudice against entering public hospital which exists in England. All classes make use of the public hospitals freely.' He explained that the hospital board and the government 'feel that anything which tends to introduce social distinctions into our hospitals is to be avoided'. To allow private practice in hospital, he claimed, would be 'contrary to the whole spirit and policy of our hospital system'.[13] The university referred Hawksworth's request to the government, which did not agree to the 'change in hospital policy' that it would entail.[14]

Both the first Labour government which had introduced social security and the National government, elected to office in 1949, were committed to the free public hospital system established under the 1938 Social Security Act.[15]

In the mid-1950s, when plans for a new purpose-built hospital were under way, the planning committee resolved that there should be no private beds in the new hospital. However, by this time senior consultant staff had become used to treating both private and public patients in the hospital, which had initially been introduced as a temporary measure because of the shortage of facilities. The staff strongly resisted the planning committee's suggestion, arguing that it was in the interests of the institution to have both sets of patients and in the interests of private patients to be near specialised facilities. Believing 'this question of "open" beds should be fought for to the last ditch',[16] in 1962 they passed a resolution that 'the senior staff of NWH are unanimously and emphatically of the opinion that private maternity beds should be retained in the new National Women's Hospital'.[17] The dual system continued.

All of the senior consultant staff at the hospital were involved in teaching. Postgraduate medical teaching in the hospital initially took two forms: six-month refresher courses for general practitioners (who did most of the deliveries in New Zealand at that time), and two years' training for those who intended to specialise in obstetrics and gynaecology, before they proceeded to England or Australia to sit their membership examinations for the RCOG. Norman Jeffcoate, professor of obstetrics and gynaecology at the University of Liverpool and later president of the RCOG, visited New Zealand in 1955 and advised that there was such competition in England for posts suitable for aspirants to membership of the RCOG that it was essential for New Zealanders to have completed their two years' training before proceeding to Britain.[18] It appears they got quality tuition at Auckland. After passing his exams in 1960, Dr Liam Wright (an obstetrical scholar) wrote back to the hospital, 'I appreciate the fact that my success in the examination was made possible by the help and training I received from them [senior staff] during my term – a very enjoyable term – at National Women's. I think all the resident staff, while at the hospital, realise that they are getting the best of both worlds – both good clinical experience and training, and good teaching. However, the fact is greatly emphasised when one meets people in similar positions over here.'[19]

Professor Spence Smyth had begun the first refresher courses for general practitioners in 1952.[20] A diploma in obstetrics was introduced in 1955, and formalised as the New Zealand Diploma in Obstetrics in 1958. Those who had completed six months' residential training in obstetrics and gynaecology, or who had delivered at least 300 babies, were eligible to sit for the diploma, following three intensive five-day courses at National Women's. Thirty-two general practitioners sat the exam in 1958, but only ten passed, indicating the high standards demanded.[21] Not only did Carey teach at National Women's, he also went on lecture tours around the country. Obstetrical consultant Dr Edwin Sayes, who worked at Northland's Whangarei Hospital, remembered hosting Carey on a number of occasions.[22] Carey also visited other small centres; for instance, in 1959 he reported that he had been the main lecturer for weekend courses in 'Christchurch, Invercargill, Hamilton, Tauranga, Napier, Whakatane, Gisborne, Lower Hutt, Masterton, Matamata, Paraparaumu and Palmerston North'. About 50 doctors attended each of these courses.[23]

National Women's also became involved in hosting doctors in training from Thailand. The Colombo Plan for Cooperative Economic Development in Asia and the Pacific had been set up in 1950 by a group of Commonwealth countries, including New Zealand. The aim was to provide assistance in the form of training programmes, loans, food supplies, equipment and technical aid to poorer countries in Southeast Asia, in order to curb the spread of Communism. As part of the plan, National Women's took junior doctors from Thailand for a year. However, there were problems, as the doctors at National Women's came to realise. In particular, they discovered that in a society where seniors were respected it was inappropriate for junior staff to criticise or question senior staff, which meant they could not introduce anything new following their return from Auckland.[24] In order to address this problem, in 1962 Carey met with senior obstetricians and gynaecologists in Bangkok, who agreed to send heads of departments rather than junior doctors. One of the first to come under this scheme was Dr Jiree Limtrakarn, director of the Department of Obstetrics and Gynaecology at Bangkok's Women's Hospital, who spent three months on the staff of National Women's in 1962.[25]

As part of his vision for the postgraduate school, Carey targeted talented young researchers to work with him. In 1956 he appointed Herb Green as his professorial assistant. Born in New Zealand (Balclutha) in 1917, George Herbert Green had completed his medical studies at Otago University in 1945, gaining his RCOG Diploma in 1948 and his MRCOG in 1950. As a registrar at National Women's Hospital from 1948 to 1950, he had written the hospital's first two clinical reports. From 1951 to 1955 he worked in hospitals in Britain before returning to New Zealand, initially to Wanganui Hospital and then National Women's. In 1961 he was promoted to associate professor of obstetrics and gynaecology. He lectured and published a textbook for maternity nurses,[26] and developed his own research interest in cervical cancer and carcinoma *in situ*. Before undertaking his medical degree, Green had completed a BA (1938) and BSc (1940) including mathematics, and developed a particular interest in epidemiology, which informed his later studies on Maori maternal mortality statistics and trends in cervical cancer.[27] An original thinker who questioned some of the more interventionist trends in modern medicine, Green was later to come to blows with some of his colleagues.[28]

In his evaluation of potential researchers, Carey appeared to show more insight than did members of the hospital board; Green commented on the 'curious situation' whereby Carey had difficulty in persuading the board to appoint as his first research assistant one of future Nobel prize-winner Professor John Eccles' protégés – for the board insisted that 'A. W. Liley, MB PhD, was far too inexperienced in research to be appointed'.[29]

New Zealand-born William (Bill) Liley had come to Auckland from Otago for his final year of medical studies in 1954, and worked as Carey's research assistant and as resident paediatric officer.[30] Carey soon earmarked him for 'his intellectual qualities, his capacity for lateral thinking, enthusiasm and depth of compassion'.[31] Liley had already enjoyed a distinguished undergraduate career, working with Eccles in Dunedin. Following graduation in 1954, he took up a research scholarship in physiology at the Australian National University in Canberra. There he continued the studies he had started with Eccles, on neuromuscular transmission. In 1957 Liley was awarded a Sandoz Research Fellowship at National Women's.[32] His teachers at Canberra were 'aghast and dismayed . . . they maintained he was throwing away a perfectly good career in basic medical research and going into one of the most unscientific branches of medicine'. 'Professional suicide', Liley said they called it.[33] In his application for the fellowship he stated that he aimed 'to investigate ways of increasing the salvage of premature infants [and] transplacental passage of antigens and antibodies'.[34]

Liley held that fellowship for one year, and was then appointed senior research fellow in obstetrics and gynaecology to the Medical Research Council of New Zealand (MRCNZ), based at the postgraduate school. In 1963, after Carey had taken up a chair at the University of New South Wales, Green, as acting head of the postgraduate school, applied to the university to renew Liley's contract. He told the registrar,

> Dr Liley has shown me letters conveying increasingly attractive offers of a position in the University of NSW. Professor Carey is well aware of Dr Liley's capabilities and I cannot blame him for trying to tempt this NZer to Australia. The plain fact and I know you are well aware of this, is that this hospital, postgraduate school and New Zealand as a whole, cannot afford to lose Dr Liley.[35]

He was right: Liley went on to put New Zealand on the world map in medical research.

Graham (Mont) Liggins also found Carey to be 'a great supporter; he gave you your head, all he wanted was that your results would be available to him when he took one of his overseas trips which he could talk about'.[36] Like Liley, Liggins was lured to National Women's by Carey. Liggins explained, 'Harvey in typical fashion said he wanted me to join the staff but he didn't really have a job, he'd get one in due course – that was how he got everybody there he wanted. And until the university appointment [senior lectureship] came along, I did various things including a year as National Women's Hospital's first medical superintendent.'[37]

Liggins was born in the North Island of New Zealand, in the mining town of Thames, and graduated in medicine from Otago Medical School in 1948. He pursued further study in Britain from 1953 and returned to New Zealand in 1959, when he was appointed temporary junior specialist to the postgraduate school.[38] In 1961 Carey secured a third full-time university post in the school which went to Liggins (the other two posts were held by Carey and Green).[39] Liggins was appointed full-time clinical lecturer at the postgraduate school from 1962, and in 1971 he was promoted to a chair in obstetric and gynaecological endocrinology. Liggins too was to bring National Women's international fame.

Carey fostered a research environment. He later reflected that his 'main contribution to New Zealand O. & G.' was to get Green back into academic medicine, to organise the administrative framework of a teaching and research unit, and to get Mont Liggins and Bill Liley started on research activities.[40] Carey's obituary noted that he was a 'great believer in academic freedom, giving every encouragement and assistance to his subordinates while at the same time allowing them to develop their own directions of research'.[41]

Hospital radiologist John Stewart said of Carey that his own talents lay in physiology rather than the practice of obstetrics and gynaecology, which caused some loss of respect among colleagues, but that he had 'a wonderful ability to motivate people'.[42]

Research was organised into teams. By 1957, Carey reported that the staff had now accepted as an established principle that different teams had a special interest in different disorders and were undertaking detailed studies. 'Under these circumstances the staff have agreed to admitting all cases suffering from the condition under study under the teams interested in that particular investigation.' Examples included 'A' team: severe toxaemia; 'B' team: pregnant diabetes and pre-diabetics; 'C' team: carcinoma of the vulva; and 'D' team: carcinoma of the cervix.[43]

From 1948, before the appointment of a professor, the staff held monthly meetings at which they discussed clinical cases and deaths at the hospital.[44] These meetings continued through the 1950s.[45] Paediatrician Jack Matthews remembered them fondly as 'great learning occasions'. He described them as 'occasions where pathologists were able to show us in detail what had happened to the babies we had been caring for and who had died. They were held at night so everyone could get there.' He also commented that visitors, 'guest professors and so on, took part in all these meetings and they themselves made comments on the very high standard'.[46]

Carey believed the meetings had important educational functions, informing students of different clinical practices in the hospital by focusing on 'controversial subjects'.[47] At some point they changed from being held monthly to weekly ('at tea-time'), but they had trouble attracting residents and students, and so they were temporarily abandoned in 1959.[48] Senior staff clearly regretted this and in 1961 Bruce Grieve (another obstetrical scholar who had been appointed to the hospital in 1950) proposed they be reinstated.[49] The following Hospital Medical Committee (HMC) meeting agreed, although it decided they should be called 'Clinical Meetings' rather than 'Tea Parties', that Green should be the convener and that the format should be 'essentially informal'.[50] These meetings had a precarious existence and again fell into abeyance; two years later, in 1963, the HMC recorded: 'Clinico-Pathological Conferences – Prof Green would like these sessions re-started.'[51]

Another feature of the hospital was the constant influx of academic visitors from overseas, from Australia, South Africa, America, Europe and Britain. In 1957 Sir James Paterson Ross, then president of the Royal College of Surgeons and surgeon to Queen Elizabeth, visited the hospital.[52] These visits enhanced the reputation of the hospital locally and internationally. Carey later explained that attracting overseas lecturers was a conscious part of stimulating interest in postgraduate obstetrics and gynaecology amongst specialists and general practitioners. He also noted, however, that the university had no funds for this, so costs were met by providing or organising private hospitality. His wife Grace had 'considerable extra work entertaining these visitors and their wives; organising social functions'. Local branches of the NZOGS also helped out. He explained that, 'In place of paying the visitors for lecturing they were taken on tours of Rotorua and the Glow Worm Caves, etc.'[53]

Maternity and Pain Relief

For all its teaching, research and hosting of academic visitors, National Women's primary function was as a maternity hospital. Many Auckland women gave birth there in the 1950s and during the following decades. Some subsequent historians have characterised hospital births in the aftermath of the Second World War as excessively interventionist. Jean Donnison wrote of North America that, 'By the 1950s, except in some remote rural areas . . . childbirth was generally hospitalised and completely doctor-controlled. Typically, normal healthy women were delivered unconscious from anaesthetic, arms and legs strapped to the delivery table, the doctor performing an episiotomy and "lifting out" the baby with forceps.'[54] According to another historian, Mary Thomas, in the post-Second World War hospital setting with obstetricians in 'total control', 'the drugged and/or anesthetized woman had almost no say in her delivery; her conscious participation was minimal at best, and . . . often unwelcome'.[55] To what extent could the same be said about New Zealand's most medically controlled and research-focused maternity centre, National Women's Hospital, in the 1950s?

The hospital's clinical reports give a good indication of medical procedures at that time. Most of the deliveries involving the use of forceps at National Women's in 1950 included the giving of deep anaesthesia, generally ether, although in just under 10 per cent local or spinal anaesthesia was given. Yet forceps deliveries constituted only 15.6 per cent (248) of all deliveries in 1950. Caesarean section, the delivery of a baby by cutting through the walls of the abdomen and uterus, constituted a further 8.2 per cent (127) of all deliveries at National Women's in 1950 and these were done under general anaesthesia. The number of 'normal deliveries' that year was 1127.[56]

It is hard to know how many of those deliveries listed as normal received some form of pain relief in labour. In a lecture delivered in the 1940s, Tom Plunkett, a senior obstetrician at the hospital, commented on the public demand for complete anaesthetics and appeared resigned to the fact that 'the parturient woman is *entitled* to . . . anaesthesia'.[57]

Certainly the pre-war clamour for pain relief in childbirth continued postwar. For instance, in 1946 a deputation representative of a local Women's Citizen Guild and the New Zealand Family Planning Association (NZFPA) met with Health Minister Arnold Nordmeyer in Wellington to discuss the question of adequate pain relief in childbirth. Mrs Ford from the NZFPA 'emphasised that the Association were not advocating any particular methods of pain relief, but were anxious that any which could give tremendous relief should be investigated'. She said that the association had the support of the NCW, which had that year passed a resolution calling for all women to have adequate pain relief in childbirth. Another member of the deputation, Mrs Hogan, who had three children, explained that her first two had been very difficult births, and that she had had very little relief, so much so that during her third pregnancy she spent nine months in fear. However, on entering the maternity home in Auckland, she was given nembutal hyoscine (a hypnotic drug) in tablet form, and almost immediately felt the effect of it. The baby was perfectly normal, and she herself slept for several hours. Mrs Hogan said that some nurses believed that mothers were unable to breastfeed their babies after receiving nembutal hyoscine, but she managed to breastfeed her baby for several months.

The deputation asked Nordmeyer to inquire into those methods that gave total relief from pain in childbirth, and into the extent to which they were available to mothers. They argued that if the need for expensive apparatus were a deterrent to the wider use of pain relief, the government should subsidise hospitals, and that if the training of personnel was a deterrent, the government should provide refresher courses for maternity nurses and doctors. They regarded pain relief as a welfare entitlement. Indeed, the deputation considered that every mother was entitled to have as much pain relief as possible during childbirth, not because women were not willing to bear pain, they explained, but because at the present time, when there was so much pain relief becoming available, mothers should not be deprived.[58]

New Zealand women were not alone in making these demands. An article in Britain in 1945 declared, 'It is no use saying our grandmothers had babies without anaesthetics. Women's standards are different today. The modern woman is not going to accept the standards of the nineteenth century. Science has proved that it can make things easier for them and they want the help that science can give them.'[59] A survey the following year of nearly 14,000 women who gave birth in Britain during a specified week found that the absence of pain relief was the most common reason for dissatisfaction with treatment during labour. The survey quoted one woman who said, 'Something should be given. I was tired out before I started. People with plenty of money don't have to suffer pain . . . . I feel scared of having another baby.'[60]

In his response to the 1946 deputation, Nordmeyer commented on reasons why pain relief might be withheld. He said that on entering maternity homes the women would be looked after by midwives, and, 'Generally speaking, most of the nurses running maternity homes were kindly people, but sometimes they were not and thought it better to make the mother tough.' Similar impressions prevailed in post-war Britain, where midwives as well as doctors were accused of a 'callous attitude to distress' and taking 'an almost sadistic joy in withholding sedatives from mothers in labour'.[61]

Finally, responding to the deputation's concern that many doctors might be out of date, Nordmeyer went on to boast about the government's new initiative in Auckland, the postgraduate school. However, he added a word of caution: although drugs would allow the mother to have a painless childbirth, he said that as a consequence she might lose her baby, and 'this had to be guarded against'.[62]

During its first decade National Women's had no full-time anaesthetist. In 1948 the HMC noted that nurses were giving ether anaesthetics without medical supervision. The committee issued instructions that the labour ward sister should call the resident immediately if she 'decided' that an anaesthetic was required. A second resident should be summoned if 'deep anaesthetics' were required; this included all forceps deliveries.[63] A decade later, nurses were still giving anaesthetics; although the HMC recorded in its minutes of 20 September 1958 that 'on no account should the nursing staff be called upon to give the anaesthetic', this was crossed out as a correction to the minutes at the next meeting.[64]

In 1948 National Women's HMC discussed accidents associated with anaesthesia. The committee pointed out that the only absolute safeguard was for each patient to be watched continuously, but realised that with the current nursing shortage this was not always possible. They considered the 'present experiment' of having particularly restless patients on a mattress on the floor an additional safeguard, but thought it most inconvenient and noted that nurses had found it impossible to lift a heavy patient to the height of the labour ward bed again. The committee recommended the construction of a bed capable of being lowered to the floor as 'the only practical safeguard' and believed that, once such a bed was provided in each labour ward, then 'every reasonable precaution will have been taken to prevent further accidents'.[65]

Yet doctors in the 1950s were generally becoming cognisant of the disadvantages of deep anaesthesia. A 1951 report on pain relief in obstetrics, compiled by a sub-committee of the NZOGS, pointed out that ether, the main form of deep anaesthesia used at National Women's, was unpleasant to the patient, produced 'gagging' and was often accompanied by vomiting. Moreover, it could lead to haemorrhage and caused more drowsiness in the baby than did light chloroform anaesthesia.[66] The previous year Dr Thomas Corkill had noted an increase of maternal deaths under general anaesthesia in New Zealand, from an average of 16 deaths per year in the early 1930s to 38 by 1950.[67]

In 1958 a newly appointed anaesthetist at National Women's, Dr Robert Coulter, conflicted with senior consultant Jefcoate Harbutt who was still advocating chloroform at the end of the second stage of labour. Coulter described chloroform as positively dangerous.[68] A second obstetrical anaesthetist, Dr Richard (Dick) Climie, who also joined the hospital staff in 1958, attempted to change the practices there. He told Carey that it had become widely accepted that general anaesthesia in childbirth was particularly hazardous and should be avoided if possible.[69] Probably under Climie's influence, in November 1958 the HMC set out to uncover the existing situation regarding deaths under anaesthesia and asked the Health Department's medical statistician Cedric Gardiner whether maternity deaths included any anaesthetic deaths. This was possibly inspired by the publication in 1957 of the first *Report on Confidential Enquiries into Maternal Deaths in England and Wales 1952–54*. This report found that 49 of the 1410 deaths associated with pregnancy and childbirth from 1952 to 1954 in England and Wales were due to complications of anaesthesia, and that in a further 20 cases anaesthesia was a contributory factor and could also have played a part in some of the deaths from haemorrhage. The inhalation of regurgitated stomach contents was the most common cause of death under anaesthesia.[70]

Gardiner responded to the HMC that death certificates referred to the underlying 'maternity cause' rather than anaesthetics as the cause of death. In 1957 three deaths classified as maternal deaths mentioned anaesthesia.

He added that there might have been others, but that this information was not available.[71] It was therefore very difficult to ascertain how many deaths were due to anaesthesia. The committee then asked him to review maternal deaths from 1949 to 1958 and to find out how many death certificates mentioned anaesthesia as a cause or associated cause of death. He found 20 instances, giving an anaesthetic death rate of one in every 22,500 births.[72]

A study in Britain around the same time showed an anaesthetic death rate of one in every 34,000 births. The author of the study, R. B. Parker, a lecturer in obstetrics and gynaecology at the University of Birmingham, commented that while this appeared low, 'because such deaths are entirely preventable, and because the victim is often a perfectly fit woman, it has an importance greater than its lowly place might suggest'. He surveyed the situation in the USA where he said, of over 4 million births annually, more than 3 million mothers received some form of anaesthesia. At the Chicago Lying-In Hospital, for instance, almost 100 per cent of the women received an anaesthetic in childbirth. Parker thought that official records might underestimate the extent of the problem of deaths under anaesthesia, in the USA as elsewhere, but he calculated that in 1955 as many as 10 per cent of all maternal deaths in the state of Michigan were due to anaesthesia. He predicted that, as other causes of death were abolished with the passage of time, the proportion of anaesthetic deaths would mount unless practices changed.[73]

In an article published in the *NZMJ* in 1960, Climie also acknowledged that the 'particular hazards' associated with anaesthesia were well recognised. He divided them into two groups: maternal hazards, nearly always the consequences of vomiting while anaesthetised, and fetal hazards, with drugs causing anoxia (breathing difficulties).[74] Concern then did not just focus on maternal risks, but also on the effects of anaesthesia on the newborn baby. One narcotic analgesic drug called 'pethidine', which had been popular since the 1930s, was later shown to be particularly hazardous for the baby's breathing; indeed it was noted that 'most of these infants required some active resuscitation'.[75]

The risks to the baby of anaesthesia had long been known. In a lecture on 'asphyxia of the newborn' in the late 1940s, National Women's consultant Tom Plunkett stated that this was probably one of the most common conditions to be encountered in the newborn baby, 'particularly in these days when the public demand fairly complete analgesia and amnesia'. He took it for granted that giving narcotic drugs late in labour 'will produce a trail of asphyxiated babies with a proportionately high mortality rate'.[76] Premature babies were particularly at risk. The hospital's first clinical report (1948–49) referred to the policy of delivering premature babies under local anaesthesia and with a minimum of analgesic drugs for the mother where possible, which the authors, Clark and Green, were confident would help to reduce significantly the mortality amongst premature infants.[77]

The 1957 UK *Report on Confidential Enquiries into Maternal Deaths* commented that chloroform was now seldom used in hospital practice, adding that local anaesthesia was increasingly employed.[78] In 1959 William Mushin, professor of anaesthesia at the Welsh National School of Medicine, University of Wales, and 'one of the most active lecturers in the world of Anaesthesia in Great Britain', visited National Women's Hospital.[79] He told Carey that the percentage of women receiving general anaesthesia in his maternity hospital in Cardiff had fallen from about 25 to less than five while the forceps rate had been rising. He predicted that local anaesthesia would be used more and more.[80]

Local or regional anaesthesia was achieved by injecting an anaesthetic agent into the pudendal canal, the caudal end of the spinal canal, the epidural space or the spine, causing a loss of sensation in that area during childbirth. A major incentive for developing local anaesthesia was to avoid the ill-effects of general anaesthesia on the newborn. Discussing lumbar epidurals in 1960, Climie enthused, 'There is no doubt that the infants in this series required a great deal less in the way of active resuscitation than a similar group of deliveries performed under general anaesthesia.'[81] As the anaesthetist, it was Climie's job to resuscitate babies; paediatricians were not attached to labour wards in the 1950s.

Climie advocated abolishing the use of general anaesthesia in obstetrics altogether, and replacing it by various local techniques.[82] He began to institute this practice at National Women's immediately upon his arrival in September 1958. Of 30 women who had forceps deliveries the month before his arrival, 16 were given local and 14 were given general anaesthesia. In October 1958 there were 30 forceps deliveries, with 21 under local and only 9 under general anaesthesia. By December 1958, 19 of the 20 forceps deliveries were done under local anaesthesia. Climie told Carey that low forceps deliveries could almost always be carried out satisfactorily under local anaesthesia.[83] By 1959, when there were 331 forceps deliveries at National Women's (from a total of 2564 births), general anaesthesia was used for only 28 women, 'many of whom had either a stillborn or abnormal infant'. His preferred method was lumbar epidurals and he reported in January 1959 that, 'So far, 15 deliveries have been carried out with this method and the results have been most gratifying.'[84] This was around the same time that epidurals were being introduced to hospitals in the United States.[85]

A mild form of pain relief given to women during labour was self-administered inhalational analgesia. During the planning of the purpose-built National Women's Hospital in 1960, Climie recommended that piped gases of nitrous oxide and oxygen be installed, as they had been at the Royal Women's Hospital in Melbourne, to give some relief during labour.[86]

Natural Childbirth and the Interests of the Newborn

Local anaesthesia and self-administered analgesia, as opposed to general anaesthesia, were not the only solutions proposed to combat the dangers of pain relief to the newborn. Harvey Carey was drawn to another solution – no pain relief at all, or 'natural' childbirth. He argued that the use of sedatives, nembutal for example, was not fair to the baby: 'My first consideration is the baby', he said, 'I don't believe in doing anything for which the baby has to pay.' Sedatives made the baby sleepy and if there was a complication in the delivery this often tipped the scales against the baby. He noted approvingly that New Zealand already had an instrumental delivery rate of only 4 to 6 per cent, compared to 50 to 60 per cent in the United States, and went on to acknowledge the contribution of the British obstetrician, Grantly Dick-Read.[87]

An advocate of natural childbirth, Dick-Read believed that women suffered pain in childbirth largely because they were afraid and unprepared. If women could be taught to relax during labour, they would not require pain relief. Some local New Zealand doctors expounded on Dick-Read's ideas in a magazine called *Woman To-day* in 1937. They were responding to feminist Vera Crowther's argument that pain relief was a woman's right. They cited an article by Dick-Read in a recent textbook edited by a prominent British obstetrician, Francis James Browne. This book ran into nine editions and was later described as 'the Bible for [those] studying obstetrics and gynaecology at the time'.[88] Dick-Read's chapter was called 'The Influences of the Emotions upon Pregnancy and Parturition'.[89] The doctors explained how Dick-Read had shown that 'fear of pain during childbirth has a retarding and generally serious effect on what would otherwise be a normal process', and that 'fear produces tension; tension, pain; and pain, increased fear. And so the vicious circle of prolonged and difficult labour is complete . . . . To develop fear in a woman is therefore causing her pain which is quite unnecessary.' As noted in the previous chapter, Crowther responded that those who feared childbirth most were the ones who had been through it before, unrelieved by anaesthesia.[90] Many women at this time were not persuaded by these doctors' arguments; as Plunkett had noted, they believed that pain relief was an entitlement.[91]

Yet this was to change as Dick-Read's teachings caught on by the 1950s. In 1951, a group of women in Wellington set up the Natural Childbirth Association (later called Parents' Centre), six years before a similar organisation was founded in Britain. By the mid-1950s there were parents' centres throughout New Zealand, and these held antenatal classes for prospective parents to prepare them for natural childbirth, as set out by Dick-Read. Some New Zealanders had corresponded directly with Dick-Read; in 1956 he wrote a letter to the *Auckland Star* in which he referred to 'your readers, from whom I have received so many letters of gratitude'.[92] A Christchurch psychiatrist, Dr Maurice Bevan-Brown, who had worked at London's Tavistock Clinic in the 1920s and 1930s, also brought back Dick-Read's ideas to New Zealand and became closely involved with the new parents' centre movement.[93]

Dick-Read and Bevan-Brown argued that it was important for women to be conscious at the moment of birth in order to initiate mother–child bonding, which would benefit the child, the family and indeed society itself. Dick-Read expounded upon his views in his manuals and voluminous correspondence. For instance, in 1950 he told one mother that a baby born by natural childbirth 'brings with it a fuller love and bondage which not only makes homes and family units secure, but spreads its influence throughout society, which within a few generations bids fair to rid this world of the hideous turmoil which robs its peoples of so much happiness and freedom'.[94] Bevan-Brown had similar utopian goals in advocating natural childbirth. At the first Dominion conference of Parents' Centres in 1957, he explained how natural childbirth with its psychological benefits for babies would lead to a better society. He declared, 'Today's big question is "How to develop a truly human society – not a race of robots or grown-up children".'[95] Natural childbirth, he believed, provided the answer.

Helen Brew, first president of the Federation of New Zealand Parents' Centres, also believed in the psychological benefits of natural childbirth. She presented a talk on 'The Parents' Viewpoint' at a conference on antenatal care at National Women's Hospital in 1958, convened by Carey. She claimed that her first qualification to speak was that she had four children and had read Dick-Read's book. But she also chose to highlight her job as a speech therapist, and referred to some case histories. She found 'a frequent pattern of traumatic childbirth – leading to inadequate early nurture – [which resulted in] speech difficulties especially stammering and associated behaviour problems'. Her husband, Quentin, had helped her prepare her talk, so that it included, she said, a father's perspective; significantly he was also a psychologist.

Helen Brew opposed hospital births. Referring to home births, she said, 'Under that system the maternal and fetal death rates were high but were not probably also the satisfactions of motherhood?' By contrast, in hospital, the woman 'often feels like a body or pregnant uterus on a conveyor belt'. She defined the problems relating to hospitals as lack of personal and individualised care for mothers and babies, assembly-line methods, lack of respect for mothers' feelings and intelligence, and all-but-complete ignoring of the father. Like Dick-Read and Bevan-Brown, Brew believed that the birth experience affected the future psychological health of the baby.[96]

Carey did not subscribe to these psychological benefits of natural childbirth, nor did he support home birth.[97] He did, however, favour natural childbirth. In 1956, he lectured on 'Taking the Fear of the Unknown out of Childbirth', emphasising in particular the advantages for the baby.[98] Melbourne professor of obstetrics and gynaecology, Lance Townsend, who was a guest speaker at a National Women's postgraduate course in 1956, agreed. Like Carey, he favoured natural childbirth, explaining that babies were healthier when delivered this way because they were not doped by anaesthetic and therefore could breathe more easily.[99] Carey told the first Dominion conference of the Parents' Centres in 1957 that anaesthetics could adversely influence the baby's chance of survival. He was averse to going back to home births, he said, because there was always a great danger of 'sudden, unforeseen haemorrhage'. In hospital, though, he did not even support local anaesthesia as, he explained, with all such methods, someone had to pay a price, the mother, the baby or both. He had no regard for the situation in America where, he declared, 'there is an idea that if the mother remembers any detail of her labour then the doctor has been negligent'.[100]

Carey saw great potential in a consumer movement that promoted natural childbirth, and he persuaded the various groups of parents' centres to federate in 1957 in order to strengthen their hand as a lobby group. The following year he organised a three-day conference at National Women's Hospital on antenatal education, and invited representatives from Parents' Centre along with another lay organisation, the Plunket Society. Following the conference, Carey asked an Auckland group which was poised to start a parents' centre to instead form a 'Parents' Hospital Committee' to work within the antenatal department at National Women's Hospital. This committee, formed in 1958, was tasked with cooperating with hospital staff to improve services for 'mothers, their babies and young children'.[101] However, the committee was not a success. Parents' Centre historian Mary Dobbie explained that Carey was often absent from the hospital and that the staff were 'politely baffled by the unsought presence' of this committee. After a while, she said, the committee moved to the 'more sympathetic' Salvation Army Bethany Hospital.[102]

When it was first introduced into National Women's with Carey's backing, natural childbirth was not particularly successful. One report stated that in 1956 only about 12 per cent of mothers at National Women's gave birth without some form of pain relief.[103] Another suggested even poorer results, referring to a survey at National Women's of 300 women, of whom only 21 persisted to the end without relief from drugs, representing 'a failure rate of over 93 per cent'. The author noted that the disillusionment involved in this type of experimentation could be extremely harmful.[104] Carey too cautioned that women who attempted natural childbirth and failed for whatever reason could have a diminished sense of achievement.[105]

By the end of the 1950s at least some women were giving birth in hospital without the use of drugs. Not all women subscribed to the natural childbirth movement, however, or felt a diminished sense of accomplishment because they had used pain-relief drugs. One woman wrote in 1956, 'I am most grateful for the fact that drugs were available and administered. I can frankly say childbirth is the most wonderful experience I have ever had.'[106] Discussing local anaesthesia in 1960, Climie thought that most mothers enjoyed being conscious but pain-free at the time of delivery, but, he added, 'many go to sleep as soon as their pain is relieved and slumber throughout the delivery'.[107]

Medical Intervention in Childbirth at National Women's

American historian Jacqueline Wolf wrote that in America in the 1940s and 1950s 'routine treatments' that included forceps replaced doctors' 'traditional "watchful expectancy" during labour'.[108] As noted above, at National Women's Hospital in 1950 about 15 per cent of all deliveries were by forceps. Hospital registrar Bernie Kyle, who compiled the clinical report for that year, considered this too high, although he also explained that it was the safest way to deliver premature infants and for those with breech presentation. In Britain

Ian Donald also discouraged the use of forceps; his 1955 textbook on obstetrics stated, 'Forceps rates over 10 per cent raise an attitude of enquiry.'[109] In the period 1946 to 1960, 11.3 per cent of the total 35,159 deliveries at National Women's were forceps deliveries, marginally above Donald's threshold.[110] Forceps were not routinely used at National Women's Hospital.

In 1929 Dr Henry Jellett had written dismissively about the glamour attached to caesarean sections.[111] Caesarean sections, which had been rare in the nineteenth and early twentieth century, had become a more viable option by this time, owing to improvements in blood transfusion and infection control. Yet even in the 1950s, with the further benefits of the newly discovered penicillin to combat infection, doctors at National Women's did not undertake this operation lightly. The rate of caesarean sections for 1950 at National Women's was 8.2 per cent (127) of all deliveries. While noting that this rate was 'higher than desirable', Kyle explained that National Women's was the only hospital performing caesareans in a population of 378,000; the incidence of caesarean section for the region was therefore 2.3 per cent, which was similar to Britain in the early 1950s.[112]

In the hospital's clinical report for 1949–50 Green had also commented on caesarean rates. He noted that, while the rate of caesareans had gone down from 14.2 per cent of all births the previous year to 9.5 that year, it was 'still too high even allowing for the fact that very few Caesarean sections are performed elsewhere among a population of 400,000 from which the hospital draws its cases'.[113] The aim was to reduce it, and Green was hopeful this would happen. He explained that the clinical policy of doing elective caesareans for suspected disproportion had been abandoned, owing to an increase in resident medical and honorary staff, with consequent closer and better supervision of labour in cases of suspected disproportion. He noted the value of improved X-ray facilities and the very high standards of radiological pelvimetry by the radiologist, Dr Anthony Crick. He warned readers that caesarean section, which was so often done in the interests of the child, was 'no guarantee of delivery of a live or healthy baby'. That year there was a 9.5 per cent infant mortality rate among those born by caesarean section. He also thought that repeat caesareans would decline with the practice of performing a hysterectomy at the time of the caesarean; in 1949, 21.1 per cent of those having a caesarean were sterilised at the same time.[114] Taking the whole period 1946–60, the caesarean rate at National Women's was 6.2 per cent, suggesting it achieved its goal of containing and even slightly reducing this rate in the 1950s.[115]

By the end of the 1950s the rate of caesarean sections was still of concern to the medical staff. In 1959 Dr H. P. (Pat) Dunn, who joined the hospital as an honorary clinical research assistant in 1958, undertook a follow-up study of caesarean sections conducted at the hospital during 1955–56, which he reported to the HMC and subsequently published in the *NZMJ*.[116] The incidence of caesarean sections in this study was 6.6 per cent of all births (276 out of 4194 deliveries).

While there were no maternal deaths in the group studied, Dunn cited an editorial comment in the *British Medical Journal (BMJ)* that 'Caesarean section is not the safe operation that some would have us believe.'[117] He referred to the *Report on Confidential Enquiries into Maternal Deaths in England and Wales 1952–54*, which stated that maternal mortality from caesarean section was approximately seven times that for vaginal delivery. He commented, 'As the overall Caesarean maternal mortality is at least seven times that for vaginal delivery, theoretically Caesarean section would be justifiable only when the foetal risk is increased sevenfold or more.' He thought fetal distress was always a nebulous diagnosis and should not be acted on too readily. He noted that many of the so-called risks were iatrogenic, that is, caused by medical interventions. Dunn also warned against the practice of surgical induction for 'disproportion, for postmaturity, and for minor indications', pointing out the many risks involved, which were also iatrogenic.[118]

Carey hoped that the electronic stethoscope to record the fetal heartbeat, introduced in 1956, would help to bring down the rate of caesarean section.[119] This was something Carey had been working on in London before coming to New Zealand in 1953.[120] He explained that this equipment provided information that was often vital in deciding whether or not a caesarean operation was necessary. He said the only current drawback with the instrument was that it required constant attention. Any movement of the mother was likely to produce false readings. But he also boasted that the stethoscope was 'above world research'; they had managed to eliminate the recording of extraneous noises such as the sound of someone walking along a nearby corridor. Among Liley's research projects for 1957 was: 'Postmaturity and foetal distress: The use of foetal heart recorder during labour'.[121]

Dunn included a survey of 256 patients' responses in his 1958 research into caesarean sections. He referred to 'perceptive comments [such] as "It's unnatural to be opened like a tin of sardines".' Of the long-term effects, he found that while some women were satisfied and appreciative, others said, 'no more babies'.[122] He recorded a high incidence of voluntary sterility following caesarean section (106 out of 121 patients answering this question), and concluded, 'In most cases caesarean section puts a stop to reproduction and complicates the rest of the patient's childbearing life.' This was clearly a concern for Dunn, coming as he did from a Roman Catholic background.

In his survey, women who commented on their hospital experience resented 'not being treated like an adult', with many stating they wanted more explanation both before and after the operation. They complained that nurses made them get up almost immediately, and that they were sent home after nine or ten days which was too soon. Dunn urged that home help be arranged, and that the mothers' incapacity be explained to their young husbands who 'in their ignorance often expected an immediate return to normal domestic and marital efficiency'.[123] This survey showed that research at the hospital was not necessarily technologically driven, ignoring the feelings and experiences of the women themselves. It also showed that women were not reticent in making their views known.

Another research project at the hospital which drew on women's emotional experience was that conducted by Dr Herbert A. (Bert) Brant and his wife Margaret in 1959, with Carey's encouragement. Brant subsequently became reader and consultant in obstetrics and gynaecology at University College Hospital, London. He had attended and given a paper on 'patient co-operation in labour' at the 1958 antenatal education conference at National Women's Hospital. He and his wife were members of the Christchurch Parents' Centre and, like Dick-Read, thought women could be taught to manage pain in childbirth without drugs. Carey invited the Brants to conduct a controlled study of the advantages of individual antenatal preparation and support involving 123 women who had booked at National Women's Hospital for their first births.

At that time National Women's had communal seven-bed labour wards and nearby delivery rooms with no sound-proofing. The Brants warned their patients that they would hear the cries of frightened women and that others in adjacent beds might moan and groan and become upset. They concluded from their study that the 'Brant treatment group' required fewer drugs, spent less time in second stage labour, had a lower incidence of operative delivery, a smaller postpartum blood loss, and were calmer and more cooperative throughout their labours. The babies of the 'treatment group' were in better physical condition following delivery as assessed by the Apgar scale.[124] Returning to National Women's twelve years later, Brant acknowledged gratefully the 'unrelenting diplomacy' on Carey's part that had made the experiment possible at National Women's – 'that hive of obstetric politics'.[125] Bert and Margaret Brant continued to work in parent education, producing *A Dictionary of Pregnancy, Childbirth and Contraception* in 1971.[126]

The End of the Carey Era

Harvey Carey's support of the Parents' Centre did little to endear him to some of the senior members of the obstetrical and gynaecological profession, who disapproved of the centre as lay interference in medicine. Indeed, his uneasy relationship with the medical hierarchy led another lay group, the New Zealand Family Planning Association, to be wary of his support; in 1960 a branch secretary wrote to the NZFPA Dominion president and secretary:

> One piece of advice [that] seems to be unanimous from all those au fait with B.M.A. politics is to keep out of Prof. Carey's way. In fact one acquaintance has even suggested that our stock would rise considerably in the medical world if we openly quarrelled! I hardly think we should go to these lengths but I do think we shall need to be extra careful just now.[127]

The NZBMA was reluctant to recognise, or give 'ethical approval' to, either the Parents' Centre or the NZFPA, that is, to allow its members to work for these organisations. Dr Alice Bush led the campaign to try to persuade them to grant such approval. Carey's wife, Dr Grace Pinkerton, held meetings of the New Zealand Medical Women's Association for this purpose in their home.[128] It was only after 'considerable discussion' at a meeting in 1961, and several avowals of the Parents' Centre's desire to 'work under medical supervision', that the NZBMA grudgingly approved.[129] As Bush's biographer noted:

> When Alice, seconded by Harvey Carey, moved, 'That this Division approves the recognition of the Federation of Parents' Centres provided there is absolute certainty of Medical Control' – surely sufficiently strong language to satisfy the most reluctant professionals – the vote was carried only by 12 to 9, with 7 abstentions. The NZFPA had fared little better with support of its recognition running at 10 to six.[130]

Carey's alliance with the Parents' Centre also put him off-side with the Nurses and Midwives Registration Board (a conflict which will be further explored in chapter 4) and hence the Department of Health, of which the board was a part. There also appeared to be a 'town versus gown' division between Carey and some of his medical colleagues. Some consultants and the Auckland Hospital Board thought it inappropriate that a university professor should have overall charge of a hospital. This led to the 1957 Hospitals Act which altered the existing arrangement authorising the professor to be the head of the hospital. Following the 1957 Act, an agreement was reached between the University of Auckland and the Auckland Hospital Board that there would be a separate medical superintendent but that the professor would still be responsible for teaching, research and the clinical running of the hospital. Dr Algar Warren was appointed medical superintendent in May 1960. Warren had been obstetrician and gynaecologist to Palmerston North Hospital Board from 1953, and had previously been a house surgeon and registrar at National Women's in 1949 and 1950. He was, according to Dobbie, a hostile critic of the Parents' Centre.[131] Before Warren's appointment as superintendent, Carey had complained to the secretary of the Auckland Hospital Board that, 'The only point put forward in favour of the proposed alterations in administrative control of the NWH was that it would give the Health Department more control over the hospital.'[132]

Conflicts arose immediately upon Warren's appointment. Warren cancelled an HMC meeting called by Carey in November 1960. In a memorandum Warren explained that, 'All committees should be convened and chaired by an impartial Medical Superintendent and not by the head of any one team or section in the hospital.' The latter, he thought, could lead to ill-feeling and friction between the various units of the hospital.[133] For his part, Carey explained his understanding of the HMC meetings. At these meetings, he said, proposals for research were discussed and approved, the results of research work were presented for the information of the hospital staff, the distribution between clinical teams of full-time postgraduate students was considered, the pros and cons and different clinical techniques were debated, and decisions were made regarding the best clinical practice. In short, he believed that the chairing of the meetings by the medical superintendent would 'seriously undermine the effectiveness of the teaching programme in the hospital'.[134] The following April Carey contested the legality of a meeting called by Warren. In response Warren referred to the medical superintendent's right to discuss with his staff 'all matters pertaining to his hospital'.[135]

Around this time, when Carey felt he was being 'driven out' of Auckland,[136] he was offered the chair of obstetrics and gynaecology at the University of

Singapore and also the newly created chair of obstetrics and gynaecology at the University of New South Wales. He accepted the latter.[137] In his letter of resignation from Auckland in July 1962, he explained that dual control of the clinical organisation of the hospital had been operating since September 1960, resulting in 'confusion, frustration and deterioration in the work of the Postgraduate School', which he did not believe was in the best interests of the patients admitted to National Women's Hospital.[138]

Harvey Carey remained as head of the School of Obstetrics and Gynaecology in Sydney until he died in 1989. There he worked on infertility drugs and contraception, and developed the Roman Catholic pill that did not suppress ovulation but rather regulated it to a particular time in the cycle, to help determine the 'safe' period. In 1963 he edited and contributed to a textbook, *Modern Trends in Human Reproductive Physiology*.[139]

In her history of the Parents' Centre, Dobbie commented that Carey's departure left New Zealand the poorer: 'The country had lost a first-class and progressive mind.'[140] Reminiscing about Carey, University of Auckland professor of medicine Sir John Scott described some of the teaching he had experienced at the medical school in Dunedin and added,

> . . . and then we suddenly came up to the old American Army hospital, met Harvey Carey and it hit us like a sledge hammer. Suddenly there were words like 'evidence', the questions, hypotheses were put to us. He was a wonderful man but he fell foul of the old general Auckland [medical] establishment.[141]

According to Bill Liley, the National Women's 'tripod' consisting of patient care, research and teaching was irreparably damaged with the appointment of a medical superintendent. He wrote an impassioned letter to the Vice-Chancellor of the University of Auckland: 'In Professor Carey's day the Professor was the Director, the hospital was the Postgraduate School and the Postgraduate School was the hospital. Everyone from laboratory technicians to visiting staff were part of the school. Certainly the biggest political sellout for the school was the appointment of a Superintendent.'[142] Doris Gordon's vision of a university hospital independent of hospital board control was at an end and the postgraduate school disempowered, a process that would eventually result in its demise.

CHAPTER 4

A WOMAN'S WORLD: MOTHERS, NURSES AND MIDWIVES AT NATIONAL WOMEN'S, THE 1950s TO 1963

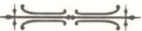

I N HER HISTORY OF MELBOURNE'S ROYAL WOMEN'S HOSPITAL JANET McCALMAN wrote, 'If male doctors and administrators ruled, the hospital none the less was a woman's world.' She explained how men passed through as doctors, visitors, cleaners and tradesmen, but that it was women – nurses and midwives – who sustained the culture.[1] The same applied to National Women's Hospital. Nurses and midwives were the mainstay of the hospital, in the antenatal, labour, delivery, postnatal and paediatric wards. A major logistical concern for the hospital was how to recruit and retain nursing staff, which in turn influenced hospital practices. The visibility of nurses and midwives also meant that when women complained of practices in hospital, it was nurses and midwives who were usually their primary target. They were the people with whom they interacted most in the hospital setting and who determined the nature of their experience. This chapter addresses that relationship and analyses how consumer groups came to ally themselves with doctors against the Nurses and Midwives Registration Board (NMRB).[2] It will be seen that the story of National Women's Hospital cannot be looked at in isolation from the broader politics of maternity care, as it both reflected and contributed to those politics.

Midwives and Maternity Nurses

In 1951 National Women's Hospital was the largest maternity hospital in New Zealand with 135 beds, but another 33 beds were unavailable because of staff shortages. The hospital had the facilities, doctors were keen to train there and women wanted to have their babies there, but to function it needed nurses. Professor Spence Smyth, the hospital's first medical director, complained in 1952 after a year in the post that the hospital board had been unable to fulfil its promise to open two more wards because of the grave shortage of nurses.[3] Commenting in the mid-1950s that 'this great institution' had been obliged to curtail its services because of an acute nursing shortage, the *New Zealand Herald* declared that, 'Provision for maternity care under the welfare state is of no value if undertakings cannot be honoured.'[4] Not only did they have trouble recruiting nurses, but in the 1950s many women who went to National Women's to train as maternity nurses did not complete their training, and there was also apparently a 100 per cent turnover of trained staff each year.[5] The hospital's suggestion of appointing male nurses to make up the shortfall was firmly rejected by the NMRB, which controlled entry into the profession.[6] National Women's was not to get its first male maternity nurse until 1979.[7]

Those responsible for setting up National Women's determined that it would not be a training school for midwives, but only for maternity nurses. St Helens would continue to train midwives. The distinction between midwives and maternity nurses had been made under the 1925 Nurses and Midwives Registration Act. This legislation rebranded former midwives as maternity nurses, and made midwifery a postgraduate training for registered nurses or maternity nurses. Maternity nurse training was six months for registered nurses and eighteen months for unregistered nurses. Once they passed the maternity exam they could take the six months' midwifery training. Maternity nurses were only able to attend a labouring woman under the direction of a doctor or midwife. If the aim of this legislation had been to increase the number of nurses able to assist doctors delivering babies in hospital, it did not work that way, as doctors were to find out. Rather, women used the eighteen months' maternity training for unregistered nurses to get into the general nursing programme, as this was accepted as an alternative to the two years of secondary school that made them eligible for entry. Some registered nurses used the maternity training for promotion, to achieve higher status within the general hospital grading. They took leave from their jobs to gain the certificate, but had no intention of practising maternity nursing.[8] Others became Plunket nurses, which also required maternity training.[9] During the Second World War some women used the training to get into military nursing – as one doctor complained, they 'couldn't wait to don their WAAF uniform for its novelty'.[10] Doris Gordon also claimed to have seen former maternity nurses 'serving in shoe stores, beauty salons, or back on the land, fruit picking'.[11] Other occupations had more appeal. Doctors could not find their handmaidens, or could not keep them.

There was a general shortage of hospital nurses in the immediate post-war years, in New Zealand as elsewhere.[12] With the post-war economic boom, new job opportunities presented themselves in manufacturing and other services. Moreover, as Gordon commented, the marriage market was buoyant, and many prospective nurses, or nurses in training, married. In Melbourne too, McCalman observed, 'Nursing shortages continued as young women married at the highest rate in modern times.'[13]

There were also problems peculiar to maternity nursing that made it particularly unattractive to young women. First were the long hours. The Hospital Boards Employee Regulations gazetted in 1947 made the eight-hour day mandatory for hospital nurses, trainees and nurse aides.[14] When National Women's medical staff discussed this the following year, they dismissed it as 'completely impracticable'.[15] In 1955 one of the hospital's doctors, Jack Matthews, drew attention to the fact that 'nurses were still working many hours in excess of their normal working week and were not being paid for it'. He thought this was 'a cause of considerable dissatisfaction and definitely was one of the causes of the ever present nursing shortage'.[16] Carey noted the same conditions in 1957 and proposed some changes to relieve the nursing shortage. Some of these suggestions give an indication of the conditions under which nurses worked and lived, such as heating the nurses' home adequately in winter and providing suitable transport for living-out staff coming off duty at 11 p.m.[17]

Another factor that deterred young women from continuing maternity nursing was the obligatory panning and swabbing of mothers in the postnatal ward.[18] This stemmed from Health Department nursing regulations, first published in 1926 and largely unmodified by the mid-1950s, which aimed to maintain an aseptic environment. Midwife Anne Nightingale recalled that nurses and midwives regarded this document as 'the Bible' well into the 1960s.[19] The regulations required nurses to pan all patients in bed four-hourly up to the tenth day following the birth, although from the seventh to the tenth day there was some flexibility: the patient was allowed to go to the toilet or be panned in bed 'according to the wishes of the obstetrician'. Regulations specified that, at least until the seventh day following the birth, even when 'early ambulation' was permitted, the mother had to 'be panned in bed by the nurse'.[20] In other words, mothers could be up and about but would have to get back into bed to be panned and swabbed by the nurse. Introduced to combat puerperal sepsis, the major cause of maternal deaths in the 1920s, the need for asepsis was reinforced in the 1950s by the introduction of a new hospital infection, an antibiotic-resistant staphylococcal aureus infection, popularly known as the 'H-bug'.[21]

In 1956, once showers were installed in the postnatal ward at National Women's, the HMC placed the matter of panning and swabbing on its agenda for a meeting and invited the matron, Miss Margaret Millar, to attend. The committee decided that 'where adequate facilities exist, showering following the use of toilet be accepted as an alternative to panning and swabbing, once the patient has become ambulatory following delivery'. In order to justify the new policy the committee pointed to a controlled trial Carey had initiated involving 1072 women in the hospital, which 'showed no increase in minor or major sepsis when showering was substituted for panning'. They noted that many women said how much they enjoyed the comfort of showering and the fact that they were no longer dependent on the junior nursing staff for pans. The committee also noted that nurses disliked panning and that it occupied an unduly large portion of their time which would be better spent on the babies and helping mothers to establish breastfeeding. Additionally, the committee believed that by making maternity nursing more attractive it would encourage more recruits and help reduce nursing shortages. Finally the committee argued, 'Once a patient is ambulatory and feeling well it is surely incongruous to put her back to bed for that specific purpose of panning and swabbing. No physiological or pathological basis can any longer be substantiated for the present arbitrary practice of making the patient use a bed pan before the 7th day and allowing her to use the toilet after this time.'[22]

Despite the extensive research into this matter and the clear reasons for a policy change, the NMRB would not budge. Frustrated, the doctors complained of the board's 'dictatorial attitude' in what, they claimed, was a 'clinical matter'.[23] Carey reduced the time of panning and swabbing to three days in his 'professorial' ward (ward 26) in 1955 and the NMRB withdrew nurse trainees from his ward.[24] National Women's was not alone in its defiance; four years later a doctor from Greymouth reported, 'At the risk of rousing the wrath of the Nurses and Midwives Board I should whisper that 36 mothers expressed the opinion that it was much nicer to be able to swab themselves and use the shower than to be "swabbed and mopped by nurse".'[25]

Another response to the nursing shortage was the introduction of 'rooming-in', which meant allowing mothers to keep their babies by their bedside rather than send them to a communal nursery. Louisa Dixon, a maternity nurse at National Women's in 1956 (and charge nurse of the postnatal ward from 1957 to 1982), remembered a big two-storeyed trolley that could carry ten babies at a time when they were taken to their mothers for feeding. She commented that 'you just had to watch you gave the right baby to the right mother'; she knew of a few times they got it wrong.[26] When Carey first introduced rooming-in in ward 26 in 1955, he told his staff this was a 'temporary administrative change' to cope with the nursing shortage.[27] In Melbourne, McCalman noted that rooming-in was extended 'to reduce the need for space and nursing staff in the nursery'.[28] At National Women's, however, it was not about saving space in the nursery: as paediatrician Dr Leo Phillips explained, ward 26 rooming-in was still 'partial', with babies being taken back to the nursery at night.[29]

Carey was clearly interested in rooming-in for more than administrative reasons. In 1956 he met journalist Mary Dobbie, who was later to play a key role in Parents' Centre. When Dobbie mentioned her interest in natural childbirth, Carey invited her to give birth in his professorial unit with freedom to try natural birth, rooming-in and demand breastfeeding, in return for providing him with a written report, recording the baby's feeding and sleeping patterns. He told her that in his ward she would have to do a lot of the childcare herself as nurse trainees had been withdrawn.[30]

The concept of rooming-in was catching on. In 1957, the HMC agreed 'that the post natal wards should be altered to enable them to function on the "rooming-in" principle and that the wards be divided into two-bedded cubicles'.[31] Rooming-in might have had administrative advantages but it was also part of the new psychology associated with the natural childbirth movement promoted by Dick-Read and others, based on the belief that maternal–infant bonding should start as early as possible.[32]

On a practical level, rooming-in was not only introduced to reduce nurses' workload, but it was also intended to reduce infection. As noted earlier, the 'H-bug' invaded New Zealand's maternity hospitals in the mid-1950s. The Auckland Hospital Board set up a sub-committee in 1955 to investigate the infection and make recommendations. The sub-committee believed that nursing staff rather than mothers, 'in the majority of cases', were responsible for cross-infection, and one of its recommendations was rooming-in.[33] In 1957 the Director-General of Health visited National Women's and approved the rooming-in principle in the new purpose-built hospital that was being planned, where women were to be given the 'option' of rooming-in.[34]

Dr Margaret Liley was a great supporter of rooming-in. She had been appointed physician for prenatal and postnatal instruction of parents at National Women's in 1957 (a position she held until 1984), having previously worked at the hospital in 1954 as resident house surgeon in neonatal paediatrics. She had married Bill Liley in 1953, and from 1954 to 1957 they were based in Australia. The couple had six children, four born at National Women's. Margaret Liley's report to the HMC on postnatal care in 1962 commented favourably on ward 26, which she later explained was run by one registered nurse and otherwise by nurse aides: 'I remember one of the aides on night duty was a Maori grandmother who could intuitively show us all what we wanted to achieve.'[35] Her report stated that, 'Ward 26 has been opened as a self-care ward with minimal staff and maximal privileges', suggesting that she regarded rooming-in, demand breastfeeding and early toileting as mothers' 'privileges'.

Liley cautioned, however, that in about 25 per cent of cases rooming-in was not feasible, explaining that 'baby may be dead, premature, unwanted, sick or for adoption, mother may be sick'. Furthermore, she believed that some patients placed in a single room for rooming-in felt victimised, as they were isolated from other mothers.[36] Communal wards promoted sociability amongst the new mothers, and anecdotal evidence suggests that some women enjoyed this aspect of their hospital stay and formed lasting friendships with those occupying adjacent beds. One woman in a communal postnatal ward in the 1960s later told interviewer Christina Jeffery, 'I had a wonderful time in there, all the ladies that were in there then, we had a ball. I was in a room with three others. The whole thing . . . was all fun. Certainly not boring!'[37]

Not all mothers supported rooming-in. In 1958 one wrote to the *New Zealand Family Doctor* about the practice and its negative effect on breastfeeding. Despite being a trained baby nurse herself, she found the responsibility of caring for her newborn baby 'quite terrifying' and argued that rooming-in was detrimental to breastfeeding as broken nights meant mothers were unable to regain their strength.[38] In 1961 the New Zealand Federation of University Women (NZFUW), an organisation of 1200 women, surveyed about 500 mothers who had recently given birth and found that only 50 per cent favoured rooming-in, and those who favoured it 'qualified their approval'.[39] A survey at Auckland's St Helens in 1962 found that only 48 per cent liked the rooming-in scheme.[40]

Another change intended to address the nursing shortage, as well as the problem of infection, was early discharge of mothers, which meant before the ninth day after birth.[41] This was, as Gordon noted, already practised in other countries that were suffering similar shortages. In 1957 Carey even suggested discharge on the third or fourth day, adding that this was feasible only if mothers had domestic help and if their home conditions were satisfactory. He also specified that such women would have to live within five miles of the hospital so that a hospital nurse could visit them daily.[42] The sub-committee on infections declared that the maximum incidence of infection in babies occurred about the seventh or eighth day and agreed that babies would be safer at home.[43]

Conditions were attached to early discharge. In 1958 the hospital appointed a midwife, Mrs Rissa Scelly, as its first medical social worker (she was attracted to the post primarily because it involved working on adoption which had until that time been the responsibility of the matron).[44] Part of her job related to early discharge. She had to interview women before they gave birth to determine whether home conditions were suitable for early discharge and 'whether the patient and her husband [were] agreeable to her going home earlier than usual'. In 'selected cases' Scelly was also to visit the home 'to ensure that conditions [were] suitable for early discharge'.[45]

Margaret Millar argued that early discharge would do little to alleviate the nursing shortage. Matron at National Women's from 1955 to 1969 (when she became Matron-in-Chief of Auckland Hospital Board), Millar demanded very high standards of her nurses. One nurse reminisced, 'she was always every inch the matron', and another that she was 'lovely, . . . fair and honest but firm'.[46] Millar opposed early discharge of mothers as it would mean, she explained, 'the registered staff would have to work far harder than they should because of the greatly increased turnover and increase in "acute nursing"'.[47] In 1957 she complained that she had received two resignations in one day because of 'overwork due to this increased turnover'.[48] In the second week of their stay mothers were generally up and about; one woman who gave birth at National Women's in 1953 remembered helping the nurses serve tea during her second week there.[49]

While there was a turnover of general nursing staff at National Women's, Dr Margaret Liley recalled that nurses ran the wards and had considerable influence over the delivery suites.[50] From 1957, when maternity was included in the curriculum for general nurse training, each trainee nurse had to deliver five babies. One doctor complained in 1960 that at least a quarter of mothers were being delivered by nurses in their third year of general training, even though the women had contracted a doctor for their confinement.[51] However, the 1961 NZFUW survey found that most mothers did not mind student nurses delivering their babies.[52] According to midwife Dorothy McAleer who worked at National Women's from the late 1950s, general practitioners who were supposed to deliver the babies would often say, 'You can deliver it, sister', and, she said, 'He would stay there and talk to the patient and just watch what was going on.'[53] One woman who gave birth at National Women's Hospital in 1953 didn't even remember seeing her general practitioner who was supposed to deliver her baby, and certainly saw no doctor in the postnatal ward.[54] Nor did this change in subsequent years, as one woman recalled the birth of her child in the 1980s: '[I] don't remember being visited by a doctor at all, just the nurses, they were very happy nurses . . . . And helpful, with bathing and anything.'[55]

Joyce Hare was charge nurse of the labour ward at National Women's from 1952 to 1976. To her the labour ward was a women's world. She explained, 'I had 22 midwives under me and a great lot they were too.' When asked about the doctors she replied, 'They didn't spend a lot of time in the delivery suite – they would only come in for the delivery.' Asked, 'How did you find the working relationship with the doctors?', she responded, 'They were quite good really – didn't see too much of them, it was quite good.'[56] Midwives who worked with her respected her. As one said, 'There wasn't anything she missed.' That midwife went on to say that at National Women's midwives 'ruled the roost', recounting a story of Hare speaking severely to a doctor about something that he had done wrong.[57]

Nor did this situation appear to be unique. At Melbourne's Royal Women's Hospital, McCalman noted, 'If doctors took the ultimate professional responsibility, the senior nursing staff none the less exercised considerable power, especially in the delivery ward.' One of her informants contrasted the situation there with America; in Australia the midwives often knew more than the young doctors and were 'more manually adept. They learnt to manage doctors.'[58] In Britain a comparable teaching hospital was University College

Hospital, London, with its own Obstetric Unit. In his biography of William Nixon, director of the unit, Geoffrey Chamberlain wrote that, 'The Queen Bee of any obstetric unit is the labour ward superintendent. At UCL during most of Nixon's time [1946–66] she was Sister Margaret Billings (or "Sister Bill"). She ruled the labour ward, the powerhouse of the Obstetric Hospital, controlling midwives, students, junior doctors, and other seniors too, with a vocative rod of iron.'[59]

Nurses also ruled in the premature nursery, as paediatrician Jack Matthews was to find out. Five days after he began work at the hospital in 1949, he was summoned to the medical director's office and rebuked 'for presuming to act outside my duties and he told me that I was causing great distress for matron as I was taking her preserves, privileges and duties'. Smyth told him that he was not to see any baby unless matron had personally asked him and he was certainly not to examine them and that, 'I'd just have to remember that I was only a young man and I didn't know nearly as much about babies as an older, senior obstetric nurse or . . . midwife.'[60] Over time Matthews clearly managed to work with the midwives. Midwife Isobel Fisher, who started work at the hospital in 1963, later reflected that he was a 'very kind nice man and, as one of my nurses said to me, he's the only one who puts the napkins on again when he takes them off!'[61]

In 1952 the hospital appointed a lactation (breastfeeding) supervisor, Miss G. Brown, who had trained with the famous British lactation consultant Dr Harold Waller of the Woolich Hospital for Mothers and Babies.[62] Sister Brown, together with obstetrician Alastair Macfarlane and Jack Matthews, set up a Lactation Department to supervise and advise mothers on breastfeeding in the postnatal wards.[63] According to Matthews, they met opposition from the midwives running the wards and abandoned the service.[64] At Auckland, as in Melbourne, midwives and nurses were the mainstay of the hospital; they were a long way from being 'doctors' handmaidens', as some histories later described them.[65] This also meant, however, that they would bear the brunt of women's complaints about hospital conditions.

Mothers Speak Out
In the 1950s mothers voiced their views on childbirth through their own consumer organisations, such as the NCW and the NZFUW, but also through a new organisation, the Federation of New Zealand Parents' Centres (commonly called Parents' Centre). At its first national conference in 1957

Dame Hilda Ross, Minister for the Welfare of Women and Children, spoke in favour of home births, as did Walter Nash, the Leader of the Opposition and soon to be Prime Minister. Nash gave a romanticised view of home birth based on his own in England (some 72 years earlier). Carey then addressed the conference. He explained that he did not support home births, but espoused three changes in childbirth services which resonated with demands made by Parents' Centre. One was rooming-in, another was demand breastfeeding, and the third was an end to perineal panning and swabbing.[66] Dobbie commented in her 1990 history of Parents' Centre: 'His audience could not have agreed more. This spare, reserved man was presenting a researcher's reasons for changes that parents centres had seen as psychologically beneficial to mother and child.'[67]

Writing of the antenatal conference Carey hosted at National Women's in January 1958, Dobbie enthused, 'After so many rebuffs from obstetrical quarters this invitation gave a great lift to morale [of Parents' Centre]. There was a sense of arrival. National Women's Hospital, centre for research, trial ground of changes in obstetrical care – where better to gain a hearing from the expectant mother's point of view?'[68] The Federation of Parents' Centres' 1958 annual report recorded, 'Such a conference at which Parents' Centres, as representatives of consumers, were invited to participate fully in a very frank and thorough exchange of views, opinions and information, marked a milestone in the history of ante-natal care in New Zealand .... its immediate and long-term importance cannot be over-estimated.'[69]

The Federation of Parents' Centres welcomed an association with doctors. Its 1959 *Newsletter* noted approvingly the formation of a 'high-level committee of specialists from various fields concerned with ante-natal education', stating that Parents' Centre was represented by Dr Wallace Ironside, head of the Department of Psychiatry at Otago University. The same year Parents' Centre set up a medical directorate, and announced at its 1959 conference that proofs of its newsletter 'should be sent to all members of the medical directorate for checking'.[70] The *Newsletter* expressed the hope in 1961 that Dr James Watt, later New Zealand's first professor of paediatrics, would be appointed Parents' Centre president, announcing that this would be 'wonderful from our point of view'. Later in the *Newsletter*, under the heading 'Publicity', branches were advised:

> As you will realise, this is a very crucial stage in the life of P.C.s, and one single well-meaning but thoughtless act on our part could alienate the medical profession

and get us thrown into outer darkness once and for all. So please PLEASE watch your step. If there's the slightest doubt – don't. Any publicity you may be thinking of publishing, please send to us first for approval by Dr Watt.... One point in particular. There is still considerable opposition to Grantly Dick-Read, so when you use the record or film leave his name out of it.[71]

This caution relating to Dick-Read was because some doctors, such as Thomas Corkill of Wellington, argued that Dick-Read set up unrealistic expectations among women about childbirth and undermined women's confidence in their obstetricians.[72]

Parents' Centre saw allying themselves with doctors as a route to public respectability, which speaks to the status of medicine in the mid-twentieth century and women's attitudes to it.[73] While representing parents, Parents' Centre was also more than ready to draw on professional expertise. Following federation it set up an Educational Advisory Council.[74] Although Carey was not a member he spent many hours discussing 'matters with members of this committee.[75] Parents' Centre gained the approval of the NZBMA in December 1958, allowing NZBMA members to work for the centres. Ethical approval was withdrawn the following September, but this proved to be a temporary hiccup; the NZBMA restored ethical status to the organisation in 1961, following the establishment of a medical panel.[76]

While Parents' Centre favoured such an alliance, so too did doctors, particularly those at National Women's. The latter saw such a partnership as useful in their running battles with the NMRB. One such battle was in relation to the revised general nursing curriculum in 1957, introduced at least partly in the hope that it would alleviate the maternity nurse shortage. Obstetric or maternity nursing was no longer a separate option but was included in the general nurse training, with six weeks in maternity wards and clinics at the beginning of the three-year course, and another three months near the end (male nurses were required to do only a total of four weeks' 'observation' in maternity to register as general nurses).[77] In this latter period, trainee nurses were to undertake 20 internal examinations of women in labour, administer ten anaesthetics ('to the obstetrical degree') and deliver five babies.[78]

National Women's HMC complained that the medical profession had not been consulted about the curriculum change: 'Obviously an important principle had been forgotten – patients commit themselves to the care of doctors, and therefore the latter must have adequate say in the training of those who provide nursing care.'[79] The doctors also objected to the requirement that nurses undertake a certain number of rectal examinations. Herb Green calculated in 1960 that no fewer than 12,000 rectal examinations were done each year at National Women's in the interests of nurse training. The doctors believed these examinations were not only unnecessary but also increased the danger of cross-infection and patient discomfort.[80] The Health Department's Director of Nursing, Flora Cameron, explained that the purpose of the student nurse's rectal examination was to enable her to tell whether she could give an enema at that stage of labour.[81] Dobbie quoted Cameron saying, 'This is a normal procedure and one cannot think entirely of patients' likes and dislikes.'[82] Parents' Centre asked Cameron whether she thought mothers had any grounds for protesting that they had not been consulted before the curriculum changed, and she replied that she could not see why mothers should be consulted, telling them, 'There was so much more in the curriculum than just mothers' point of view.'[83]

Not only Parents' Centre but also the NCW came down firmly on the side of Carey and National Women's in the disputes with the NMRB. In 1956 the Auckland branch of the NCW wrote to the NMRB explaining that its executive had been greatly impressed with the work of Carey and his staff in their efforts to make maternity safer and more comfortable for patients and less arduous for nurses. A meeting of the Auckland branch, attended by representatives of 56 women's organisations, resolved: 'That the National Council of Women request the Nurses' and Midwives' Board to allow more latitude for the staffing of wards in connection with research and new techniques at the National Women's Hospital.' The branch added that this request came from 'a body of responsible women, interested in the welfare of both patients and nurses, and which is impressed with the work which Professor Carey is now doing in Auckland'.[84]

In 1959 the Auckland branch sent a remit to the Minister of Health asking him to investigate the functioning of maternity training hospitals 'in regard to the rights of the individual doctor to prescribe medical treatment for his own patients'.[85] They declared that they now realised that until reforms were instituted at the top level, mothers' needs could not be met, and reiterated that progress was related to the 'right of the individual doctor to prescribe treatment for his own patients'.[86] Green welcomed this initiative, declaring that he was 'glad to realise that some of the difficulties inherent in the new basic curriculum have percolated through to the people they affect most, that is the patients'.[87] Doctors and mothers appeared to be firmly allied against the NMRB.

In 1960 the Wellington branch of the NCW produced a report called 'Maternity Services in New Zealand', based on interviews with mothers. This report was concerned primarily with hospital births, noting that 93 per cent of all European births and 90 per cent of all Maori births now occurred in hospital. It referred to the current understanding of the 'psychosomatic approach to childbirth' and the 'vital effects upon later family life' of childbirth experiences; this included mother–child and marital relationships. It declared that many organisations were concerned about the long-term effects of hospital experiences during childbirth. These organisations included 'nursery play centres, adult education councils, the League of Mothers, kindergarten and Plunket mothers' clubs, parents' centres, family planning associations, family/marriage guidance councils, workers' educational associations, parent–teachers associations, numerous church women's organisations, and teachers' colleges'.[88] Modern parents saw childbirth as part of the process of establishing good family relationships, influenced by the popular psychology emanating from Grantly Dick-Read.

The NCW report's main target for criticism of childbirth experiences in hospital was not doctors but rather nurses. Mothers had complained that if they 'made a fuss' as a result of panic or pain, they were 'slapped, threatened or criticised' by nurses. The report included as an appendix a document from the Oamaru Mothers' Group, a particularly activist group. One of its complaints was the 'virtual refusal by the hospital authorities to let a mother see her doctor at the time of confinement except at the discretion of the nurses in charge'. They claimed that in many cases when a mother wanted her doctor to be sent for, the hospital staff refused, and contact with her doctor was restricted by the fact that she could not see him to discuss any problems without a nurse being present.[89] The Auckland branch of the NCW demanded a government inquiry, stressing that this was an area 'peculiarly our own'.[90]

The NCW invited Carey to address one of its meetings in March 1960. As Dobbie wrote, 'Unperturbed by the chilly presence of 8 of New Zealand's most senior nurses', he outlined his concerns regarding the new nursing curriculum, the intransigence of the NMRB relating to new maternity nursing techniques and the 'difficulties at Wairoa Hospital'. According to Dobbie, 'A quiet and authoritative speaker, accustomed to talking to women on medical matters, he was given an attentive hearing.'[91]

Other women's organisations joined the battle against the NMRB. The Combined Auckland Housewives' Associations explained in the *Auckland Star* that they had grave misgivings about the revised nursing curriculum, quoting 'a Dunedin doctor' that it produced 'droves of young inexperienced girls in labour rooms'.[92] The 'difficulties at Wairoa Hospital', which Carey referred to, were related to the installation of bidets for mothers to use following childbirth. Over 1100 women signed a petition to the local hospital board asking it to support the NZOGS recommendation that the Health Department give permission for bidet installation. 'Surely our statistics, the supporting work at National Women's Hospital, the installation at Charing Cross Maternity Hospital [London] and the Obstetrical and Gynaecological Society's recommendations is sufficient to justify your Department allowing installation to proceed on an experimental basis.'[93] Cameron, who opposed bidets, apparently retorted, 'Bidets! They're used in *France – by prostitutes!*'[94]

Carey and his deputy Green were fully supportive of the NCW and Parents' Centre in their demands relating to childbirth services. Dobbie commented on the 'determination of those close to Miss Cameron to discredit the parents' centre movement, linked, as they saw it, with their severest critics at National Women's Hospital'.[95] For his part, Green told the Parents' Centre president that he believed the NMRB interference was affecting patient welfare, and assured her that 'any move by organisations such as yours – who represent patients – to improve the standard of maternity services in New Zealand will meet with my unqualified support'.[96]

The government managed to defuse the situation by setting up a new committee, the Maternity Services Committee, as a sub-committee of the Board of Health. Director-General of Health Harold Turbott suggested in June 1960 that this was the best way of short-circuiting the agitation for an inquiry and counteracting criticism.[97] The new body included Carey along with Professor Lawrence Wright, professor of obstetrics and gynaecology at Otago, and representatives from the RCOG, the NZOGS, the NZBMA and the NMRB, as well as the director of Maternal Welfare in the Department of Health and the superintendent of a St Helens hospital.[98] This move, according to Dobbie, 'took the wind out of Parents Centre sails'. The Auckland branch of the NCW withdrew its call for an inquiry.[99]

However, women's organisations criticised the absence of a consumer representative on a new committee whose 'findings vitally affect the welfare of all mothers'.[100] Helen Brew, as president of Parents' Centre, declared the omission 'deplorable'.[101] The Parents' Centre dominion executive unanimously resolved to support the National Consumer Council, the NZFUW and the Christchurch branch of the NCW in their request for a consumer representative on the Board of Health committee, and to make representations to the government. Echoing Doris Gordon, the executive also commented that if mothers had been represented from the beginning in the planning and functioning of New Zealand maternity services, many current causes of dissatisfaction might have been avoided.[102]

At the beginning of 1962 the Board of Health confirmed to the NCW that its nominee, ex-nurse Mrs Gwen Stacey, had been appointed to represent the interests of mothers on the Maternity Services Committee.[103] The Oamaru Mothers' Group had recommended to the director of Maternal Welfare that the consumer representative should be 'in no way connected with the medical or nursing profession', and objected to the appointment of Stacey because she was not a 'lay person'. Health Minister Don McKay replied that the committee's work was concerned with matters of a professional nature and 'a representative could feel embarrassed and inadequate if he or she did not possess sufficient background knowledge to enable full participation in the committee's discussions'.[104] The Oamaru group appeared to accept this argument as the matter ended there and Stacey remained the consumer representative for at least the next ten years.[105]

The 1961 NZFUW survey of the childbirth experiences of 500 women revealed women's views on hospitalised childbirth around the middle of the twentieth century. The report showed that only a 'small minority' were dissatisfied with the maternity services, and that most had confidence in their doctors. Criticisms were 'almost entirely related to intense personal feelings and the difficulties of reconciling them with the hospital routine'.[106] Despite opposing hospital routines, only 50 per cent favoured rooming-in and some of those only supported it during the daytime. Once again, nurses bore the brunt of the criticism. Some mothers felt that they were not treated as intelligent human beings, and others considered nurses to be indifferent or even callous. Again, the report regretted that there was no opportunity to talk privately with the doctor, as visits tended to be formal, with staff in attendance.

The survey found that most women did not favour home births; about 18 per cent liked the idea, but only if circumstances were suitable, and they believed that New Zealand conditions were generally unfavourable because of the lack of domestic help. Many mothers welcomed the stay in hospital as a break from domestic duties. The report noted that a more representative cross-section of mothers would probably show an even greater preference for hospital births as domestic circumstances would be even less favourable.[107] Hospital births were there to stay, but mothers wanted a more homely atmosphere whilst in hospital. As historian Judith Leavitt found in America, 'women wanted the psychologically comforting practices of their traditional birthing rooms [or, it should be added, their imagined traditional birthing rooms] to be incorporated into the modern practices in the birthing rooms of medical science'.[108]

Another Parents' Centre demand was to allow men into the labour and delivery wards to support their wives. This was based on the ideas of Grantly Dick-Read, who argued that the father's presence promoted marital happiness and better long-term family relationships (as will be further discussed in chapter 9). When Christine Cole, one of the founders of Parents' Centre, asked an eminent obstetrician if her husband could be present at the birth of their baby in 1950, she was apparently told, 'Indeed not – never heard anything so extraordinary!'[109] At National Women's in the early 1950s there was a marked rise in requests for husbands to be present during labour and delivery. This ran counter to a 1953 hospital directive expressly forbidding any person other than medical or nursing staff to attend the birth. The HMC remarked, however, that this directive had obviously been drafted to prevent lay members of the hospital staff witnessing deliveries and was not originally intended to refer to the husbands of patients. The committee decided to clarify the ruling: 'Throughout the Labour Wards of the NWH, husbands and other lay people be not allowed in the precincts of the labour suites except in very special circumstances and then only after permission had been obtained from 1. the patient herself, 2. the medical officer in charge of the case or his deputy, 3. the supervising sister of the Labour Ward or her deputy.'[110]

The issue did not, however, go away. By 1960 the *New Zealand Herald* reported a recent British Ministry of Health recommendation that, 'Husbands who want to stay with their wives in the first stages of childbirth should be allowed to do so.'[111] At National Women's at the time the medical consensus was that it was good in principle for husbands to be with their wives during the first stage of labour, but as a result of the prevailing conditions in the labour ward it was preferable to retain the existing policy.[112]

At this time, at least some mothers shared the hospital's reservations about their husbands attending deliveries. A writer to the local press in 1960, who rejoiced in the nom de plume 'Mama minus papa, Mt Roskill', explained, 'I do feel childbirth is a woman's task. No man however hard he may try can understand the emotions involved in a woman's mind, nor can he ever know the joy and fulfilment of new life. That he is denied, as likewise he is spared the pain.'[113] Similarly, a 1962 study at Auckland's St Helens Hospital found that more than half the 265 women surveyed did not want to have their husbands present through the entire labour.[114] This was to change in later decades.

A Medical Institution?
National Women's Hospital as a medical institution enjoyed an international status in the world of obstetrics and gynaecology. It was set up to be doctor-run and doctor-controlled and to train doctors and maternity nurses but not midwives. However, it is clear that the day-to-day running of the hospital was very much a midwives' and nurses' affair. There were some career midwives who stayed for many years and ran the wards. It was harder to attract and retain women to perform the day-to-day chores in the labour, delivery, postnatal and paediatric wards, although they too were essential. Changes to obstetric practice had as much, if not more, to do with the demands of nursing administration, in particular the problem of staff shortages, than with new scientific ideas. Practices in the postnatal wards, such as showering and toilet arrangements, length of stay and rooming-in, were primarily responses to nursing shortages. The curriculum change for general registered nurses in 1957 to include maternity was also at least partly a response to the nursing shortage. As a nurse who experienced the new curriculum, Joan Dodd, later recalled, the six weeks of 'junior obstetrics' in the nurse-training programme was 'totally hands-on, we were actually the work force', doing everything apart from delivering the babies.[115] Huge demands were placed on these new trainees.

In their efforts to improve their hospital experience, mothers saw doctors as allies, albeit from a distance. In the 1930s women had fought in alliance with doctors for the right to pain relief; now in the late 1950s, equally in alliance with at least some of the doctors at National Women's, they fought for the right to refuse it, and more generally called for a less regimented and more caring environment. A study of National Women's cannot be divorced from the politics of childbirth at a national level. Yet at National Women's and elsewhere, those women who publicly complained about services were probably a minority. Women chose to go to hospital to have their babies and many enjoyed their stay, making friends with other new mothers in the postnatal wards. Although midwives and nurses bore the brunt of patients' complaints, relationships between midwives, nurses and mothers were not all bad. Most of the views expressed came through white middle-class women's organisations, such as the NCW, the NZFUW and Parents' Centre. As consumer organisations they fulfilled a function of keeping a watching brief over conditions under which women gave birth, just as Doris Gordon had hoped they would.

CHAPTER 5

FROM PREMATURE NURSERY TO PAEDIATRIC DEPARTMENT, 1950s TO 1963

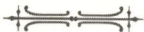

When Auckland's new Women's Hospital was being planned, Dr Helen Deem, medical adviser to the Royal New Zealand Plunket Society, raised the question of provision for premature babies. Dr Doris Gordon reassured her that this was certainly visualised: 'We cannot be a model post graduate teaching Hospital without the best infant work we can evolve . . . . Want someone of the Alan Moncrieff type [professor of child health at the University of London] on senior staff giving daily lessons to students and doctor grads on the problems of the new born.'[1] Internationally, the 1950s was a time when the care of the newborn was medicalised and this can be traced clearly through an examination of developments at National Women's Hospital, where events would propel New Zealand medical research onto the world map.

Care of Premature and Sick Newborn Babies before 1950
In the early twentieth century, maternity and general hospitals did not normally have facilities for the medical treatment of premature and other sick newborn babies. Appreciating this gap in hospital services, Dr (later Sir) Frederic Truby King set up an infant hospital in 1907. He envisaged this as a part of an infant welfare movement to be managed by the newly established

Society for the Promotion of the Health of Women and Children (subsequently the Plunket Society). The society's main function was to employ nurses to advise new mothers. These nurses were trained in the infant hospitals, called Karitane hospitals, after Truby King's holiday home at Karitane near Dunedin, the site of the first unit. By 1927 there were six Karitane hospitals, located in Dunedin, Invercargill, Christchurch, Wanganui, Wellington and Auckland.[2]

The Karitane hospitals were premised on the confident belief that premature and other weak babies could, and should, be saved. Plunket Society publications in the 1920s declared that the society was fighting public criticisms that its activities were instrumental in saving 'better dead' babies. It asserted that most of the so-called weakling babies, if given the correct care and treatment from the beginning, grew up to be strong normal children.[3] Anne Pattrick, director of Plunket Nursing from 1920 to 1934, explained, 'In theory it is easy to say "they are better dead". In practice, babies do not always die when people want them to, even if neglected, and is there any justification whatever for wittingly causing a baby suffering until that suffering in turn causes death?'[4]

In a public appeal for donations for these voluntarily funded hospitals, a *New Zealand Observer* writer in 1931 claimed the fathers were proudest of all when their babies began to gain weight. He added: 'Many of them are most attached to their delicate children, but simply don't know what to do with them. An extremely worried and frightened father arrived at the Karitane Home, not long ago, carrying his tiny son and heir in a cardboard shoe-box.'[5] Again in 1946, noting that some people openly questioned whether such babies were really worth saving, a *Weekly News* reporter pointed out that some of these babies 'turned out to be the brightest of the brood'.[6]

Truby King followed the latest international trends in advising the care provided at the hospitals. At the 1922 Plunket Society conference, he explained that preparation for the premature baby should be made before it was born, in order to conserve and maintain its heat directly after birth took place, 'without a moment's unnecessary delay'. Pointing out that half the babies who died in New Zealand did so in the first ten days, he maintained that the records of the Karitane hospitals showed that 'provided the infant is not actually moribund on admission', it would survive as a result of the careful attention given.[7] That same year American paediatrician Dr Julian Hess (later described as the father of American neonatology)[8] set out guidelines for the care of premature babies. He recommended that they be isolated to avoid infection, that their temperature be carefully controlled, that the cots be heated by four hot water bottles in canvas pockets with one changed every hour in rotation, and that careful attention be paid to their nutrition.[9] The Karitane hospitals put these practices into effect, with each premature baby having its own nurse. As the matron of the Auckland Karitane Hospital explained in 1926, 'minute attention to detail must be given: the temperature of the ward regulated, and hot water bags frequently refilled. This, together with the feeding and general care of these wee mites, takes up almost the whole of one Nurse's time.'[10] The society was very proud of its successes, although the nurses did tend to get depressed by the high death rates.[11]

By the 1940s a growing profession of paediatricians began to demand better facilities. The Paediatric Society of New Zealand was set up in 1947, and in 1948 Dr Samuel Ludbrook, the society's founder and first president, told Deem, 'I have been simmering with suppressed rage for some years over the neglect of the Newborn but it has been like butting your head against a brick wall.'[12] The following month he wrote to Deem about the inadequate facilities for premature babies in Auckland, commenting that most maternity homes did not even provide adequate care for healthy newborns. But he also told Deem that there were plans to set up a unit for premature babies at the new women's hospital in Auckland and he hoped she would support this, 'so that there could be co-ordination with any developments at Karitane'. He pointed out that the 'premature population' at the new hospital was about twelve and growing.[13]

Ludbrook was invited to attend early meetings of Cornwall Hospital's HMC to help organise the 'Paediatric Department'. The committee anticipated that the hospital would provide a premature infant service for the whole of Auckland.[14] When the hospital opened, Dr Alice Bush, a visiting paediatrician to the Karitane Hospital, agreed to be a visiting paediatrician for Cornwall Hospital as well, and the following year Dr Macky Hercus took over. In 1948 Dr Renton Grigor was appointed assistant paediatrician to look after the premature ward, with obstetrician Dr Tom Plunkett acting as senior paediatrician.

Dr Jack Dilworth Matthews was appointed to the hospital in 1949 and worked there until 1983. Matthews had gained his Diploma of Child Health in London, and held a residency in 1948 with Alan Moncrieff at Great Ormond Street Children's Hospital. Prior to leaving London, Matthews had spent time at the Hammersmith Hospital Intensive Care Unit for Neonates, which had been set up and supervised by Moncrieff. According to Matthews, this was the first real neonatal unit in London and made him interested in neonatology.[15] Matthews returned to New Zealand in 1948 and set up in private practice before accepting the post at National Women's Hospital. Despite holding the London diploma, when Matthews was appointed in 1949 he was assistant paediatrician to obstetrician Tom Plunkett.

A Premature Unit

The early clinical reports at National Women's Hospital noted that prematurity remained the principal neonatal problem.[16] In 1950, 77 per cent (37 out of 48) of the neonatal deaths were of premature babies. A premature infant at that time was defined as one weighing 5 ½ lbs (2500 g) or under at birth, irrespective of the length of gestation. Infants weighing 2 ¾ lbs (1250 g) and under were classed as pre- (or non-) viable; one of 17 in this group survived in 1948, 6 of 21 in 1949, and 9 of 26 in 1950. What caused babies to be born prematurely was often unknown. Toxaemia of pregnancy was the most significant known cause of prematurity while multiple pregnancy also rated high in the list of known causes. However, in 1950 no cause for premature birth was ascertained in 65 cases (41.1 per cent).[17]

National Women's opened a new premature unit with 22 cots in 1950. In the hospital's *Second Clinical Report*, Herb Green enthused that it was a 'really up-to-date properly designed premature unit . . . [which] may be expected to improve survival rates still further'. He also noted, however, that the shortage of nurses experienced in handling premature babies might hinder progress.[18] When asked to discuss the development of the premature ward, Matthews identified nursing as the major problem, arguing that ideally there should be 24-hour coverage by nurses specially trained in the field. The HMC agreed, stressing the urgent nature of the nursing, in which two or three minutes were often of vital importance; it deplored the 'easy acceptance of premature deaths as compared with deaths in other age groups'.[19]

Matthews later explained that the major problem for premature babies was infection, especially respiratory infection. For that reason, 'the gowning and isolation techniques [in the premature ward] were so strict as to be unbelievable'.[20] As parents were not allowed to handle their premature babies (also called 'cot cases'), intensive nursing was required. A decade later, in 1962, a newly appointed assistant paediatrician, Dr Ross Howie, also pinpointed the standard of nursing as the most significant factor in the care of premature babies.[21]

Apart from avoiding infection and keeping the babies warm, medical treatment in the premature ward consisted of giving oxygen. Matthews later explained that oxygen was given to most premature babies: 'For a long time we had known that intrauterine oxygen lack caused brain damage with subsequent mental defect and cerebral palsy so we were increasingly realising the importance of preventing and dealing with postnatal anoxia even in relatively minor degrees.'[22] There were oxygen points in the ward before Matthews arrived, and babies received oxygen by nasal catheter or an 'oxygen tent'. Matthews described such a tent devised by Mont Liggins who started as a resident at National Women's three weeks before Matthews arrived in 1949. He had made an oxygen tent out of X-ray film, placing it over the baby's head and packing bedclothes closely around it.[23]

Premature babies were also brought to the hospital from other locations. In 1948 there were 51 such admissions, but more than a third of them died. The clinical report for that year noted, 'Many of them suffer from over handling before admission', and referred to a recently established system whereby a trained nurse collected the baby in an ambulance equipped with a special premature carrying cot with oxygen attached.[24]

Matthews aimed to get incubators into the ward, for isolation purposes and for oxygen treatment. Incubators had first been introduced for premature infants in the 1880s by a French obstetrician, Stephane Tarnier. As they did not appear to increase chances of survival they went out of fashion until Hess converted the incubator into an oxygen chamber in America in 1934. Matthews described the situation when he arrived at National Women's: 'The incubators in those days were relatively crude but the latest ones from Oxygenair Vickers in England were really thought to be quite something and I had great difficulty getting these and indeed had to resort to improper means in order to get their purchase approved.' He maintained that getting their first three incubators in 1954 'opened a whole new ball game in the management of babies in Auckland, and I think, in New Zealand'.[25] In 1955 the Department of Scientific and Industrial Research designed and built an 'automatic respirator' at its Auckland laboratory.[26] Howie later commented that its tank-like structure made access to the baby difficult.[27]

Matthews also noted that there was little control over how much oxygen was given to babies at that time, and that this inadvertently caused an epidemic of blindness among the babies (from retrolental fibroplasia).[28] The connection between giving oxygen and retrolental fibroplasia had been made in

Melbourne in 1951. Melbourne's Royal Women's Hospital neonatal paediatrician Dr Kate Campbell and ophthalmologist Dr Hugh Ryan investigated the high rate of retrolental fibroplasia among premature infants in their hospital compared to the nearby Queen Victoria Hospital, and came to the conclusion that the differing use of oxygen was the cause.[29] A similar study was carried out in Auckland by an eye, ear, nose and throat specialist, George Fenwick, in 1953. He examined the eyes of 212 premature babies at the Auckland Karitane Hospital and National Women's Hospital. He found no cases of retrolental fibroplasia at the Karitane Hospital, but at National Women's, only four miles away, he discovered that 23.7 per cent of infants with a birth weight below four pounds (1840 g) were affected. Fenwick observed that staff at the Karitane Hospital rarely used oxygen, while National Women's employed oxygen routinely.[30] Walter Hope-Robertson, an eye specialist in Wellington and president of the Ophthalmological Society of New Zealand from 1956, recommended that oxygen should not be used routinely under any circumstances other than for cyanosis (where babies turned blue from low oxygenation).[31] This was a problem throughout the Western world; in his history of Dublin's Rotunda maternity hospital, Alan Browne described the overuse of oxygen at this time as a 'well-intentioned but misdirected therapeutic intervention' leading to retrolental fibroplasia. He added, 'Compounding such therapeutic misadventures was the imposed isolation of the premature infant because of the risk of infection, separating infants from their mothers and families.'[32] The belief that isolation harmed the baby related to the new psychology developed by Dick-Read, as previously discussed.

In the mid-1950s, in order to enhance teaching and research relating to prematurity, Harvey Carey organised a visit by Dr Mary Crosse from Birmingham, England. Crosse had been responsible for setting up the first ward for premature babies in Britain, at the Sorrento Maternity Hospital, Birmingham, in 1931.[33] She subsequently published a textbook, *Premature Baby* (1946), which reached seven editions by the time she died in 1973. Matthews described her as the doyen on premature baby nursing and management and said that her unit in Sorrento was 'a must' for anybody interested in this area.[34] Crosse held appointments with the World Health Organization (WHO) to advise on aspects of prematurity, and the WHO recognised her unit as a training centre in the care of premature infants.[35] In 1962, after she had retired from her appointment in Birmingham, Crosse visited National Women's again for one month as a temporary honorary neonatal paediatrician.[36]

As the 1950s progressed the hospital's paediatricians extended their work beyond prematurity to encompass other medical problems. In 1956 the HMC announced the commencement of Clinico-Pathological Discussions of all Stillbirths and Neonatal Deaths, held on Saturday mornings once a month. The neonatal period was defined as the first four weeks of life. Paediatricians Jack Matthews and Leo Phillips attended these meetings with pathologist John Sullivan, and they hoped that other staff would also come along.[37] The following year the HMC announced that 'premature ward 24' should now be 'regarded more as a paediatric unit'.[38]

Rhesus Haemolytic Disease

Writing about the history of the care of the newborn in the UK, British paediatrician Professor Peter Dunn commented that during the first half of the twentieth century, nursery nurses, midwives and junior obstetricians generally looked after newborns in hospital. He pinpointed one medical intervention that established an entry for paediatricians into maternity hospitals – the introduction of the umbilical exchange transfusion for Rhesus haemolytic disease.[39] Another British paediatrician exclaimed more dramatically that with the introduction of exchange transfusion, 'the hitherto passive attitude to neonatal care expressed as, "Let's provide babies with tender loving nursing care, a bit of warmth and as much milk as you could" was swept away and thereafter it became morally justifiable to undertake active therapeutic intervention'.[40]

The identification of Rhesus haemolytic disease and its treatment were relatively new developments when National Women's opened, related to advances in haematology (the study of blood). In 1901 Karl Landsteiner had identified different blood types and ascertained that blood transfusion had to be from a compatible blood type – antigens 'A' and 'B' and their absence labelled 'O'. His ABO system enabled blood types to be matched. However, occasionally blood transfusion proved to be disastrous, and when the blood types of the donor and recipient were checked, no reason was found for the apparent mismatch. The mystery was solved in 1940 when Landsteiner and Alexander Wiener identified the Rhesus factor (named after the monkeys on which this research was done). The Rhesus factor, also known as the D antigen, is a thin coating of chemicals that surrounds the red blood cell. About 85 per cent of people have this and their blood is called Rh-positive. Those with only a partial coating or with no coating on their red blood cells are called Rh-negative. People with Rh-negative blood cannot tolerate

Rh-positive blood. If blood with D antigen (Rh-positive) is transfused into a patient without that factor (Rh-negative), the D antigen acts as an unwanted invader. Antibodies are formed to destroy it. A subsequent transfusion of Rh-positive blood will then provoke a transfusion reaction.

In 1931 American paediatrician Dr Louis K. Diamond identified various cases of stillbirths and serious brain damage as having the same cause.[41] Ten years later American physiologist Philip Levine showed the cause to be the incompatibility in the blood of the mother and the baby, as a result of an Rh-positive father and an Rh-negative mother. He found that the disease (also subsequently known as 'erythroblastosis fetalis') occurred when there was an Rh-negative mother whose baby inherited Rh-positive blood cells from the father. The mother built up Rh-antibodies against the baby's blood cells or became what was described as 'sensitised'. This did not affect the first pregnancy, but in subsequent pregnancies the mother's antibodies might attack the baby's red blood cells causing stillbirth, or, if the baby survived, severe jaundice, which could lead to cerebral palsy.

From the time National Women's opened, every patient admitted to the hospital, obstetrical or gynaecological, had her blood typed for ABO and Rh grouping. If a woman was found to be Rh-negative, her husband was typed. If he was Rh-positive, other children of the marriage and the father's parents were typed where possible.[42] With this knowledge the hospital staff felt they would be ready to act upon the birth of an affected baby.

The action taken was 'exchange transfusion' through the umbilical cord vein immediately following birth. In 1946 Diamond and his colleague Fred Allan in America successfully carried out the first umbilical exchange transfusion to treat Rhesus haemolytic disease in a newborn baby.[43] The aim was to wash out the child's infected blood and to replace it with Rh-negative blood, through a polythene tube inserted into the umbilical vein. The process was repeated as many times as was thought necessary over several days. It was heralded as a revolutionary treatment. Nevertheless, the infant death rate due to the disease was still about 40 per cent of those affected. Already in 1950, Green, who had carried out the first exchange transfusions at the hospital together with Renton Grigor, commented, 'there is a growing feeling that replacement transfusion as a form of therapy has not fulfilled the expectations once held of it', citing a recent article by Diamond.[44]

There was a second problem with the new development, according to another hospital obstetrician, Bruce Grieve. He believed that the public had become too conscious of the Rh factor, which was causing undue fear. He explained in 1954 that it was very important to explain to a young woman having her first child, who was found to be Rh-negative with an Rh-positive husband, 'that her first baby will almost certainly not be affected; that there is only a five to ten per cent chance of her ever having an affected baby – and much less of that infant not surviving. That she may have six or more children without ever becoming sensitized.'[45]

Nevertheless, exchange transfusion was regarded as a new and progressive medical intervention, and became a key part of the work of the paediatric department of the hospital. By the time the baby was born, however, it was sometimes so badly affected that it was too late to rescue it. In 1956 the HMC noted that recent reports in the literature indicated that there was a definite place for premature interruption of pregnancy in cases with a history of previous stillbirth due to haemolytic disease. The committee moved that a 'panel of the obstetric and paediatric staffs of this hospital be set up to review cases where a Rh-sensitized mother had had a stillbirth . . ., with a view to deciding whether premature interruption of pregnancy might not increase the chances of survival of the subsequent children'. The panel members were Carey (chair), Grieve, Matthews and Phillips. The consultant or practitioner referring the case to the panel and any other interested practitioners were also invited to join.[46] The following year the 'Rh Sub-committee' (now including Carey, Grieve, Matthews, Phillips and Green, who had recently been appointed professorial assistant) proposed to extend the policy of early induction to include cases where the disease in successive infants became steadily worse, to the point where it could be reasonably assumed that the next one would be a stillbirth.[47] Later commenting on his impression that it was relatively rare in other places for obstetricians and paediatricians to collaborate, Ross Howie pinpointed the importance of this committee in fostering close relations between the disciplines at National Women's, a development which would lead to other important advances in perinatal medicine (see chapter 7).[48]

When he was appointed National Women's first research fellow in 1957, Bill Liley specified the refining of prenatal diagnosis of the severity of haemolytic disease as one of his research projects. For this he used paracentesis (later called amniocentesis), a technique to extract and examine liquor from membranes, which Drs Douglas Bevis and A. H. C. Walker of Manchester, England, had developed in the early 1950s. Liley was aware of Bevis's recently published work relating to methods of detecting which babies were likely to develop kernicterus (brain damage due to jaundice following haemolytic disease).[49]

Liley began a systematic study of Rh-sensitised pregnant women to determine whether he could refine the method to calculate the severity of haemolytic disease. In 1959 Grieve noted that Liley's investigations of the amniotic fluid had helped the Rh committee to decide on early inductions.[50] In 1961 Liley produced a report entitled 'Liquor Amnii Analysis in the Management of Pregnancy complicated by Rhesus Sensitization'. In it he pointed out that he did not approve of routine induction of premature labour in Rh-sensitised patients, but thought that premature delivery obviously had much to offer, both in the prevention of stillbirth and in the avoidance of the severely anaemic and moribund neonate. He believed that liquor analysis could provide much of the information on which to base such a decision.[51]

The consequent policy of selective induction based on amniocentesis reduced the perinatal mortality from haemolytic disease at National Women's Hospital from 22 per cent in 1957–58 to 9 per cent in 1962.[52] By 1962 Liley was using amniocentesis to gain prognostic information on other causes of intrauterine deaths apart from haemolytic disease, testing women with pre-eclampsia, hypertension and diabetes.[53] He put forward an additional research proposal in 1962 on the biochemistry of amniotic fluid: 'in view of the success obtained with ante-natal prediction of haemolytic disease he wished to ascertain if something similar could be done in cases of placental insufficiency'.[54]

Prenatal testing was becoming established, and Liley's work was regarded as having great potential. In 1963, urging the university to grant research leave for Liley, the acting head of the postgraduate school Herb Green told the registrar that Liley's achievements 'include the fact that his work has halved the perinatal mortality from haemolytic disease of the newborn, [and] has increased [the] international stature for this hospital and school'. He added that some current work being done at Columbia University stemmed directly from Dr Howard C. Taylor's 1960 visit to Auckland and his appreciation of Liley's research into amniotic fluid.[55] Taylor was chairman of the Department of Obstetrics and Gynecology at the Columbia-Presbyterian Medical Center, and was in the process of founding the Columbia University International Institute for the Study of Human Reproduction, opened in 1965. Liley was granted leave and went to New York in 1964–65, where he was based at the Columbia-Presbyterian Medical Center.

Meanwhile, a month after Green's letter to the registrar, Liley made international headlines for conducting the first-ever successful intrauterine blood transfusion. The possibility of intrauterine transfusion of Rh-negative blood, in order to gain time for the severely afflicted fetus to develop in utero, occurred to Liley as a result of a mishap. While doing an amniocentesis he accidentally needled the distended fetal abdomen instead of the amniotic space, leading him to consider penetrating the abdomen on purpose. Yet for intraperitoneal blood transfusion to be successful, he needed to know whether blood cells would pass into the fetal circulation. He received the answer to this from a young English geneticist who was visiting the hospital on her way back home from Nigeria. In Africa she had been involved in the treatment of sickle cell disease anaemia in infants and this involved the introduction of normal red blood cells into their peritoneal cavity. Liley viewed her slides which showed 'floods of normal cells in their peripheral blood'.[56]

Liley decided to try intraperitoneal transfusion in fetuses who had severe haemolytic disease early in the third trimester of the pregnancy and who were predicted to die in utero. He developed a technique to outline the fetal gut, thus identifying the peritoneal cavity, by injecting contrast medium into the amniotic cavity and relying on the well-known ability of the fetus to swallow amniotic fluid and concentrate dye in the lower bowel. As a reporter for the *New Zealand Herald* put it, 'For the doctor's guidance – just as necessary in directing a needle to an unborn baby's stomach as in aiming a space probe at Venus – radiologists provided a finely developed x-ray technique.'[57] This allowed intraperitoneal blood transfusion.

Liley's great success story was the baby of 32-year-old Mrs Edna McLeod from Fern Hill, Hastings, whose first-born in 1957 had survived but whose next three (a baby in 1960 and twins in 1962) were lost to haemolytic disease. She had been admitted to the hospital at 30½ weeks when she was mildly hypertensive. She and her husband Rex, a farmer, were very keen to have a second live child. They were told of the prognosis for the fetus, the possibility and uncertainty of an intrauterine transfusion, and the potential hazard to the mother (that is, of infection). Liley carried out the first intrauterine transfusion at the beginning of the 32nd week of pregnancy. Eight days later, his attempt to repeat the transfusion failed but two days after that he succeeded. Thirty-four weeks was thought to be the earliest time it was safe to induce the baby, and so at 34 weeks and 3 days, on 20 September 1963, the baby was born following an induction.[58]

At birth the baby weighed 2560 g; he was pale and very jaundiced and had a huge umbilicus and a very large spleen. He was transferred to the paediatric team for further transfusions. Liley explained the importance of this, using as a metaphor New Zealand's national sport, rugby: 'It's no use getting a good pass away from the scrum if you're going to drop the ball in midfield.'[59] Within a few hours of birth the paediatricians carried out an exchange transfusion, although by this time the baby had developed moderate respiratory distress syndrome. They performed a second successful exchange transfusion at nineteen hours. Apart from being slow to feed and regain his birth weight, the baby progressed well. As Moira Tretheway, who nursed him in the neonatal ward, later commented, 'we weren't allowed to take our eyes off him'. He stayed in the ward for three months before going home.[60]

Mr and Mrs McLeod christened him Grant Liley McLeod, and his birth and survival made world headlines.[61] The local press later described Grant's story as a 'Miracle of Modern Medicine'.[62] Writing on the history of fetal medicine, American historian Monica Casper stated:

> As news of this breathtaking achievement spread across the globe in 1963, the 'unborn patient' became a new clinical and social entity . . . . Given the rich and evocative meanings of *whenua*, it seems fitting that fetal surgery began in New Zealand. This exquisite island nation ably plays the part of paradise in the origin story of the unborn patient.[63]

Casper was not the first to romanticise the story and the environment in which it occurred. In 1971 John Stallworthy, professor of obstetrics and gynaecology at Oxford and a New Zealander by birth, gave the oration for Liley when he was elected to a fellowship *ad eundem* of the RCOG:

> Professor Liley comes from a chain of small islands in the South Pacific which on the map look so small, in the midst of such vast oceans, that foreigners have been known to wonder what the inhabitants do when the tide comes in. It is perhaps therefore not surprising that even as a young professional man Dr. Liley became interested in the waters, and . . . started to take a submarine interest in the activities of the unborn foetus as it swam around in its portable goldfish bowl. But his approach was that of a physiologist, not a deep sea fisherman, nor of a detective, like many of his scientific contemporaries in other countries who were busy devising new techniques for bugging the activities of the innocent, lonely and

unsuspecting foetus. But he like them wanted to know what was happening and why.... This dramatic development [transfusion] captured the imagination of the press, radio and television and almost overnight Dr. Liley became world famous. In the midst of the drama many overlooked the full significance of his great contribution to medicine. He had focussed attention on the possibility of active therapy for the unborn child.[64]

Liley became an international star following this achievement. Casper commented in relation to Liley's 1964–65 sabbatical in New York where he worked with Vincent Freda and Karliss Adamson that their combined efforts shaped reproductive and fetal medicine for the next 30 years.[65] Liley was much sought after during this sabbatical leave – he was a guest speaker at twelve conferences, participated in nine symposia, was a guest lecturer at 46 institutions and visited eight other centres. Most of his talks were in the United States and Canada, but he also gave an address on intrauterine transfusion and haemolytic disease at the Tenth Joint Congress of the International Societies of Haematology and Blood Transfusion in Stockholm in September 1964.[66] At a 2003 Wellcome Witness Seminar in London on 'The Rhesus Factor and Disease Prevention', Charles Rodeck, professor of obstetrics and gynaecology and director of the Fetal Medicine Unit at University College London Hospitals, was to comment, 'I think that Liley's work, both diagnostic and therapeutic, is a beacon and was way, way ahead of his time.'[67] Remarking on the international significance of Liley's prenatal work in the 1960s and 1970s and crediting him with 'inaugurating the practice of fetal medicine, or fetology', a recent historian incorrectly stated that he moved to America in 1964.[68]

Liley continued as a senior research fellow at the postgraduate school until 1968 when the Medical Research Council of New Zealand agreed to fund his elevation to a personal chair, as Research Professor in Perinatal Physiology, on condition that the university assume responsibility for funding after five years.[69] Dennis Bonham (who had succeeded Carey as professor in 1964) noted that this appointment was the first occasion on which the MRCNZ had supported the establishment of a personal chair in a New Zealand university. He declared, 'Both the Council and the Auckland University regard this as a progressive step in the promotion of medical research.'[70]

Neonatal Paediatrics
Neonatal paediatrics was becoming established internationally by the late

1950s. In his history of Dublin's Rotunda Hospital, Alan Browne noted that the term 'neonatology', meaning the study and science of the newborn, was first coined in the 1950s, and reported the opening in his hospital of a neonatal operating theatre in 1956.[71] Writing on the history of paediatrics in Britain, Peter Dunn pointed out that there were practically no resident paediatric staff in British maternity hospitals in the 1950s (even though nearly half of childhood deaths occurred in the first three days of life) but believed that the founding of the Neonatal Society in 1959 signalled a turning point.[72] By 1960 neonatal paediatrics was incorporated into general MRCOG training.[73]

At National Women's the HMC recognised the new trend of extending the role of the paediatrician. It noted in 1956 that the Paediatric Committee of the Royal College of Surgeons had 'generally felt that the Pediatricians [sic] should have responsibility for the normal neonate, rather than as hitherto being called in by consultants only for the sick baby'.[74] Routine medical checks for newborn babies had taken off following a system devised in America by Virginia Apgar in 1953.[75] An anaesthesiologist, Apgar was interested in assessing the effects of obstetric anaesthesia on babies. She devised a score for assessing their physical state, including heart rate, respiration, muscle tone, reflex response and colour. Staff administered the tests one minute after birth and five minutes later, in order to ascertain whether intervention was necessary.

As the 1950s progressed, paediatricians at National Women's gained confidence and began extending their authority beyond the paediatric ward. In 1960 Matthews complained that some babies had been discharged early when still losing weight, and asked that resident staff and the matron be advised that this should not happen without paediatricians' approval.[76] Paediatricians were not, however, involved in the resuscitation of newborn babies in the labour wards, which was still the responsibility of the anaesthetist or the obstetrician. Hospital anaesthetist Dick Climie complained in 1961 that he had been appointed to give anaesthetics only but had begun to resuscitate babies by default. Climie told the committee that although he had taken the initiative to organise equipment in the labour ward for the resuscitation of neonates, 'they were primarily obstetrical responsibilities, and that his position was rather obscure'.[77] Carey asked him to continue with that responsibility, adding that Matthews would be on call if required.[78] The Paediatric Department gained an additional member of staff in 1962 when Dr Ross Howie accepted the position of paediatric registrar on condition that he would have time to work on his MD thesis.[79]

In 1962 Matthews took a proposal to the HMC to expand the work of the Paediatric Department. He thought they should take in babies from other institutions suffering from 'asphyxia neonatorum, acute respiratory syndrome and jaundice'. Algar Warren, the medical superintendent since 1960, told him that the hospital did not have the nursing staff and facilities to do so.[80] The hospital continued its practice of admitting only premature babies and Rh babies for exchange transfusions.[81]

Also in 1962, the hospital trialled a new test for newborn babies in the labour ward. In 1945 a Cambridge University immunologist Robin Coombs had devised a procedure for the detection of Rh agglutinins in newborns (called the 'Coombs test' in his honour). Bruce Grieve referred to this in a 1954 article on haemolytic disease of the newborn, but it was not until 1962 that Liley suggested that the hospital undertake a trial for its routine use. In asking for permission to do so, Liley pointed out that it enabled 'a closer check on antibodies in new born babies . . . especially rarer antibodies like anti-Kell and anti-Duffy'. Importantly, he said, 'Milder cases of ABO Haemolytic Disease – at present probably missed – would be picked up' and 'unrecognised cases of Haemolytic disease would be picked up where the mother did not have [an] ante-natal test'.[82] The task of collecting the cord blood specimens would fall upon the nursing staff in the labour ward and the main concern was whether they could cope with this extra work. The HMC agreed to the collection of cord blood specimens from all babies born in the hospital for a trial period of three months, providing that charge nurse Sister Hare was satisfied as to the practicalities.[83]

As National Women's Hospital was about to open its new purpose-built premises in the early 1960s, the newborn baby was becoming an increasingly important consideration in the services the hospital offered the public. The 'neonate' had become a patient in his or her own right, and even the fetus was poised to launch its career as a patient, resulting in fresh social and moral dilemmas over the ensuing decades. Liley was internationally renowned for having created a new patient, the 'unborn child'.

CHAPTER 6

A BRIGHT NEW AGE: ADVANCES IN REPRODUCTIVE MEDICINE, 1964–1980s

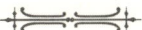

IN 1984 AUCKLAND'S *METRO* MAGAZINE FEATURED A STORY ABOUT NATIONAL Women's Hospital entitled 'The Glamorous Gynaecologists'. The journalist, Carroll Wall, portrayed the doctors at the hospital as dashing and dedicated, gynaecological equivalents of the debonair TV soap star of the 1960s, Dr Kildare. She described her visit to the hospital as an awe-inspiring experience. The two decades following the opening of the purpose-built hospital in 1964 had witnessed major advances, in particular in fertility (assisting to bring about pregnancies) and perinatal medicine. This chapter sets the scene for the dawn of this new era and then addresses the first of these 'advances'. Of the fertility services at the hospital Wall wrote, 'There can be few stories more romantic than that of the brilliance, the dedication, and the daring and the ethical recklessness that will bring these tiny lives into the world against infinite odds.'[1] This was an age of technological wonders, but also one that raised new moral and ethical issues relating to reproductive medicine. At the same time, the glamour of modern medicine enhanced public expectations which could not always be met.

A New Hospital and a New Professor
On 14 February 1964 the new National Women's Hospital, situated on the

slopes of Auckland's One Tree Hill, was officially opened in front of an audience of a thousand people. Her Majesty the Queen Mother, who had opened Wellington's Karitane Hospital 40 years earlier, was to have presided but had to cancel her visit owing to illness. The Governor-General Sir Bernard Fergusson took her place and paid tribute to the efforts of women's organisations in bringing the hospital to fruition. Sir Douglas Robb, Chancellor of the University of Auckland, also spoke, referring in particular to National Women's international status owing to Liley's antenatal blood transfusions.[2] With a sparkling new hospital, further advances were eagerly anticipated.

The hospital – eleven floors high and described in the *New Zealand Nursing Journal* as a 'skyscraper'[3] – had a smaller three-storey extension for accessory services and medical staff quarters. There were four postnatal obstetrical wards of 33 beds each (seventeen single-bed rooms and four four-bed rooms), an antenatal ward of 38 beds, and two gynaecological wards of 34 beds each. A nursery accommodated 54 premature and sick babies. There was also a large outpatient department, a suite of delivery rooms and four theatres with a recovery area. Features 'not previously seen in New Zealand' included 'a liquid oxygen plant with piped oxygen to most parts of the building and a fully centralised sterile supply system with automatic delivery to the various ward units'. The isolation block still under construction had been a late addition owing to the 1950s H-bug. This block was also to include facilities for radium treatment of gynaecological cancer, which was to be kept separate from the hospital's main services.[4]

At the end of the hospital's first year, New Zealand television aired a documentary extolling its virtues. The documentary praised the size of the new institution, enthusing that each month more than three thousand women either gave birth there or were treated, examined or instructed. In its first year around 4500 women had their babies there, and over 1000 major and 2500 minor gynaecological operations were performed.[5] As midwife Dorothy McAleer, who was working there when the new hospital opened, later said, 'Everybody wanted to have their baby at National Women's.'[6]

Thirty-nine-year-old Dennis Bonham, the new professor of obstetrics and gynaecology and head of the school, arrived from London in December 1963, two months before the hospital opened. While teaching facilities included a lecture hall, museums and accommodation for doctors attending postgraduate courses, Bonham found that the hospital did not possess a separate unit for the university staff, which he sought to remedy. The opening of a professorial unit, five years later, was officiated over by Sir John Peel, president of the RCOG, who had supported Bonham's appointment to the chair and was visiting at the time.[7]

English-born Dennis Bonham had qualified MA MB BChir at the University of Cambridge in 1948 and gained his MRCOG in 1956 and his FRCS (England) in 1958. Prior to coming to Auckland he had been a lecturer since 1960 in Professor William Nixon's Obstetric Unit at University College Hospital, London. Nixon inspired him with enthusiasm for obstetrics and gynaecology and suggested he take up the Auckland post. Nixon's biographer wrote, 'It was Nixon's ambition that all his assistants should fly the nest as professors and consultants in other parts of the UK and the world. They would be missionaries of his philosophy and few of them did not so succeed .... Several record being called to his office to be told that a professorship had been arranged for them in some other part of the world.'[8] During the appointment process for the Auckland chair Bonham was described as:

> ... a man of plump build with dark receding hair. At interview he was poised and confident but showed no signs of aggressiveness though from what members know of him he is not lacking in firmness. The committee is especially impressed by the warmth with which Professor Nixon writes of him and it believes that the experience which he has acquired under Professor Nixon's direction gives him some strong claims to appointment. His reputation as an original worker is high.[9]

In his inaugural lecture in 1964, Bonham spoke of the difference between a clinical chair and a 'normal three-legged university chair'. These three legs were teaching, research and administration. The clinical chair, he told his audience, had an 'extra, very sturdy leg, the responsibility for clinical care of patients ... day and night throughout the year'.[10] Sir John Scott, professor of medicine at the University of Auckland, later suggested just how seriously Bonham took that role: 'Undergraduate and graduate students, nurses and staff at National Women's regarded him with awe and elements of fear, but equally with recognition that here was a man who got things done, a man on the University payroll who walked the wards and attended the clinics day and night.'[11] Other evidence corroborates this assessment; for instance, a 'message' from Bonham was recorded at a 1979 delivery staff meeting: 'All A team patients to have a doctor present at every delivery (without fail) day or night. If unable to contact H/S [House Surgeon] then get Registrar otherwise call Prof Bonham.'[12] One woman whom Bonham delivered by caesarean section in 1985 found him 'really nice' but commented that the theatre staff were all 'jumpy' in his presence. On that occasion he ended up shouting at the paediatrician and the patient described his booming voice reverberating through the theatre.[13]

The postgraduate school maintained the international status it had begun to build up under Harvey Carey. The annual report for 1967, for instance, listed the large numbers of conferences attended and overseas visits by staff members and also identified 158 distinguished overseas visitors to the school that year.[14] Bonham's wife Nancie remembers entertaining many of these visitors in their home, and the gifts of appreciation they received over the years.[15]

In New Zealand Bonham introduced a national register of maternal mortality and was largely responsible for the 1968 Maternal Mortality Research Act that sought to improve standards in maternity services (see chapter 9). Immediately upon arrival he was appointed to the Board of Health's Maternity Services Committee. He also became involved with the WHO from 1968, appointed to its Advisory Panels on Maternal and Child Health and on Perinatal Mortality. He spent two weeks of his 1969 sabbatical leave in Geneva drafting and taking responsibility for the final revision of a WHO report on perinatal morbidity and mortality.[16] He was the founding president of the New Zealand Perinatal Society in 1980.[17] One of his other tasks upon arriving in New Zealand was to chair a Senate Advisory Committee that met weekly for two years to prepare the ground for the Medical Faculty of the University of Auckland, which admitted its first students in 1968.[18]

At National Women's Hospital, Bonham standardised record-keeping and insisted on monthly meetings to discuss perinatal mortality. Staff were required to attend and the discussions clearly impressed visitors.[19] Academics from other parts of the university regarded him highly; in his 1983 history of the University of Auckland, Sir Keith Sinclair described Bonham as 'a human dynamo and a great success', responsible for 'an excellent centre of research'.[20]

In his 1964 inaugural lecture Bonham highlighted two areas of research that he said were attracting international attention. He noted that Herb Green 'led an authoritative team for the management of carcinoma in situ and invasive cancer of the cervix, [while] the research team inspired by Dr A.W. Liley have established a world reputation in the management of Rhesus isoimmunisation'.[21] That same year, putting forward a request to the hospital board for dedicated accommodation for research and office space for the professorial unit, Bonham asserted that these two areas had given the hospital a reputation for work of the highest quality. He argued that, in order to maintain New Zealand's lead in world research, 'as indeed we must', they required a much larger budget.[22] In his first two annual reports for the school, he again referred to a 'powerful research programme initiated by this School some years ago [which] has been continued with increasing momentum', specifically Liley and Green's research.[23]

While Bonham stressed Liley and Green's work as the cornerstones of National Women's international prestige, they were not the immediate cause of the next 'famous moment' for National Women's. Just over a year after opening, it was home to the birth of the Lawson quintuplets facilitated through its fertility services, which made national and international news. Mont Liggins recalled, 'Our success in achieving pregnancies was quite good but nothing prepared us for the world media hype that followed the birth and survival of the Lawson quintuplets in 1965. National Women's Hospital had definitely arrived on the global map and we were inundated with visitors, sabbatical professors, invitations to travel to USA and Europe.'[24]

Fertility Services

National Women's Hospital provided fertility services from the outset. These were initially conducted in the 'Sterility Clinic', renamed 'Infertility Clinic' in 1950.[25] In providing such a service it followed international trends. In 1926 American gynaecologist John Rock (who was later instrumental in developing *in vitro* fertilisation) initiated what was to become an important infertility clinic in America, at the Harvard-affiliated Free Hospital for Women. By the late 1930s most major American cities had established such clinics.[26] In Australia, Sydney's Crown Street Hospital set up an infertility clinic in 1937, and Melbourne's Royal Women's Hospital followed in 1945 (although, as McCalman noted, the 'starkly named Sterility Clinic' did not adopt the name 'Infertility Clinic' until 1968).[27] American historians Margaret Marsh and Wanda Ronner argued that by the 1940s, infertility was no longer a subject whispered about behind closed doors and had become a staple of popular journalism. The American Society for the Study of Sterility was founded in 1944, and established its own journal in 1950. According to Marsh and Ronner, this growing interest was not so much related to medical developments as to the pronatalist movement (the desire to encourage large families) in the wake of the Second World War and the boundless confidence that science could cure all health problems, including infertility.[28]

In New Zealand, too, gynaecologists were paying attention to problems of sterility by the 1950s. In 1951 a Wellington gynaecologist, Ed Giesen, wrote of the treatment of sterility, 'It is a surprising thing that in a modern community, one of the most common complaints which brings a patient to a gynaecologist is infertility . . . . the sterile woman patient is often quite pathetic in her longing for a child of her own and it is a great satisfaction one is able to do something to help her to achieve this goal.' He advised gynaecologists first to check the patient's hymen, observing that, 'Complete and satisfactory coitus is obviously essential for conception and yet it is not uncommon to encounter an intact hymen in a patient complaining of sterility.' He cited a 1948 study by John Stallworthy of 581 patients seeking help for sterility: 5 per cent of their marriages had not been consummated. Another problem that was often overlooked, according to Giesen, was male infertility. He pointed out that 30 per cent of infertile marriages were the result of faulty spermatogenesis.[29] From the outset, National Women's remit included male infertility as well as female.[30]

The understanding of infertility was largely dependent on developments in endocrinology, the study of hormones, following the discovery of estrogen in the 1920s, which had led to a 'vogue for glandular preparations' to treat infertility.[31] In the 1950s a Swedish doctor, Carl Gemzell, developed an injectable form of the human pituitary gonadotrophin hormone, which stimulated ovulation and conception.[32] The problem with using the hormone was that it often caused hyperstimulation and multiple pregnancies. In 1962, when the future of National Women's Hospital's endocrine laboratory came up for discussion at an HMC meeting, the chairman advised that 'Dr J. B. Brown, known to be one of the outstanding men in this field, wanted to return to New Zealand and would be interested in a position at National Women's, provided suitable remuneration could be arranged.' Salary appeared to be a major difficulty as Brown was not medically qualified and would therefore be employed on a lower technical salary scale; in England he was on the same salary scale as those medically qualified.[33]

James Brown had an MSc from the University of New Zealand (1940) and an Edinburgh PhD (1952). He worked on the application of hormone assays in the identification of the phases of fertility and infertility during the menstrual cycle. In Edinburgh, where he was based from 1949 to 1962, he was involved in the development of the first accurate hormone assays for estrogens, pregnandeiol and total gonadotrophins in urine. Auckland would not meet Brown's salary demands, but Melbourne did. McCalman described how that hospital made a 'major intellectual investment' in endocrinology with the appointment 'from Scotland of J. B. Brown'.[34] As Liggins later recalled, Brown was involved from his position in Melbourne in the successful treatment of the mother of Auckland's famous Lawson quins. He produced gonadotrophin for clinical use in Australia, New Zealand, Singapore and parts of Canada.[35]

On 28 July 1965 *The Times* of London reported that 26-year-old Mrs Shirley Ann Lawson of Auckland, the wife of a fish shop owner, had given birth to quintuplets, four girls and a boy, at National Women's Hospital. The babies were in incubators and were doing well. Their weights ranged from 3lb 3oz to 4lb 3oz (1500 g to 1900 g). Mrs Lawson, who already had a five-year-old daughter, was sitting up in bed two hours after the birth. The babies, delivered at 33 weeks, were the fifth surviving set of quintuplets in the world and the first in New Zealand.[36]

Medical superintendent Dr Algar Warren wrote in his annual report that the birth 'created world-wide interest and it was several weeks before the invasion of enquiries, by telephone and letters, press, photographers, writers, lawyers and business firms, eased off'. He added that the quintuplets progressed very well and were discharged from hospital on 6 October 1965. Later that year, quadruplets were born at the hospital; they too did well and were discharged after a two-month stay.[37]

The three doctors involved in this area at National Women's were Mont Liggins, Richard Seddon and Kaye Ibbertson. The latter had been granted honorary university status in 1964 'to enable him to use beds in the Professorial Unit for endocrine investigations'.[38] Seddon had been appointed senior lecturer in obstetrics and gynaecology in 1965. The school's 1966 *Annual Report* stated that:

> The first series of 20 women treated with human pituitary gonadotrophin [HPG] resulted in 10 pregnancies with a high proportion of multiple pregnancies. In the second series the scheme of administration was altered to produce a higher incidence of single ovulation. This appeared to be successful in 10 cycles but only one pregnancy resulted. The third series is coming with the use of a single large injection of HPG to enable repeated administration on an outpatient basis.[39]

A word of caution emerged amidst the excitement: gonadotrophin could be used only to overcome sterility caused by deficiencies of the pituitary glands. This applied to 5–10 per cent of women who were infertile. Most cases of infertility were caused by other factors, such as congenital problems and the after-effects of disease.[40] The other fertility drug to stimulate ovulation that appeared around the same time was a synthetic preparation, clomiphene citrate, used for cases of polycystic ovary syndrome.[41] In 1977 the MRCNZ's National Hormone Committee (set up the previous year) recommended that HPG be used only after clomiphene or another new drug, bromoergocryptine, had failed, because of the increased risk of multiple ovulation with HPG.[42]

Numbers attending National Women's Infertility Clinic increased steadily over the years, from 243 in 1951–52 to 859 by 1972–73. Most of this increase came after 1967, once news had spread about the effects of gonadotrophin and clomiphene citrate. A 1969 article in *Thursday* magazine enthused that research was continuing at National Women's, and that 'the department bristles with optimism'.[43] A further technological advance came in 1972 with the introduction of laparoscopy, allowing better observation of the uterus, ovaries and fallopian tubes.[44] The laparoscope was a lighted miniature telescope 1.5 cm in diameter that was inserted through a tiny incision below the navel under general anaesthesia. While laparoscopy was seen as a great advance, as an invasive procedure requiring general anaesthesia it was not entirely risk-free. As an article published in the *NZMJ* in 1971 noted, this was a significant consideration as the patients were 'normal healthy women pre-operatively'.[45] Nevertheless, over the following years it gained in popularity in New Zealand as elsewhere. It was used in other procedures relating to sterilisation and *in vitro* fertilisation, and was increasingly conducted under local anaesthesia.[46]

While male infertility was included within the remit of National Women's Infertility Clinic, Dr Bernard Shieff, who was in charge of the clinic from 1961 to 1978, reported in 1975 that this had not been successful. He noted resistance from men to investigations because of the 'time commitment', and concluded that the investigation and treatment of male infertility were at a 'very low ebb'. He hoped that the recent appointment of a part-time urologist might improve the situation.[47] Marsh and Ronner found a similar situation in America. Those treating infertility tried to involve husbands but 'they proved elusive creatures', something Marsh and Ronner attributed to the continued association in men's minds between their masculinity and fertility.[48] Similarly, at National Women's, it is likely that more than time commitments prevented men from attending.

Artificial Insemination by Donor Sperm

In 1972 Bonham, together with a number of his university colleagues, began a small private artificial insemination by donor sperm (AID) service at National Women's in response to patient demand, charging a token fee.[49] The reason they kept it private, as the Dean of the Medical School Professor David Cole later explained, was opposition related to 'religious issues'.[50] When Bonham attempted to expand the services to the public sector in 1982 he met resistance from the Auckland Hospital Board to his request for funding sperm-freezing equipment; he thought this had been blocked by a 'small group' for 'religious or other reasons'.[51] New Zealand was not alone in this. In America, too, Catholics in particular opposed AID, and others saw it as an attack on the traditional family.[52]

In an attempt to promote fertility services, Bonham referred in 1982 to concerns about the 'shrinking size of the population'.[53] He also pointed to the humane goals of helping couples who 'through no fault of their own' were unable to conceive, and claimed that, despite what some people said, those who advocated fertility services 'really [did] believe in family life'.[54] There were growing demands for the new services, based on public expectations arising from medical developments. A 1982 article in the *NZMJ* commented on the 'immense newsworthiness' of the developments, noting that AID was now 'extraordinarily fashionable'.[55]

From the mid-1980s National Women's programmes, now available through the public system, at any one time incorporated 30 couples for AID and 30 for AIH (artificial insemination by husband) and they had another 60 on the waiting list for each programme. According to a 1986 report in the *New Zealand Woman's Weekly*, having made it to the top of the list, couples on AIH had three treatments with a 7–10 per cent success rate per cycle. Under AID a couple was allowed ten treatments, with a 60 per cent success rate. The *NZWW* commented, 'With hundreds of couples waiting, and hundreds more not eligible for treatment, frustration levels among both medical staff and infertile couples are high, sparking plans for New Zealand's first private fertility clinics.' The article reported that one of the hospital doctors working in this area, Richard Fisher, hoped to have a private clinic ('Fertility Associates') operating by mid-1987.[56]

The hospital had trouble recruiting donors, as did most AID programmes. According to one national survey in 1985, medical students and the husbands of obstetric patients were the most common donors.[57] Initially, anonymity was considered important. Bonham's private fertility programme of the 1970s received publicity 20 years later when Rebecca Hamilton, conceived in 1976, attempted unsuccessfully to trace her father and made a film about it, screened on national television in New Zealand in 2001.[58] From 1982 National Women's kept a record of every donor, which Fisher believed to be 'way ahead of the rest of the world'.[59] Bonham noted in 1984 that, while anonymity was preserved, they now kept separate registers of donors so that, ultimately, tracing would become a possibility. He commented that the law appeared to be lagging in providing full protection and rights for 'insemination children'.[60] Those opposed to anonymity included Catholic gynaecologist at the hospital, Pat Dunn, who pronounced, 'If AID donors choose to create new lives, they should be made to support them, and the profession should not protect them from this duty.'[61] The 1987 Status of Children Act addressed AID, specifying that the donor, unless he married the mother, did not have 'rights and liability of a father', which meant that donors might be less reluctant to be identified. From 1993 the private clinic started by Fisher, along with Freddie Graham and John Peek, elected not to take donors unless they agreed to be identifiable, not from concerns about the moral duties of the father, as expressed by Dunn for instance, but because of concerns about the rights of the children conceived.[62] Eventually, the 2004 Human Assisted Reproductive Technology Act secured the rights of children conceived through these means.

In Vitro Fertilisation (IVF)

In 1978 Louise Brown, the world's first 'test-tube baby', was born in Britain, at Oldham General Hospital, with *Daily Mail* headlines announcing the birth of 'the baby the whole world is waiting for'.[63] Louise was conceived through *in vitro* fertilisation, following twelve years of research and experimentation by Dr Patrick Steptoe, a gynaecologist, and Dr Robert Edwards, a Cambridge University specialist in reproductive physiology. An egg taken from Mrs Brown's ovaries had been successfully fertilised by her husband's sperm in a petri dish, and kept alive for two and a half days before being implanted in her uterus. A baby conceived through IVF was born at the Melbourne Royal Women's Hospital in 1980.[64]

New Zealand's first test-tube baby was born in Christchurch on 15 March

1983 (with the actual fertilisation occurring in Melbourne). The following month Bonham asked the Health Department to let him start a test-tube baby programme at National Women's. At that time New Zealand couples wanting treatment had to spend $5,000 going to Australia. Auckland Hospital Board chairman Frank Rutter declined to fund a new service, declaring that instead the government should pay for couples to go to Melbourne. Hospital Board Superintendent-in-chief Dr Leslie Honeyman also opposed the introduction of local services, commenting that there were ethical questions in relation to 'manipulating life in a test tube'.[65] Another hospital doctor, Professor Colin Mantell, told the press that it was 'incongruous' that the hospital board spent $300,000 a year on an abortion service, but was unable to find $100,000 for a test-tube baby clinic.[66]

The doctors went ahead without hospital board support. As journalist Carroll Wall enthused, 'Like so many programmes mounted by the Postgraduate School, the IVF project was led by Dennis Bonham, a man not known for asking permission about anything, a man who rips through the red tape of the Hospital Board with devastating speed and undeniable results.'[67] In early 1984 Bonham explained in the *NZMJ* that the pilot IVF programme being developed in Auckland was 'designed to be the spearhead of a national programme in keeping with the national concept of the Postgraduate School and the National Women's Hospital'.[68] The following year the Department of Justice, in a paper entitled 'New Birth Technologies', noted that National Women's was operating New Zealand's only IVF programme.[69]

The first IVF at National Women's was performed in July 1983. Certain criteria were laid down for the selection of couples. For example, they had to be in a longstanding and stable relationship; the woman had to have irreparable tubal damage and be under the age of 40; and couples with no children were given priority. Between July 1983 and February 1984 the hospital admitted 36 couples into the IVF programme. All were legally married and were counselled prior to their acceptance.[70] Two of the 36 couples were successful: in December 1983 the hospital announced its first test-tube babies were due to be born at the end of June 1984.[71] *Metro* journalist Carroll Wall saw symbolism in the Christmas announcement, 'when everyone was full of good cheer and thoughts of miracles and the birth of Christ'.[72]

The *Auckland Star* pronounced on 14 July 1984 that the *in vitro* team was as proud as parents of their babies. Two healthy babies had been born during the previous two weeks using IVF. 'The long-haired dashing Doctor

Freddie Graham', as Wall described him,[73] led the IVF team of biochemists and clinicians, radiographers and nurses, headed by Bonham. The team also included a social worker, Joy Ellis. According to the *Star*, Freddie Graham, 'a native Scot, has a wildfire enthusiasm for National Women's IVF unit and insists it is providing a service much in demand from the public . . . . "The feeling I get is just indescribable," he says. Or perhaps, just a little like God', the reporter added, without any sense of disapproval implied in the simile. The *Star* further explained that Graham saw infertility as a hidden disease, seldom talked about, which caused distressing emotional problems.[74]

At that time 60 women were undergoing treatment at National Women's, another 60 were waiting their turn, and a further hundred were awaiting assessment. Graham appealed for public money to finance the unit's Infertility Research Trust and acknowledged the financial support from the Auckland Infertility Society, which he had been instrumental in setting up in 1981 and which had 400 members by 1984.[75] Those accepted into the programme were not required to contribute to the costs, as these fell within the public health system. Between July 1983 and July 1985, a hundred couples were treated, and 22 succeeded in having a baby.[76]

By 1986 the popularity of the service had grown immensely. The hospital continued to provide the only IVF programme in the country and the waiting list was six years long, so no more couples were being taken on. Hospital funding catered for only 50 couples a year. New techniques using ultrasound instead of laparoscopy were being introduced as well as a new treatment known as gamete intrafallopian transfer.[77] Public interest in 1986 was such that Opposition health spokesperson Paul East asked the Health Minister what steps were being taken to ensure more women had access to IVF. He believed that six years was 'an inexcusable delay'. He noted that in an attempt to lower the waiting list, women had to be under the age of 32 to apply. Pointing out that large numbers of New Zealand couples of childbearing age were unable to have families because of infertility, he maintained that 'in a modern society such a situation should not be allowed to continue'.[78] Services struggled to keep up with demand.

In the face of inconsistent funding and growing waiting lists, from 1987 Graham, Fisher and Peek offered a private service – Fertility Associates – while also working in the public clinic at National Women's until 1996. That year competitive tendering for public-health funding led to almost all the money for Auckland's services being awarded to Fertility Associates. In response

National Women's rebranded its unit, calling it 'Fertility Plus', and managed to win back some funding in 2000 when government spending on fertility services increased.[79]

Not everyone supported the new development, as Fisher later noted.[80] Within National Women's there was opposition to both AID and IVF from Pat Dunn. His religious convictions led him to believe that 'the transfer of the germ cells between husband and wife must be confined to the normal loving marital embrace as designed by the Creator'. To illustrate how the procedure was a travesty of marriage, he declared, 'it is quite possible that an ovum could be extracted in Auckland while the husband is ejaculating in Hamilton and his semen delivered, still viable, by courtesy of NZ Couriers Ltd'. He thought that the reputation of the profession was at stake, for allowing such unethical behaviour. He also referred to the 'longsuffering' taxpayers who were required to pay for the services even though morally they might not approve of it.[81]

Concerns were also expressed by those who defined themselves as advocates for the 'unborn child'. Dr Norman MacLean, president of New Zealand Doctors for Life which represented 330 registered medical practitioners, made a case for the rights of the embryo. He believed that IVF was 'one of the most dramatic technological advances in modern medicine' and that it 'confirmed beyond question the uniqueness of individual human life from conception'. For him, the right to life of the embryo was the central issue. He was not opposed to IVF but worried about uses of the embryo other than to facilitate pregnancies.[82] Graham reassured MacLean, pointing out that in the Auckland IVF programme they did not 'experiment or dispose of embryos, practise embryo cryopreservation', and furthermore that 'routine amniocentesis and possible abortion are not part of the clinical protocol'.[83]

Despite opposing voices, IVF was here to stay. In Britain an influential report had appeared in 1984 on the subject of 'human fertilisation and embryology' chaired by philosopher Mary Warnock (later Baroness Warnock).[84] As *The Times* declared, 'The unanimous decision of the Warnock committee to support IVF as a clinical service has been seen as representative of a considerable shift in public opinion in England since Steptoe and Edwards were criticised for collecting human eggs and sperm in 1969.'[85] New Zealand too had seen that sea change.

Yet IVF did raise ethical issues, relating in particular to the status and the rights of the embryo. One commentator referred to embryo freezing and research as a 'legal minefield'.[86] The potential fate of surplus embryos was aired in the *NZMJ*.[87] In a 1984 article Bonham assured his readers that no one had accepted the cloning of embryos and expressed his view that discussions on cloning were 'essentially red herrings from the Pandora's box of horrors offered by those who fear rational discussion of help for the childless'.[88]

Dramatic advances in infertility services were creating moral dilemmas, debated well beyond the specialism of obstetrics and gynaecology, and contributing to the development of the new discipline of bioethics.[89] In this formative period of medical developments in infertility, the 1960s to the 1980s, National Women's was at the centre of the action for New Zealand, providing a national service. While this was a contested development, it was also considered eminently newsworthy and even heroic medicine, with National Women's gynaecologists being described in *Metro* magazine for example as glamorous.

CHAPTER 7

THE NEW PATIENT AND PERINATAL MEDICINE

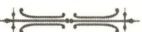

T HE GLAMOUR WITHIN REPRODUCTIVE SERVICES WAS NOT RESERVED FOR those involved in fertility. In her 1984 *Metro* article, journalist Carroll Wall wrote:

> While [Freddie] Graham and his team are working to get pregnancy started, the paediatricians are working to save the babies that have been expelled from the uterus too soon. It's here that those scraps of bone and arms and legs, hooked up to every conceivable kind of monitor, little hearts pumping wildly, struggle to stay alive, watched over, often for 12 weeks at a time, by teams of extraordinarily dedicated men and women.[1]

William Liley's successful antenatal blood transfusion in 1963 heralded the start of a new era in fetal medicine. Referring to this in an article on New Zealand medicine in *The Times* in 1966, the University of Auckland Chancellor Sir Douglas Robb declared, 'In clinical work New Zealand is perhaps best known abroad for her embryotics or foetology at the National Women's Hospital.'[2] In 1968 Liley was appointed research professor in perinatal physiology; the founding of such a chair was indicative of the new importance attached to perinatal medicine. In 1980 there was further evidence of the maturing of the discipline when the New Zealand Perinatal Society was founded, 'to encourage training and research', with Bonham as chair.[3]

Neonatal paediatrician Professor Jane Harding later described the 1960s and 1970s as the golden age of perinatal medicine in Auckland.[4] Another National Women's paediatrician, Associate Professor Ross Howie, calculated that New Zealand's perinatal mortality fell by nearly 80 per cent from 1950 to 1980.[5] While acknowledging the contribution of broader social factors, Howie believed that improvements in the survival rate of babies from the early 1950s was 'one of the greatest success stories of public health in this country and arguably the greatest achievement of the hospital'.[6] This chapter will investigate the development of perinatal medicine during these formative decades.

Respiratory Distress Syndrome and Ventilation

In the 1960s the leading cause of death for newborn babies was respiratory failure. In 1969 Bonham explained that respiratory disorders accounted for approximately half of all neonatal deaths in New Zealand (amounting to around 300 per annum), and featured prominently in disorders requiring neonatal intensive care.[7] New Zealand was not alone; a paediatrician at Scotland's Glasgow Royal Maternity Hospital reported that same year: 'The importance of respiratory distress cannot be over-emphasised. Between 60 and 70 per cent of all neonatal deaths are associated with respiratory distress in one form or other.'[8] Premature babies were at particular risk of respiratory distress syndrome (RDS).

The 1960s saw the development of mechanical ventilators for newborn babies with respiratory failure, and in 1966 National Women's Hospital purchased the latest model, the Bird Mark VIII ventilator. Britain's Sorrento Maternity Hospital, world-famous for its premature ward, purchased such a ventilator the very same year, suggesting just how much National Women's kept up with international trends.[9]

While the Bird Mark VIII was regarded as a technological advance, it was labour-intensive, requiring almost full-time supervision by a special trained nurse, paediatrician, registrar and laboratory assistant. According to paediatrician Jack Matthews, much of the work fell on Ross Howie.[10] Howie himself had some reservations about the value of the innovation. He later commented that it was useful for babies 'with relatively normal lungs, but was not especially effective in the majority (especially premature babies) who had immature lungs'.[11] He reported in 1968 that during the previous year only two out of seventeen babies so treated at National Women's had survived. He commented that this was similar to the results at the Cardiovascular

Research Institute, San Francisco, where 10 per cent of RDS babies treated on a respirator survived. He thought that better results reported from other centres might be due to 'more liberal indications for treatment'.[12]

Graduating from Otago Medical School in 1956, Howie had been a paediatric registrar at National Women's in 1962–63 and then went to England where he met Bonham before the latter took up his post as professor in Auckland. Howie was impressed when Bonham encouraged him to return to Auckland, commenting, 'To have an obstetrician who actually valued a paediatrician, well, I think there were some at National Women's but at other places they just didn't seem to talk much with each other.'[13] The Auckland Medical Research Foundation funded Howie as a research fellow in neonatal paediatrics from 1963 to 1966, after which he was appointed senior research fellow at the postgraduate school in 1967, senior lecturer in neonatal paediatrics in 1973 and then an associate professor from 1977 until he retired in 1995.

In 1969 Howie complained about the shortage of staff required for continuous supervision of premature babies, in particular for monitoring oxygen therapies. He explained that precise regulation of oxygen therapy was important: too much and the baby could be blinded from retrolental fibroplasia; too little and he or she might die of hypoxia. Howie came to the depressing conclusion that assisted ventilation had only a small place in the treatment of the newborn, noting that of 24 treated in 1968 only three had survived.[14]

A breakthrough came in 1970, when the practice of continuous positive airways pressure (CPAP), developed by George Gregory in San Francisco, was introduced to National Women's. Mont Liggins brought back the ventilator from his travels abroad even before the technique had been publicised.[15] In his history of newborn care in the UK, Peter Dunn commented that CPAP, introduced in 1971, was the most exciting advance in the field ever. As a result RDS mortality had dropped 'precipitously overnight from over 30% to 5%'.[16] In Auckland, too, Howie said that with CPAP the RDS mortality 'fell from 30–40% to about 10% overnight'.[17]

In his 1974 report Matthews again paid tribute to Howie who had borne 'the major burden in developing and providing this service', commenting that Howie had personally provided 24-hour supervision of babies on CPAP and other respirators. As some of these babies had required respiratory care for over a week, Matthews said this had placed a very great physical strain on Howie.[18]

Between 1975 and 1980 there was a sudden upsurge in the survival of premature infants, which was attributed to this new technology. Along with CPAP respirators, in the mid-1970s a second generation of ventilators arrived, incorporating PEEP (positive end-expiratory pressure).[19] Unfortunately, prolonged use of the ventilator sometimes caused lung damage, resulting in chronic lung disease. A report two decades later noted, 'Sometimes an infant would survive the early complications of prematurity often still dependent on a ventilator, only to die some months later from respiratory failure.' It was with this in mind that a new method of neonatal physiotherapy was introduced in 1985, which became the source of a later dispute.[20]

While there were definite advances in keeping alive babies by respiratory support, Howie also became involved with an important research project which attempted to prevent the condition from arising in the first place. In this project he collaborated with Mont Liggins, appointed professor of obstetric and gynaecological endocrinology in 1971, and knighted for his achievements in 1991.[21]

Liggins, Howie and Corticosteroids

Discussing the research which led to his international fame, Liggins explained that early in his career he had sought advice from Liley who told him to pick a 'hot topic' that had the potential to be solved. Liggins chose to study premature birth as the outstanding problem, adding 'what's more I was naïve enough to think that I could solve it'.[22]

Like some of his contemporaries overseas, Liggins decided to use pregnant sheep for his research, because of their relatively long gestation (145–147 days), large bodies, mostly singleton pregnancies and the comparative rarity of miscarriage following fetal surgery.[23] He appealed to his friend Dr Robert Welch, a scientist at the Ruakura Agricultural Research Station, a 'world-famous animal research station'[24] located in a farming region 130 kilometres south of Auckland. Liggins' research agenda fitted well into the station, and from 1963 he spent two days a week at Ruakura researching pregnant sheep.[25] In order to test a hypothesis that the pituitary gland played an important part in initiating labour, he learnt to remove the pituitary gland of fetal sheep.[26]

In 1965 Liggins started work under Bonham's supervision on a PhD thesis, on the physiology of the fetal adrenal, which he completed in 1969. During the first year of his thesis Liggins won a Lalor Foundation Fellowship to the University of California Davis, where he worked in the Department of Physiological Sciences at the School of Veterinary Medicine for ten months. There he continued his work on pregnant sheep. At the same time he was appointed research associate at the Cardiovascular Research Institute of the University of California Medical Center, San Francisco, where researchers were studying fetal and neonatal lung physiology. He spent the last two months of his leave in Britain, at the Agricultural Research Council's Unit of Reproductive Physiology and Biochemistry under Roger Short, who later became foundation director of the UK Medical Research Council's Unit of Reproductive Biology in Edinburgh and still later (1982) professor of reproductive biology at Monash University, Australia.

At Davis, Liggins affirmed that surgically removing the pituitary gland from the fetal sheep led to the pregnancy continuing weeks past term until the fetus died in the womb. He concluded that the fetal pituitary played an essential part in the initiation of labour in sheep.[27] Attempting to discover which pituitary hormone was the key, he infused adrenocorticotrophin (ACTH, a hormone produced in the pituitary glands) and cortisol (a steroid hormone made in the adrenal glands) into the fetus and found that both brought on labour. After he returned from his sabbatical, in February 1968 the UK Wellcome Trust provided him with a research grant of £15,000, 'to investigate the mechanisms responsible for the initiation of human parturition'. He continued to work primarily on sheep and rabbits, and acquired a derelict hut in the grounds of the adjacent Green Lane Hospital for this purpose. In 1971 the Wellcome Trust awarded him a further grant of £23,050 for a 'study of the hormonal control of ovine parturition'. From 1975 the MRCNZ funded his research.[28]

Liggins was developing an international reputation and his interaction with the international community was to prove important to his own research career. In 1968 he gave talks at Cornell Medical College, New York, and at the Universities of Leeds, Wales, Cambridge and Copenhagen, at the Blair Bell Society in London, and most crucially at a London Ciba Foundation Symposium.[29]

The Ciba Foundation had been established after the Second World War to promote international collaboration in medical and chemical research.[30] Geoffrey Dawes, director of the Nuffield Institute for Medical Research in Oxford since 1948 and internationally known for his work on fetal and neonatal physiology, organised the 1968 Ciba Symposium which he called 'Foetal Autonomy'.[31] The editors of the proceedings explained, 'The control exercised by the mammalian foetus over its own growth, development and security is now being studied by workers in so many different fields, that quite apart from its intrinsic interest, it seemed a particularly suitable topic for a

Ciba Foundation symposium.' They acknowledged that the original stimulus for the meeting came from reports of Liggins' work on the role of the fetal adrenal in determining the onset of parturition in sheep.[32]

At this symposium Liggins revealed another finding from his research. During the discussion following one contributor's paper on the development of the fetal lung, Liggins reported that, much to his surprise, lambs delivered at around 120 days that had been given an infusion of ACTH about 48 hours prior to birth survived without apparent respiratory distress. He explained that this was 'probably indicative of a fair degree of surfactant activity and an earlier maturity than would be expected'. (Surfactant is a complex soap-like substance that prevents the lungs from spontaneously collapsing from the forces of surface tension.) He concluded that it was 'reasonable to suggest that premature induction of surfactant had occurred as a result of corticosteroid activity'.[33]

Another participant at the Ciba Symposium was Dr Leonard Strang, who had set up the Department of Paediatrics at London's University College Hospital Medical School in 1963 and was researching the adaptation of the fetal lung to air breathing. He became very excited by Liggins' pronouncement, declaring: 'This is a very extraordinary and vital finding indeed. Are you really sure of the gestational age?'[34]

Still focusing his attention on the question of parturition, Liggins later explained, 'I didn't have time to pursue this lung problem any further.'[35] Back in New Zealand he attended a meeting in Christchurch of the NZOGS at which the guest speaker was Mary Ellen Avery, professor of paediatrics at McGill University, Montreal, a leading figure in RDS and the first to confirm that surfactant was necessary for lung expansion. At this meeting, Liggins again described his findings. He later commented, 'She couldn't get back to the US fast enough to set up [animal] experiments . . . and produce the definitive paper on the effects of corticosteroids on lung maturation.'[36] She published on this in 1970.[37]

Meanwhile, Liggins lost no time in setting up his own trial, taking his proposal for a randomised controlled trial on preterm infants at National Women's to the HMC in February 1969 for approval. He later explained that the main purpose was to let the staff know what was going on and to enlist their cooperation. The trial was to run within the clinical care of each mother and no funding was required. He told the committee that verbal consent would be obtained.[38]

Liggins sought Howie's help in conducting this trial. Howie later described as a highlight of his career the day Liggins handed him the lungs of twin lambs, prematurely delivered, one of whom had been infused with cortisol and the other not. The lungs of the infused lamb were pink and floated in water, in contrast to the lungs of the other which sank. Howie said that, having spent far too many nights trying to ventilate babies with respiratory problems, he found this very exciting, not to mention 'the possible benefits to babies in sparing them the tender mercies of intensive care'.[39]

With the approval of the HMC, in December 1969 Liggins and Howie launched their double-blind randomised controlled trial administering prenatal corticosteroids (using the synthetic corticosteroid, betamethasone) to mothers in whom premature delivery threatened or was planned before 37 weeks' gestation. Betamethasone proved to be a serendipitous choice, as Liggins' biographers later noted, with subsequent studies confirming its benefits over other glucocorticoids.[40]

The results of the trial were soon clear – more babies were surviving and staying healthy in the treated group. Results from the first 282 infants delivered at less than 32 weeks' gestation, whose mothers had been given betamethasone therapy at least 24 hours before delivery, showed improved survival and a considerably reduced incidence of RDS and pneumonia. The first results were published in 1972.[41] A subsequent report on 717 mothers confirmed earlier findings and also revealed a lower incidence of intraventricular cerebral haemorrhage in treated babies.[42] By 1979 they had carried out ten separate studies, involving 3407 mothers.[43]

Liggins later claimed, 'It really did hit the world', as evidenced by the fact that the findings were submitted to the specialist journal *Pediatrics* on 22 June and accepted on 5 July, which he said was unheard of.[44] Yet the response of *Pediatrics* was in sharp contrast to that of the British medical journal, *The Lancet*, which had previously rejected the paper. According to Liggins, *The Lancet* had not even sent it out for review, on the grounds that it lacked general interest.[45] The editors of the specialist journal clearly thought differently.

As early as 1973, Howie reported that their research was attracting the interest of the WHO.[46] The following year, through its Human Reproduction Program, the WHO asked Howie to lead an international multicentre controlled trial on prenatal steroids. He persuaded them instead to fund a follow-up study in Auckland. Conducted by Dr Barton MacArthur from the University of Auckland's Department of Education, this ran from 1975 to

1979; MacArthur followed the first 318 children born during the trial to the age of six or seven years. The children underwent detailed medical and neurological examinations, which showed no evidence of any long-term hazards from the therapy.[47] This study was supplemented 30 years later by a follow-up, which again showed no long-term adverse effects.[48]

In the meantime a multicentre trial had started in the UK in 1974, and the National Institutes of Health (NIH) in America conducted a Collaborative Group Study, published in 1984.[49] The use of antenatal steroids for preterm births received a setback in 1982 when one of the contributors to the NIH Collaborative Study published an editorial in the *British Medical Journal* questioning its applicability across all sectors of the population.[50] Patricia Crowley, a consultant obstetrician gynaecologist at Dublin's Coombe Women's Hospital and a supporter of prenatal steroids from the 1970s, began to collect data on various trials in order to refute these negative reviews, particularly by the NIH Collaborative Group. Her study, a systematic review of eight large trials of antenatal steroids, was the first to be entered onto an Oxford Database of Perinatal Trials. A graphic representation of this study became the logo of the Cochrane Centre set up in Oxford in 1992. One of the centre's founders, Sir Iain Chalmers, explained that they wanted to make the point that this very important information had been available more than a decade earlier, yet had often not been acted upon. In their brochures and in talks on the centre, Chalmers and others stressed that tens of thousand of babies had suffered and died unnecessarily (and cost health services more than they need have done) because information had not been assembled in a systematic review and meta-analyses had not been used to show the strength of the evidence.[51]

In 1994 an NIH conference reached a consensus on antenatal steroids, which was endorsed by the American College of Obstetricians and Gynecologists.[52] In Britain the RCOG published guidelines in 1992 on the use of antenatal steroids, and invited Crowley to update them in 1996. She later determined that, 'By the late 1990s 70% of preterm babies delivered in the UK were being treated with antenatal steroids prior to delivery.'[53] Liggins himself wrote in his autobiography that 'no treatment other than vaccination can have had such a favourable cost-benefit ratio', pointing out that a few cheap injections could save tens of thousands of dollars in intensive neonatal care and long-term care of handicapped infants.[54] And yet it took until the 1990s for it to be incorporated into general practice.

This delay was discussed at two medical historical 'witness' seminars in London in 1999 and 2004, on the origins of neonatal intensive care and the introduction of prenatal corticosteroids respectively.[55] Some commentators believed the delay was because paediatricians focused on management of the baby following birth, using mechanical ventilation, whilst obstetricians were more interested in preventing premature labour than in improving the outcome for infants born prematurely.[56] The commentators thought that a lack of dialogue and even territorial jealousies between obstetricians and paediatricians prevented them from collaborating. Howie pinpointed National Women's Rh sub-committee, set up in 1956, as important in bringing together specialists from different fields, which, he said, did not happen overseas.[57] Yet by the time of Liggins' and Howie's research such collaboration was not uncommon. For instance, in 1969 the *Scottish Medical Journal* reported on the 'increased awareness of the necessity, not only for practical co-operation between obstetrician and paediatrician, but for a pooling of information between the clinical disciplines and those working in the fields of foetal and neonatal physiology and pathology'. This had resulted in the formation that year of the European Society of Perinatal Medicine.[58] New Zealand itself did not set up its Perinatal Society until 1980, as noted earlier.

Other commentators at the seminars thought the delayed recognition related to scientific snobbery and disbelief that a significant finding could come from a 'colony', or 'this rather primitive backwater'.[59] Yet New Zealand – and National Women's Hospital – was part of an international network. For instance, Dawes visited Liggins' laboratory in 1969 and the following year Liggins went to Dawes' department in Oxford, which Liggins described as the 'hub of the universe' in terms of fetal physiology.[60] In 1974 Liggins made the return trip to the northern hemisphere no less than six times. At the 2004 Wellcome seminar some commentators speculated about professional rivalry. Chalmers told the seminar, 'I had the impression that he [Dawes] was very annoyed that he hadn't made the discovery that Mont and Ross had made.'[61] It was a tight international community, of which New Zealand was a part despite the tyranny of distance, but at the same time it seems that national and personal rivalries abounded.

Locally, corticosteroids were a source of great pride, particularly focused on National Women's. In 1980 the hospital witnessed the arrival of the first quadruplets born there for fifteen years. They featured on the front page of the *New Zealand Herald*, which declared that they appeared 'screaming their heads off and clearly unaware of how lucky they were'. The mother, flown in from Samoa, gave birth prematurely to four identical sisters under the supervision of a team of 22 staff, including paediatricians, obstetricians, midwives, nurses and an anaesthetist. She had been given a course of steroids before giving birth. The celebratory reports noted that the work done here was now practised internationally and that New Zealand was 'justly proud' of it.[62]

In 1971 Liggins had been given a personal chair in obstetric and gynaecological endocrinology at the University of Auckland, a position he held until he retired in 1987. Other honours followed. In 1976 he was elected a fellow of the Royal Society of New Zealand, and in 1978 an honorary fellow of the American College of Obstetricians and Gynecologists. He became a fellow of the Royal Society of London in 1980 (nominated by Dawes and Short, a further display of the international network), and was knighted in 1991.

At the opening of the University of Auckland Liggins Institute in 2002, the public was reminded of the legacy of the man whose discovery of antenatal steroids for lung development of premature infants had 'saved the lives of literally hundreds of thousands of premature babies around the world'.[63] Likewise, various obituaries that followed Liggins' death in 2010 highlighted his discovery, which had helped prevent the disability or death of countless premature babies.[64] Yet Liggins himself had never abandoned his first and related research project, the mechanisms for bringing on labour. This was funded by the MRCNZ which had reported in 1973:

> The aim of this work is to study the physiological mechanism by which labour is initiated at term in various species. The sheep serves as the principal mode but in addition, certain aspects of mechanism have been studied in rats, rabbits, guinea pigs and women. Previous work by the group in sheep has demonstrated the dominance of the fetus in the regulation of the complex hormonal changes leading to the onset of uterine activity.[65]

When Liggins was asked to reflect on his contributions to science after his election as a fellow of the Royal Society in 1980, he did not focus on RDS. Rather, he chose to concentrate on his work relating to the onset of labour, which he described as 'the greatest mystery in obstetrics'. He explained that 20 years previously it had been generally believed that unborn babies were docile passengers afloat in a warm, dark sea, who had as little control over their own birth as the toothpaste did over the moment when it emerged in response to irresistible forces squeezing it. Through his research on sheep he made the 'great discovery [that] labour is initiated by the unborn baby's hormone message'. For example, he said, 'Among animals that suckle immediately on being born, one of the last tasks of the unborn creature's adrenal gland is to shoot off a message that says "I'm coming" to the mother's milk-making glands. A minute later the little animal is swallowing the hot drink it ordered on the way out.'[66] In other words, he was giving the fetus agency.

Liggins had identified the trigger for the onset of labour in sheep but not humans. He believed, however, that it was only a matter of time and 'hard work' before the one led to the other. He predicted in 1976 that they would have a 'complete understanding of human birth' within five years.[67] By 1991, when Liggins was knighted, the secret had still not been uncovered, but this did not curb his enthusiasm. Under the headline 'Mystery Solver Rewarded', he explained, 'I was lucky enough to solve a problem that puzzled the philosophers ever since before Hippocrates. Is it the mother or the baby who initiates labour?' Again he drew attention to his work on unborn lambs, showing that the fetus was like a 'co-pilot' of its own growth and birth, with its pituitary and adrenal glands acting as triggers to birth. He admitted that human babies did not have the same amount of control as lambs, and that it would take a few more years' research to solve fully the riddles of human birth,[68] but, as one of his obituaries noted, this mystery had still not been solved at the time of his death in 2010.[69]

While still hypothetical, Liggins' idea had captured the imagination of the scientific community in the 1960s. Dawes, inspired by Liggins' work, concluded the 1968 Ciba Symposium with the following graphic account:

> The foetus has been likened to a spaceman: passive, insulated and preserved from stimuli – which is only half true. On the contrary one could think of the mammalian embryo as a hitchhiker with a large pack on his back getting into a rather small car; he is a friendly fellow who chatters away all the time and is prepared to do some driving if given half a chance – he takes you off your route and tells you when and where he would like to get out.[70]

This conceptualisation had significant implications for obstetrics. As Bonham declared in 1967, obstetricians were moving towards accepting the 'unborn baby' as not just a passenger in the womb, but rather as the patient and in charge of the case. He said that Liggins' research had 'proved that all conditions associated with pregnancy were governed by the foetus from the beginning'.[71]

Other technological developments contributed to this new trend of giving the fetus agency. As Clare Hanson explained in her 2004 history of childbirth, the age of the fetal portrait was inaugurated with the 1965 publication in *Life* magazine of Lennart Nilsson's dramatic photographs of the embryo in the womb. Nilsson and Lars Hamberger published *A Child is Born: The Drama of Life before Birth* in 1966. Nilsson's imagery likened the fetus to a spaceman, which is what Dawes had alluded to.[72] This concept, whether as spaceman or hitchhiker, was aided by the new technology of ultrasound scanning. The pioneer of ultrasound, Ian Donald, professor of midwifery in Glasgow, described how prior to ultrasound the 'developing human being' had been hidden from the medical gaze, shielded behind the 'Iron Curtain' of the maternal abdominal wall.[73]

Diagnosing the Fetus

Ultrasound as a means of diagnosing fetal problems had its origins in the research conducted by Ian Donald in the 1950s. By 1956, working with Tom Brown, an engineer, he had created a device which appeared to provide new and useful diagnostic information about the female abdomen.[74] Ultrasound had originally been developed to track submarines during the First World War. The basis of ultrasound was that, when subjected to an electric charge, certain crystals emit high-frequency sound-waves which travel through water, sending back echoes when they encounter a solid object. Donald applied his knowledge of the naval echo-sounding technique of 'sonar' (an acronym for 'sound navigation and ranging') to create ultrasound technology. He himself declared in 1969, 'There is not so much difference after all between the fetus in utero and a submarine at sea.'[75]

One of the reasons why this new technology attracted interest was concern about the effects of X-rays on the fetus, that arose primarily from the work of Dr Alice Stewart in Oxford in the 1950s. Subsequent technological developments made ultrasound even more attractive. A major breakthrough came in the 1970s when real-time imaging replaced static images, utilising cheaper, lighter and smaller equipment which 'universalised' ultrasound, so that by the end of the decade this was the most common method of monitoring fetal development in the UK.[76] In his history of Dublin's Rotunda Hospital, Alan

Browne described the introduction of ultrasound to the Rotunda in 1976 as 'one of the most exciting periods in the history of perinatal care'.[77]

As early as 1964 National Women's Hospital expressed interest in adding ultrasound to its X-ray Department.[78] In 1967 the hospital began to consider the purchase of 'an ultrasound pulse monitor' from either America or the UK, and the following year it bought a monitor from Britain. The HMC noted, 'There is no doubt that the fetal pulse machines working on the ultrasound principle are a great advance in obstetrics. For continuous monitoring, the problem of aiming the ultrasound crystal at the fetus as it moves about has not yet been solved.'[79]

A major advance on such fetal pulse monitors were ultrasound imaging devices. By 1970 National Women's had such a machine on hire from an American manufacturer and was considering purchasing its own. That year Dr Florence Fraser had returned to National Women's, following two and a half years' postgraduate training in Britain. Whilst in Britain she had become particularly interested in the new technology and contacted Ian Donald in Glasgow 'for the opportunity to learn a technique not yet used in New Zealand but hoped for in the near future'.[80] Donald provided her with residential accommodation in the Queen Mother's Maternity Hospital in Glasgow for six weeks. On her return to New Zealand, Fraser persuaded National Women's to purchase a Scottish product called a Diasonograph, which was used in Donald's ultrasound unit in Glasgow.

In their application to the hospital board for funding the Diasonograph (costing $23,000), the HMC referred to its usefulness for fetal transfusions, for which the hospital was so famous. It noted that ultrasound was 'safe, painless and may be repeated with impunity – without the danger of irradiation'. It also gave examples of clinical situations other than fetal transfusions where ultrasound would be valuable: these included the early diagnosis of multiple pregnancies, the assessment of fetal growth, the detection of antepartum haemorrhage, haemolytic disease and all gynaecological tumours, and the diagnosis of ectopic pregnancies and some types of threatened miscarriage.[81]

It was successful in this application, and the first Diasonograph scanner arrived in early 1973. Bill Faris, who had also studied ultrasound overseas, publicly announced that 'the diagnostic value of ultrasonic scanning made it one of the great obstetric advances of the decade'.[82] At the same time the hospital created a new post, a whole-time specialist obstetrician and gynaecologist for 'haemolytic disease and diagnostic ultrasound', to which Florence

Fraser was appointed. The X-ray Department became the 'Department of X-raying and Ultrasound Scans'.[83]

In the 1970s scans were not yet routine at National Women's. In 1976 Bonham cautioned, 'The final place of ultrasound scanning as an alternative to radiology, particularly for the diagnosis of twins, placenta praevia, and fetal health growth is not yet certain.'[84] In 1979 the HMC suggested caution in the use of this new technology, recommending that ultrasound only be performed 'if indicated and ordered by a registrar at least – preferably in consultation with a senior'.[85]

The early 1980s, however, saw new moves to make ultrasound scans routine in pregnancy. Fraser resisted this trend on the grounds that it negated the 'use of brains, hands and clinical skills and reduces patient contact'. She warned that a number of abnormalities would not show up at 20 weeks and that even if several ultrasound examinations were done after that date, it would not guarantee a normal baby.[86]

In 1982 the HMC recommended the restriction of ultrasound imaging to cases where there was a medical indication. Obstetrician Tony Baird explained that many patients were requesting scans, often because friends had had them, either to ensure everything was all right or to determine the sex of the child. While he accepted that unexpected benefits could accrue from a scan, he could not see the justification for conducting scans on 'principally social grounds'.[87]

This was discussed again at the next HMC meeting. Bonham felt that ultrasound teaching should be incorporated in the training of registrars and that all antenatal patients should be scanned before sixteen weeks' gestation. The committee agreed to 'work towards the progressive provision of some type of ultrasound facilities' at the hospital and to engage specialists when required.[88] Six months later Baird now agreed that women should be scanned twice during pregnancy.[89] Scans were fast becoming standard practice.

National Women's had two scanners by 1983, a static scanner and a real-time scanner. The Department of X-raying and Ultrasound Scans reported that recent developments had been related to the real-time equipment; static scanners were becoming outmoded. The hospital board approved a new position in ultrasound radiography, and authorised structural alterations to provide a 'proper ultrasound room'.[90]

The new women's health movement, which generally regarded medical technology with suspicion, questioned the enthusiasm for the new procedure, both in New Zealand and overseas. In 1986 British sociologist Ann

Oakley noted that ultrasound had been introduced before its effectiveness and possible hazards had been scientifically evaluated. She pointed out that the first controlled trial of obstetric ultrasound was reported in 1980, fourteen years after the obstetric ultrasound caseload at one centre had been described as 'unmanageable'.[91] Such unbridled enthusiasm had not been evident at National Women's in the early years of ultrasound.

In 1989 the *New Zealand Woman's Weekly* ran a feature article on the safety of scans. It cited Lynda Williams, then patient advocate at National Women's Hospital and a spokesperson for Fertility Action, who told the reporter that many women were unhappy about the number of ultrasound scans being performed and about not being told of the possible risks. 'Many pregnant women report a lot of foetal movement after a scan, and feel their baby didn't like it. A lot of women are now choosing to have their babies naturally and refusing to have ultrasound scans . . . . Ultrasound just hasn't been proved completely safe.' Williams referred to the miscarriage support programme at National Women's Hospital, for women who had had more than three miscarriages. These women were entitled to weekly scans, an offer which most of them accepted, but a procedure that Williams described as 'dreadful'.[92]

The following year Williams broadened the objection to include concern at the disempowerment of women through the use of technology like ultrasound. She believed that technology undermined women's confidence in, and knowledge of, their own bodies, and that, 'Women have been sold on the idea by the medical profession.' The West Auckland Women's HealthWatch agreed: 'Ultrasound represents the latest in a series of medical technologies applied to mass populations without any scientific proof of benefit and with considerable evidence of risk.'[93]

Some doctors had resisted the move towards routine scans and using scans for social reasons, claiming that pressure from patients had encouraged the trend. By contrast, some feminists believed the pressure came from the doctors as part of their unerring love of technology and their goal to control childbirth. Who was driving the trend? Two obstetricians from Donald's base in Glasgow argued in favour of both: 'In our experience all obstetricians provided with this service have found it most valuable; mothers have found fascinating and reassuring the sight of their fetuses moving on the real-time display.'[94] This was probably a realistic assessment.

Donald and others had for some time been involved in studying the safety of ultrasound; a 1970 study concluded that it did not appear to adversely affect the fetus.⁹⁵ In their history of ultrasound, Malcolm Nicolson and John Fleming wrote that by the mid-1970s it was widely accepted that ultrasound did not damage chromosomes but the possibility of some other harmful effect remained, and indeed was never quite laid to rest.⁹⁶ At National Women's, in 1982 Dr Murray Jamieson referred to considerable dissension in the USA as to whether it could cause tissue damage.⁹⁷ In 1984 a consensus panel of the National Institutes of Health concluded that the available evidence did not justify routine use; by contrast, that same year a working party of the RCOG in Britain supported the routine use of ultrasound.⁹⁸

A further technique introduced to National Women's in the 1980s was Doppler ultrasound. In the early 1980s Lesley McCowan, who had completed her Diploma in Obstetrics and Gynaecology at National Women's Hospital in 1976, worked in a new unit specifically dedicated to looking after women with difficult or complicated pregnancies. In 1985 she was awarded a two-year fellowship at the Mt Sinai Hospital in Toronto, Canada, where she researched the use of Doppler ultrasound. As McCowan later explained, the technology allowed the researchers to monitor the blood flow from the baby into the placenta, detect problems at an early stage and induce the mother early to save the baby from dying in the womb.⁹⁹ Returning to Auckland in 1986, McCowan lobbied for a Doppler to be purchased for National Women's Hospital. Following a successful fundraising campaign which she led, National Women's acquired a Doppler ultrasound machine in 1987.¹⁰⁰

The 1970s and 1980s were decades of technological advances in fetal diagnosis, not only in ultrasound, but also with amniocentesis and fetal heart monitoring. Indeed, Australian neonatal epidemiologist Judith Lumley claimed that fetal heart monitoring was the story of obstetrics of this era 'in microcosm'. This story included, she believed, the powerful professional urge to use ever more expensive equipment, under commercial pressure, the devaluing of clinical skills, debates about risk management and the efficacy of intensive care, as well as 'the explosion of malpractice suits and defensive practices'.¹⁰¹

The story of the introduction of ultrasound to National Women's shows a close monitoring of international trends and links with overseas workers, medical enthusiasm for technical advances tempered by expressions of caution, and simultaneous patient demand and public debate. While New Zealand did not have an 'explosion of malpractice suits' owing to its Accident Compensation legislation introduced in 1974, by which complainants received income-related accident compensation for injuries in exchange for foregoing the right to sue, it was not immune from a critical environment. While some feminists believed doctors were all too ready to embrace modern technology, at least two women complained publicly of the opposite. In their 1988 letter to the *New Zealand Herald* these women expressed the view that women's health did not determine practice at National Women's Hospital. They complained about the hospital's policy of withholding amniocentesis, a prenatal test for detecting Down's syndrome, from women under the age of 37, calling this a 'neglectful practice'.[102] The practitioners of new medical technology were treading a fine line, whether they gave it or withheld it.

Neonatal Intensive Care Unit

New prenatal diagnostics and treatments led to more babies ending up in the paediatric department. Reflecting the maturing of this specialism, in 1969 the 'Premature Baby Unit' was officially renamed the 'Neonatal Intensive Care Unit'.[103] Parents' expectations rose as new technologies became available.

Exchange transfusion had been an important factor in establishing perinatal medicine in the 1950s, as discussed previously. Its importance continued into the 1960s. Browne reported from the Rotunda Hospital in Dublin that the management of Rhesus haemolytic disease 'formed a major part of the work of the paediatric department' in the 1960s.[104] In Auckland, too, exchange transfusion continued to occupy much of the time of neonatal registrars and residents at the hospital.[105]

In 1967 paediatrician Jack Matthews produced a report complaining about staff shortages in the unit. Discussing Rhesus haemolytic disease he pointed out that there had been a 76 per cent increase in the number of affected babies treated there since 1957. At the same time the mortality rate from haemolytic disease had declined from 26 per cent in 1957–58 to 9.3 per cent in 1966–67. While he welcomed this decline, it also meant more babies to look after and more pressures on the unit.[106]

Liley's prenatal transfusion had attracted world acclaim but had not offered the ultimate solution to Rhesus haemolytic disease. In the eighteen months following Liley's first successful fetal transfusion in 1963, 35 fetal transfusions were performed at National Women's, and thirteen babies survived.[107] In 1967 an editorial in the *British Medical Journal* reported on 92 intrauterine transfusions, with a 50 per cent survival rate. This report also warned that the procedure could be hazardous.[108] A *Scottish Medical Journal* article the same year agreed. The authors noted that babies might be transfused unnecessarily and that it could cause premature labour with all the attendant problems. They concluded that it was 'a potentially dangerous technique both to mother and foetus', requiring 'a skilled team of workers – obstetrician, radiologist, haematologist, paediatrician – and specialised facilities not readily available in all centres'.[109] Liley's contribution through this particular intervention to international practice was more symbolic than actual.

Meanwhile in New Zealand, the hundredth survivor of fetal transfusion was born at National Women's on the day Liley was knighted in 1973.[110] In the mid-1970s Liley carried out between 24 and 30 fetal transfusions each year.[111] The number of prenatal transfusions continued to decline so that by the time Neil Pattison took over from Liley in the 1980s, they were only doing about four to six per annum. The number of exchange transfusions being carried out postnatally also declined from a hundred babies per annum to 50 in the 1970s and continued to decline thereafter.[112]

The main reason for the decline was probably a new vaccine for mothers of at-risk babies introduced to National Women's in 1968.[113] This vaccine, devised in the UK by Cyril (later Sir Cyril) Clarke, professor of medicine at Liverpool University, was given to at-risk mothers after the birth of their first baby or to at-risk pregnant women to destroy the Rh-positive cells in their blood (that is, to prevent them becoming 'sensitised') so that the next baby would not be affected. Assessing the vaccination scheme after five years, Liley considered it beneficial but warned that it could not replace the existing antibody screening, or diagnostic/therapeutic services for haemolytic disease. 'Opening a second front in the war on haemolytic disease', he cautioned, 'does not eliminate the first.'[114] He reported to the MRCNZ that after five years of using the vaccine the rate of sensitisation had only dropped by 40–45 per cent.[115] Howie later assessed the immunisation programme, explaining that it was commonly said to be 98 per cent effective in preventing rhesus sensitisation, without mentioning that with no protection at all 95 per cent of mothers at risk never became sensitised. So, he said, 'the difference it makes is less impressive than it is commonly made out to be'.[116]

Howie thought another innovation of the 1970s was equally important in reducing the need to transfuse babies. That was phototherapy (or 'light energy') for jaundiced babies, introduced to National Women's in the early 1970s by paediatrician John Martin.[117] Neil Pattison thought smaller family sizes might also have contributed to the decline as the condition worsened with each successive pregnancy. Discussing fetal transfusions he explained that improvements in ultrasound allowed blood samples from the fetus to be taken more easily, reducing the number of unnecessary transfusions.[118]

Decline in the practice of exchange transfusions for haemolytic disease did not reduce the overall workload of the neonatal intensive care unit, however. In his 1967 report, referred to earlier, Matthews complained that over the previous ten years there had been a 74 per cent increase in the number of babies treated per annum in the unit (from 2727 to 4774), with no increase in staff. Admissions to the premature unit had increased by 109 per cent and to the paediatric follow-up clinic by 111 per cent.[119]

From the 1970s the resources in the unit were stretched even further. Howie recalled how during his absence overseas in 1974 two relatively large preterm babies died of RDS. When he heard, he 'hit the roof and sent in his resignation'. He was persuaded to withdraw his resignation by the offer of additional support. Susan Sayers was appointed the first neonatal tutor specialist in 1975.[120]

By 1976, Howie had two colleagues, Sue Sayers and Stephen Wealthall, to assist him with ventilation, and they treated 56 babies that year.[121] Yet problems persisted. In 1977 Sayers described to the acting medical superintendent the conditions in the ward: 'You suggested that I document these instead of reporting the major accidents as we have done in the past with the three massive haemorrhages occurring from catheters that have come apart.' Leaving the meeting with the superintendent at 2.45 p.m., she decided to document 'the more minor events over the next 24 hours that would demonstrate our acute situation'. She began her study at 3 p.m. and only one hour later, by 4 p.m., concluded that the point might well be taken from one hour's observation rather than 24 hours.[122]

Sayers' report provided a graphic description of conditions in the unit. The first case she listed was an Rh baby who was receiving his ninth exchange transfusion with no nurse available to assist the registrar; the second was a preterm baby with RDS who had his head out of the head box and was breathing air instead of the prescribed 40 per cent oxygen. Also at the same time (3 p.m.) another preterm baby in a ventilator 'had head box twisted' and was also receiving 30 per cent oxygen instead of the 40 per cent needed. At 3.05 a preterm baby in a ventilator 'had CPAP mask unattached and the baby was blue and apnoeic and required positive pressure ventilation by myself'. Two minutes later 'Dr Cairns was preparing his own IV trolley'. So the list went on. At 3.30 Sayers noted that a preterm baby on three-hourly feeds was still waiting for the three o'clock feed. An exchange transfusion baby was 'completely unattended while doctor checked result on the teleprinter'. Another baby was being cared for by a nurse whose second day it was in the unit, and Sayers discovered that its IV fluids had double the amount of K+ ordered, with no water in the humidifier supplying oxygen to the baby, and that the umbilical catheter tubing was caught in the incubator door. By four o'clock the baby she had noted an hour earlier with his head box twisted was 'now completely out of the head box breathing air'. She concluded, 'this list seems like an indictment against nurses, and I would like to emphasise that it is not so, it is to the credit of the nursing staff that the unit can function to the capacity it does with so few major catastrophes'.[123]

Shortage of nursing staff, a problem since the 1950s, became of even greater concern in the context of new therapeutic developments. In order to promote recruitment into this field, Matthews had persuaded the NMRB to set up the country's first neonatal intensive nursing care course, commencing in 1966 and run by Penelope Dunkley.[124] This was a six-months' post-basic certificate course. Over the next nine years about a hundred nurses took the course, including some from the Pacific Islands and Australia.[125] However, in 1973 the Nursing Council of New Zealand (successor to the NMRB) replaced the course with in-service training, to be funded by hospital boards. Medical superintendent Algar Warren complained that the Nursing Council made the decision without consulting National Women's. Faris also objected to the reduction in the length of the course from six months to thirteen weeks, and thought hospital boards would be reluctant to release nurses to attend the course in any case. In fact there were only two applicants for the new course in 1977, and so it was abandoned.[126] The hospital matron Verna Murray told the HMC in 1977 that she advertised frequently for neonatal nursing staff, 'but applications were not being received'.[127]

One innovation in 1979 was the setting up of a group of staff and parents to provide support for parents whose babies were in the unit and to provide feedback to the hospital as consumers.[128] Chaired by Dunkley, it held its first meeting in November 1979. The support group included fathers; a press report around this time declared, 'Miss Dunkley stresses the importance of the baby–father relationship. "Worried fathers of babies in the unit are encouraged to ring up at any time day or night".'[129] They also provided practical support: one parent, whose baby had been born at 28 weeks following steroid treatment and was in the unit for six months, remembered they ran cake stalls to help fund things like transport costs for parents to visit their babies in hospital.[130]

In 1980 Bonham asked professor of paediatrics John Dower and Dr Matt Spence, director of the Department of Critical Care at Auckland Hospital, to report on National Women's Neonatal Intensive Care Unit. Dower and Spence concluded that the nurse staffing was 'inadequate by far'. By whatever yardstick, it was 'grossly below either Australian, European, or North American standards'. They noted that it was hard to recruit nurses, which they thought was not surprising since the morale of the professional staff in the unit was so low. They attributed this partly to the nature of the work which, while challenging, carried a high emotional impact. But, they added, morale was also low because staff realised they could be doing a more effective job if they were given the human and equipment resources. The range of equipment by international standards was inadequate and makeshift. Vital apparatus frequently broke down and periods of down-time were extremely long. They noted that several of the neonatal paediatricians were expert in operating the equipment necessary for intensive care nurseries, and that because of their interest and dedication much of it, even when it was archaic, had been kept in running order. They concluded that in a unit that demanded vigour, they saw fatigue; in a unit that required optimism, they saw demoralisation. They recommended a commissioning grant, and stated that the immediate appointment of a full-time neonatal paediatrician as director of the neonatal intensive care unit was 'imperative'.[131]

Following Dower and Spence's report, things went from bad to worse. In September 1980 it was reported that during the previous week five mothers and babies and one pregnant woman expecting premature twins had been transferred to Waikato Women's Hospital in Hamilton (which had opened in May 1980),[132] and another premature baby was flown to Wellington (where the Women's Hospital, called the Grace Neill Block, had opened in 1978). Two premature babies were transferred to St Helens Hospital, Auckland, and a further two were sent to Waikato. 'Auckland's reputation as a centre of excellence in medical care is not improved when premature babies have to be shipped urgently to other centres because of a shortage of respirators and staff at National Women's Hospital', the daily press warned in September 1980.[133] Howie later claimed, 'This episode I think still holds the record for intense and sustained publicity of any issue of lack of health resources in this country: it hit the headlines for 19 days.' He collected 148 news items published on the episode.[134]

From 1977 Howie had also been involved in constructing a report on newborn services for the Maternity Services Committee, which was published in 1982.[135] He believed that this report was more influential than most of its kind because of the publicity during the 1980 crisis in the neonatal unit at National Women's. He also considered that together 'the crisis and the report could be fairly said to have been crucial in developing special care services for the newborn in the whole country' in the following decades.[136] The report put forward the case for more resources for neonatal services nationally.

In 1984 David Knight was appointed full-time paediatrician upon Matthews' retirement (and in 1989 was to become clinical director of newborn services). Facilities continued to be limited in the 1980s, however: in 1986 the *NZMJ* reported continuing concern over the number of babies and mothers being transferred to other units from National Women's intensive care unit.[137]

Meanwhile, from the patients' perspective, it appears that those who came to the hospital still appreciated the services. In 1979, shortly before Dower and Spence's damning report, one grateful mother wrote enthusiastically to the press,

> I was fortunate enough to have a lovely room to myself overlooking Cornwall Park, the spring lambs adding to my delight. For the most part I found the sisters and nurses very helpful . . . . My baby was in intensive care for three days . . . . For my part there was intimacy and beauty and most important of all, there was our beautiful son who just might not have survived without the care and attention he received at National Women's.[138]

Costs and Benefits

In his history of newborn intensive care, American professor of paediatrics Jeffrey Baker wrote that these units had 'become an oft-cited example of runaway technology; their critics have charged that physicians are engaged in a relentless quest to rescue ever smaller premature infants', causing long-term physical and psychological problems.[139]

Survival rates of low-birth-weight babies at National Women's dramatically improved over the decades. From 1959 to 1976, almost 9000 low-birth-weight babies (2500 g or less) passed through the neonatal unit at the hospital. Death rates, standardised by weight, dropped from 22.5 per cent in 1959 to 12.5 per cent in 1976.[140] In a 1973 report to the MRCNZ on 'Neonatal and Infant Health', Bonham and paediatrician Professor Bob Elliott noted that rapid advances in perinatal care during the previous fifteen years had undoubtedly contributed to a general improvement in immediate survival, but that they still knew little of the quality of survival.[141] Dr Barton MacArthur of the Department of Education was carrying out research into the development of low-birth-weight babies, which was eventually formalised when National Women's set up its Child Development Unit in 1986.

The ethics of 'rescuing' very small babies was becoming subject to popular debate. The 1982 report on *Special Care Services for the Newborn in New Zealand*, of which Howie was a joint author representing the Paediatric Society of New Zealand, included a section on 'Some Popular Misconceptions about Special Care for the Newborn'; this was reminiscent of the arguments that the Plunket Society confronted in the 1920s about 'better-dead babies'. The authors of the 1982 report firmly believed that intensive care of newborn babies was not only allowing more low-birth-weight babies to survive but also to make it much less likely for these survivors to be permanently damaged. They declared that over 90 per cent of the survivors of the most intensive newborn care turned out to be normal. They thought that damage was not a problem of premature birth but rather of 'larger infants beset by obstetric complications in labour and delivery'. The emphasis then should be on better perinatal care to prevent handicap.[142]

Despite the upbeat tone of the report, not all medical commentators were convinced. In a leading article in the *NZMJ* in 1983, John Clarkson from the Paediatric Department of Dunedin Hospital noted that the effectiveness of neonatal intensive care had been a source of continuing controversy in New Zealand as well as overseas, including the high costs of such programmes.[143] The following year a position paper in the *NZMJ* stated that retrolental fibroplasia, which had come to the fore in the 1950s when newborn babies were first given oxygen, was still a problem to be reckoned with, and might even have increased. This was owing to the enhanced survival of very low-birth-weight babies (less than 1500 g) resulting from modern advances in neonatal intensive care.[144]

'How small is too small?' asked Dr Brian Darlow, then senior lecturer in the Department of Paediatrics, University of Otago, Christchurch, in 1985.[145] He pointed out that current data from several major units around the world showed that overall survival of infants with a birth weight of 1000–1500 g was about 85 per cent, whilst that of infants weighing 500–1000 g was 50 per cent. He believed that preterm labour at 24 to 27 weeks should be just as actively managed as it was at longer gestation, accepting a 50 per cent survival rate for infants less than 1000 g or 24–26 weeks' gestation, and that perhaps 30 per cent of those surviving would have a functional handicap as the worst scenario.[146] Responding to this article, Dr Stephen Munn found it 'sobering to think . . . that while 50% of infants between 500 and 1000g are being saved in the neonatal unit, not far away perfectly healthy babies of similar weight are being aborted "unmonitored and . . . unsupported on a gynaecology ward"'. He added, 'In their desire to relieve maternal distress doctors have had to ignore and subconsciously suppress the kind of information that Dr Darlow presents. Abortion is not a matter of choice but rather a denial of pre-, peri-, and neonatal physiology.'[147] Doctors were being drawn into the moral and ethical issues relating to abortion, as a result of advances within perinatal medicine and survival rates, something that will be further explored in the next chapter.

American historian David Rothman has observed that premature infants always constituted the great majority of babies treated in newborn intensive care units and provided most of the ethical and policy problems encountered there. Nevertheless, he said, another group attracted undue attention and became the focus of a new battleground in the 1970s and 1980s: those with Down's syndrome and spina bifida. Public attention was heightened in America by the celebrated 1982 'Baby Doe' case, in which the parents of an infant with Down's syndrome elected with their doctor to allow the infant to die rather than undergo corrective surgery.[148] This case led to a law change in America in 1984 setting out guidelines for the treatment of seriously ill or disabled newborns, regardless of the wishes of the parents. At National Women's Hospital, paediatrician Simon Rowley reflected in 2005 on a strong push from the disabled community against discrimination in the 1970s and 1980s which had led to a rethinking of the way children's disabilities were viewed. He explained that paediatricians would no longer withhold treatment if a newborn had Down's syndrome or spina bifida as they might have done in the past.[149] Newborn babies and even 'unborn' babies were now being conceptualised as patients in their own right, separate from their parents. This chapter has shown how National Women's contributed to this new conceptualisation internationally through its ground-breaking research but also how it struggled to keep up with the new public demands. David Knight, who graduated at Oxford and came to New Zealand in the 1980s, reminisced in 2004 on how he had been inspired to come to National Women's partly because of the reputation of Liggins and Liley, explaining that he thought it was going to be 'this hot place and in fact it was a bit of a sleepy New Zealand place'.[150] The glamour of the hospital's international reputation did not translate into resources at ground level. Yet, while Knight might have found it a 'sleepy place' in the early 1980s, it would soon be jolted awake, propelled once again into media attention, although not this time because of its international fame, as will be seen.

CHAPTER 8

CONTRACEPTION, STERILISATION AND ABORTION

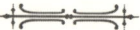

FERTILITY CONTROL IS IMPORTANT TO WOMEN'S HEALTH AND WELLBEING, and part of the scope of any modern women's hospital is to deal with the issues surrounding fertility. As providers of services, doctors at National Women's by necessity had to confront this socially sensitive issue and, as a consequence, their own value systems. The feminists of the 1970s regarded reproductive rights as integral to women's liberation. To them fertility control signalled much more than health concerns and was allied to women's control over their own bodies and self-determination. In doing so they sometimes regarded the predominantly male medical establishment as 'the enemy'. However, issues relating to reproductive health did not create a binary division between doctors and women. This chapter will show how the views of doctors working at National Women's Hospital were as varied as those of the women they served.

Sex Education and 'Family Planning'
In 1964, speaking at a Federation of New Zealand Parents' Centres conference, Professor Dennis Bonham lamented that many parents were not providing adequate sex instruction for their children.[1] In the 1960s there was widespread resistance to sex education in schools. Many people believed this

to be a private family affair, and in any case that too much knowledge amongst young people would lead to sexual experimentation or promiscuity.[2] Bonham, more liberal than many others, supported the widespread availability of sex education and contraception, and saw sex education as a way of reducing unwanted pregnancies. He added his weight to public debate by advocating sex education in intermediate and secondary schools.[3]

In 1966, two years after taking up his professorial post, Bonham proposed to the HMC, seconded by Herb Green, that the hospital set up a clinic to provide contraceptives and to train medical students in their use. Bonham was possibly inspired by his former mentor, William Nixon, who had established such a clinic at University College Hospital, London, in 1949.[4] The HMC rejected Bonham's proposal, although it agreed to incorporate 'Family Planning' into the existing postnatal and gynaecological clinics.[5]

Five years later, in 1971, signalling a changing social climate, Richard Seddon, who had been appointed senior lecturer in obstetrics and gynaecology the previous year, persuaded the HMC of the need for such a clinic. He explained that both the students' tutor and the students themselves had considered their knowledge of family planning inadequate. He also noted a growing public demand for contraception, stating that 25 per cent of women referred to the 'A team' gynaecological clinic during the previous three months had come with problems relating to contraception. He added, 'The all-too-common situation of the woman who has had quite inadequate contraception being referred at a stage when nothing short of sterilisation or (as is more pertinent to today's scene) abortion will suffice, represents in our society a failure of patient-education and professional assistance with contraception.'[6] The hospital's Family Planning Clinic was opened in February 1972, directed by Dr John Taylor.

The New Zealand Family Planning Association was originally set up as the Sex Hygiene and Birth Regulation Society in 1937 but changed its name in 1939 to affiliate with its British counterpart. It opened its first clinic in 1953, although it was not until 1961 that the NZBMA allowed its members to work in the clinics. In the 1950s the NZFPA had enjoyed the support of Bonham's predecessor at National Women's, Harvey Carey.[7] Before coming to New Zealand, Bonham had been president of a local family planning branch in Britain, and once in New Zealand was also supportive of the NZFPA. Historian Helen Smyth described him as 'a consistent friend and champion of FPA'.[8] He helped the association to acquire films for health education.[9] He included NZFPA professionals in postgraduate obstetrics and gynaecology courses, and was responsible for organising the first state-sponsored family planning forum, held at National Women's Hospital in 1971. The following year the NZFPA set up a medical advisory council chaired by Bonham.[10]

While the NZFPA agreed to extend contraceptives to unmarried as well as married people in 1970, NZBMA policy opposed the supply of contraceptives to the unmarried.[11] In 1971 the Board of Health's Maternity Services Committee, of which Bonham was a member, tackled this stand and recommended that 'the most suitable method of birth control including surgical methods should be readily available free to all who need it'. The committee appealed to the NZBMA to re-examine its ethical rules in relation to doctors prescribing contraceptives for the unmarried.[12]

While Bonham was on the side of making contraceptives readily available, other members of his staff approached family planning differently. In 1968, when the abortion debates were beginning to rage internationally (see below), Pope Paul VI issued the encyclical *Humanae Vitae*, prohibiting Roman Catholics from using contraceptives. The only form of contraception he sanctioned was the so-called rhythm method. In 1970 *Zealandia*, a local Catholic newspaper, announced that the Catholic bishops of New Zealand were providing $12,000 for a three-year research programme at National Women's Hospital, led by Dr John France, to improve rhythm methods of birth control. The aim of the project was to find a way to predict ovulation at least six days in advance, in order to develop more reliable methods of family planning whilst working within the Catholic Church's teaching. Cardinal Delargey, Bishop of Auckland, declared, 'One is proud too, that the work will be carried out at the world-renowned National Women's Hospital . . . . It's a heart-warming collaboration of the Church with the best of modern medical science. I know that Catholics will pray for a successful outcome to the research, because it could be of great benefit to couples throughout the world.'[13] This project was written up in the NZFPA magazine, *Choice*, in 1971.[14] Following his research, in 1972 France announced that cervical mucus test kits to predict ovulation were to be made available through 'Catholic family life clinics and family planning clinics'.[15]

In 1975 John France along with Dr John Crowley and Ngaire Walsh set up the Natural Family Planning Association.[16] That same year another National Women's gynaecologist and Catholic, Pat Dunn, published his study of 600 private patients using natural family planning, noting its advantages over conventional contraceptive techniques 'despite its bad press'.[17] A decade later there were about 60 natural family planning clinics around the country.[18]

Mont Liggins, another member of the NZFPA medical advisory council, began to study a relatively new form of contraception in 1965, a hormonal oral contraceptive. The 'Pill' had been developed by American biologist Gregory Pincus, with trials in Puerto Rico from 1956, and was approved for use in the USA in 1960. It was introduced to Britain in 1961 and around the same time in New Zealand, where it quickly became popular amongst women and doctors alike.[19] Bonham pointed out that 30 per cent of married women were on 'the Pill' by 1968, and that New Zealand had the highest utilisation of oral contraceptives in the world (comparable rates were 24 per cent for North America, 16 per cent for the UK and 2 per cent for 'the World').[20] In 1973, applying for an MRCNZ research grant to support Liggins' work, Bonham stated that over 150,000 women used hormonal contraceptives in New Zealand, making it important to examine their efficacy and side-effects. The aim of the research was to 'study improved safer regimes and monitor adverse reactions more fully with the co-operation of Family Planning Clinics throughout the country'.[21] This echoed international concerns about possible side-effects of the Pill, following the publication in 1969 of *The Doctor's Case Against the Pill* by American feminist journalist Barbara Seaman. Other studies too in the late 1960s and 1970s were suggesting possible links between the Pill and some forms of cancer and other life-threatening conditions.[22]

In 1980 Liggins launched 'The New Zealand Contraception and Health Study', a prospective observational study following three groups of 7500 women using Depo-Provera, intrauterine devices (IUDs) or the Pill for five years. Not only the Pill, but these other forms of contraception had become controversial by this time. Depo-Provera was a hormonal injection that inhibited ovulation for three months. It had been developed by an American multinational pharmaceutical company, Upjohn, which contributed funding to Liggins' study.[23] When questioned by feminist Phillida Bunkle about his link with Upjohn, Liggins 'vehemently' maintained that the study was 'independent and was initiated by him'.[24]

The US Food and Drug Administration had banned the use of Depo-Provera in the United States by this time, but it was still available and was being tested in developing countries.[25] New Zealand women could access it from 1968, and by 1980 there were about 35,000 women using it. Some health professionals apparently favoured it because it was easier for women to use than the contraceptive pill. Feminist activists Sandra Coney and Sue Neal launched the Campaign Against Depo-Provera in 1980 as they believed it was unsafe and that New Zealand women were being used as guinea pigs: 'From our observations it is used particularly on Maori and Pacific Island women (who are most at risk from some of its side effects), women in lower socio-economic groups and mental patients. Health activists overseas have described it as "the contraceptive for second-class citizens".'[26]

Others were also suspicious of Liggins' research links with a drug company. Writing in a local feminist magazine, *Broadsheet*, on his research, Dr Ruth Bonita accused the MRCNZ of 'encouraging the production of pseudo-scientific facts for financial gain by a multi-national corporation'.[27] While Liggins had been researching contraception before he got funding from Upjohn, the extensive public criticism of the links with Upjohn led the MRCNZ to suggest that Liggins ask its Standing Committee on Therapeutic Trials to assess the protocols of the 1980 study. Headed by Auckland University professor of medicine John Scott, the committee saw no problem with drug company sponsorship, provided the protocol was sound, as it thought it was in this instance. It commented, however, on the 'lack of objectivity' in public discussion of the study, calling it a 'trial by media'.[28] This was, according to a 1980 *New Zealand Listener* article on Depo-Provera, the result of the attitude of 'a section of educated, liberated women . . . to pharmacologically based, largely male-dominated medicine'. This article ended with the comment by one 'activist woman' that 'if men had to take a hormonal contraceptive the Pill would still be under test in a laboratory'.[29] The Depo-Provera story reveals the conviction amongst some feminists that doctors experimented upon women's bodies for profit, and that such experimentation was possible because their subjects were women.

Reproductive health was high on the agenda of the new women's liberation movement, which had reached New Zealand in the early 1970s. Sandra Coney was a leader in the movement, and together with feminist sociologist Phillida Bunkle, she founded a women's health advocacy group called Fertility Action in 1984. This group was the instigator of the 1987 Inquiry into the Treatment of Cervical Cancer at National Women's Hospital (the Cartwright Inquiry; see chapter 10).[30] In its submission to that Inquiry, Fertility Action included a section on Depo-Provera, indicating its belief that the investigation was about much more than the research programme of Associate Professor Herb Green who was ostensibly its focus but who was not involved in this research. This section of their submission was labelled 'Drug Company Funded Research – Upjohn's Contraception and Health Study'.[31] Fertility Action criticised the study for its lack of independence from Upjohn, and the fact that Depo-Provera was not approved in the drug company's home country. However, it failed to mention that the manufacturers of Depo-Provera had been granted a long-term British licence in 1984.[32]

Controversy also surrounded intrauterine contraceptive devices. A 1977 *NZMJ* editorial estimated that some 50,000 New Zealand women used an IUD for contraceptive purposes at that time. The major device marketed in New Zealand from 1970 to 1975 was the Dalkon Shield, but it was subsequently withdrawn. According to the editorial, there were two possible major complications: ectopic pregnancies and pelvic inflammatory disease.[33] In America, the Dalkon Shield, manufactured and marketed by A. H. Robins, was reported to have caused at least eighteen deaths and in excess of 200,000 cases of miscarriages, hysterectomies, uterine infections and 'other gynaecological complications', as well as birth defects, paving the way for a lawsuit filed by more than 300,000 women and a $2.5 billion settlement.[34]

In 1984 Phillida Bunkle wrote an article for *Broadsheet* on the Dalkon Shield. Having found two papers written by National Women's Hospital gynaecologist Ron Jones in 1974 and 1975 supporting the Dalkon Shield, despite the fact that it had by then been withdrawn from the American market, she phoned him. She reported that she found him 'hostile' and 'affronted' that she should ask him questions about his work.[35]

In 1985 the Labour government's Health Minister Michael Bassett, and Ann Hercus, newly appointed Minister of Women's Affairs, met with representatives of the manufacturers A. H. Robins, who agreed to pay for a medical check for women still wearing an IUD fitted in the 1970s and to fund a publicity campaign to warn women of its dangers.[36] Fertility Action placed a letter in the *NZMJ* alerting doctors to the right of women who had suffered symptoms from using the Dalkon Shield to lodge claims in the United States courts against A. H. Robins, announcing, 'We have the facilities to assist women with these claims and to offer support.'[37] By September 1986 Fertility Action was in contact with 360 women who had complaints about the Dalkon Shield, and over 200 with complaints about other IUDs.[38] In 1993 Sandra Coney reported that 258 claims had been sent to attorneys in the USA; she did not provide details of the outcome, but stated that payouts had begun in 1991.[39]

In December 1986 a group of women obstetricians, gynaecologists and family planning doctors formed a committee called 'Contraceptive Choice', based at National Women's Hospital. The group, including Helen Roberts, Lesley McCowan, Christine Roke, Hilary Liddell, Lynda Batcheler and Jennifer Wilson, got together because of their concerns with the negative publicity in the lay press about various forms of contraception, which they thought was causing unnecessary fear and anxiety and possibly unwanted pregnancies and terminations. They argued that, contrary to the adverse publicity, the copper IUD was 'an effective, safe and appropriate form of contraception for many women'. There had also, they said, been much scaremongering relating to the contraceptive pill and its supposed links with breast cancer, which had not been proved. They added:

> We are also concerned that a woman's relationship with her doctor may be undermined by constantly portraying medical practitioners as uncaring about their women patients. Conversely the majority of doctors who advise women on contraception are well informed and highly motivated to find the best method for each individual. We support the concept of informed consent about all methods of contraception, but believe it can be provided in a balanced way to emphasise the relative risk and benefits for each woman.[40]

Coney was critical of Contraceptive Choice, arguing that it did not place enough emphasis on the possible dangers of some contraceptives.[41] The debates continued to be played out in the *NZMJ*. Some observers believed that these debates contributed to an increased demand for sterilisation.[42]

Sterilisation

In 1972 Richard Seddon commented on the growing number of 'tubal ligations' (a form of sterilisation) performed at National Women's.[43] Sterilisation was not subject to law in the same way as abortion, which was illegal unless the woman's life was in danger, but was still considered a moral issue for doctors. In 1953 the editor of the *NZMJ* had commented that voluntary sterilisation was a new problem faced by doctors, owing to the 'economic considerations of recent years combined with the aims and aspirations of modern society'.[44] Yet it was not entirely new. In 1932 the New Zealand Obstetrical Society had expressed concern about women demanding sterilisation 'for purely selfish reasons' only to be told by the Director-General of Health that it was not illegal.[45]

Willingness to perform this operation varied widely. Elsie Barnes, a receptionist at National Women's from 1957 to 1961, later commented, 'We all knew which doctors we hoped that patients who needed a tubal ligation wouldn't end up in front of. I mean we had Roman Catholic doctors on the staff and if a woman really needed a tubal ligation for social reasons, we would hope that they would get someone who was sympathetic to their problems.'[46]

During the second half of the 1960s the number of tubal ligations at National Women's trebled. This was probably related to the greater demand by women to control their own fertility and because contraception (at least for married people) was socially acceptable and even an expectation. A course on family planning and gynaecology at National Women's in 1974 included discussion of tubal ligation. One doctor referred to the 'difficult problem' posed by demands from a comparatively young woman, with perhaps one or two children and a shaky marriage, to which Bonham replied that 'there was no easy way out. Each case had to be judged on its merits. And it was the responsibility of the doctor to be the judge.'[47]

Unlike doctors in America, New Zealand doctors did not tend to suggest hysterectomy as a form of birth control, as Bonham later explained.[48] Even in the USA, however, in the 1970s tubal ligations were increasingly replacing hysterectomies as the preferred method of sterilisation. The number of tubal ligations in America doubled between 1970 and 1975. This was partly a result of improved technologies, specifically laparoscopy, which enabled ligations to be performed under local anaesthesia. While one American historian, Ian Dowbiggin, noted the importance of laparoscopy as 'a major breakthrough in women's health care', he also argued that the increase in tubal ligations in the 1970s resulted from consumerism and lifestyle choices and not just technological advances.[49] Two contributors to the *NZMJ* in 1976, discussing the relative benefits of tubal ligation and hysterectomy for contraception, came up with a third option. They noted that the mortality rate for vasectomy was 'virtually nil'.[50]

By the late 1960s vasectomy, the severing of the male's duct through which sperm pass from his testicles, was being seriously considered as a form of birth control for the first time. In 1970 articles in the *British Medical Journal* declared vasectomy to be not only legal but also a 'simple, safe, aesthetic, efficient and cheap method of achieving permanent family limitation'.[51] From 1972 it was available under the National Health Service.[52] In America too vasectomy was becoming more popular: in 1968 the *Journal of the American*

Medical Association called vasectomy 'safe, quick and legal'; and 1970 saw America's first National Conference on Vasectomy. One 1972 estimate claimed that every year 'over 300,000 married American men' had vasectomies, leading some to declare that America was in the grip of a 'vasectomy revolution' and others to speak of 'vasectomania'.[53]

Public demand for male sterilisation also increased in New Zealand from the late 1960s. In 1970 a writer to the *NZMJ* pointed to the growing demand for vasectomy from the public because of publicity through the daily press and television, while also noting continuing concerns, for instance, relating to popular confusion between castration and vasectomy and about the 'demasculinising potential' of the latter.[54] Wellington urologist Donald Urquhart-Hay, who returned to New Zealand from his studies in London in 1967, claimed to have performed the first voluntary contraceptive vasectomy in New Zealand that year.[55] Urquhart-Hay stated in 1970 that this was the most effective method of contraception for married couples. He stressed that he had both husband and wife sign a consent form which he witnessed, confirming that they fully understood the nature and effect of the operation.[56]

At National Women's in 1970 Bonham persuaded the HMC to ask Auckland Hospital to perform vasectomies in cases where family planning was desirable but female sterilisation was 'unduly hazardous' for some reason. Auckland Hospital's medical superintendent Dr Alexander Warren responded that, despite acknowledging the ease of the operation in males as opposed to females, the hospital's policy was not to undertake male sterilisation unless the man was subject to a clinical condition which made the operation 'clinically desirable. . . . This would include the transmission of genetically determined abnormalities through the male with a high risk of the children being affected and where the disability was likely to be seriously detrimental to health.'[57]

Nevertheless, Auckland Hospital found itself increasingly under pressure to perform these operations, from National Women's and from the public. A 1971 article in the women's magazine *Thursday* described vasectomy as the 'most effective and simple means of birth control possible'.[58] Two years later, the same magazine cited 'an Auckland doctor' who warned of the consequences of vasectomy: 'In one or two cases, the women either wore their men out in the first few weeks or they lost interest completely because the danger element of pregnancy was no longer present.' Bonham remarked around the same time, however, that, 'It is interesting that wives do not appear to mind their husbands being sterilized.'⁵⁹ In any case, despite the Auckland doctor's misgivings, the *Thursday* article described the operation of vasectomy as 'booming', with more than 200 men in Auckland alone having the operation each month.⁶⁰ In 1972 the NZFPA magazine *Choice* similarly observed that there had 'literally been an explosion in the numbers being done in the past three years in New Zealand'.⁶¹

The Board of Health's Maternity Services Committee discussed male sterilisation in 1971. Given that demand for this operation was increasing, the committee thought it should be publicly available.⁶² Sterilisation on demand for contraceptive purposes was finally made legal in New Zealand under the 1977 Contraception, Sterilisation, and Abortion Act. The *New Zealand Listener* reported in 1980 that the growing popularity of sterilisation was causing a drop in the number of contraceptive pill users.⁶³

Despite increased demands for male and female sterilisation, doctors at National Women's remained uneasy about sterilising younger women. As gynaecologist John Taylor explained in 1979, a large and growing number of women later regretted their decision (he said that Ron Jones had recorded a hundred between 1973 and 1979). Taylor, who was generally liberal in his views on contraception, sterilisation and abortion,⁶⁴ said he had just declined five requests for tubal ligation from women under the age of 25, and upon consulting several members of the senior staff, he found that most were opposed to sterilisation on socio-economic grounds for women under the age of 30. He proposed a circular be sent to general practitioners advising them that this was hospital policy. He added that two of the five patients he had declined were irritated that they had waited several weeks for an appointment and for an hour in the clinic before being seen. They asked why their doctors had not been advised that requests for sterilisation on socio-economic grounds at the age of 25 were usually, if not always, declined.⁶⁵ Bonham did not think such a circular to GPs would be sensible as it might be 'misconstrued'; he thought it was better to inform GPs about hospital policy by way of the letters sent to them in reply to their referrals.⁶⁶ While he thought doctors had a responsibility to act in what they considered the best interests of their patients, he clearly did not wish the public to think they were being judgemental.

Research confirmed that not all women remained happy with their decision to be sterilised. In 1980 gynaecologist Peter Jackson wrote a report on 831 women who had been sterilised by tubal ligation at National Women's in 1972–73. Nineteen per cent regretted their decision and eight patients sought reversal of the procedure. He reported that following the operation, 10 per cent of the Europeans and 45 per cent of Maori reported decreased libido. Menorrhagia was a common complaint after sterilisation and 7.5 per cent had a hysterectomy within five years. He and his co-researcher concluded that tubal ligation should not be undertaken lightly despite its increasing popularity. They gave the example of one patient who postponed her sterilisation for three months after the delivery of her second child in case it failed to survive the neonatal period; the baby died of sudden infant death syndrome three days after its mother's sterilisation.[67] These doctors found themselves in the position of having to help women make difficult personal decisions and choices that went far beyond the realms of medicine.

Abortion and National Women's Hospital, 1940s to the 1970s

Doctors at National Women's became caught up in the abortion wars of the 1970s when this emerged as the biggest social issue of the decade. National Women's did not present a united front but spanned the full spectrum of views in the debates.

Gynaecologists at National Women's Hospital had performed terminations of pregnancy on medical grounds since the hospital opened. Under the Crimes Act 1908 (reaffirmed in section 182 of the Crimes Act 1961), abortion was illegal unless the woman's life was in danger. The ruling in a famous rape case in Britain in 1938, brought to law by gynaecologist Aleck Bourne, extended the grounds for abortion to include mental as well as physical dangers to the health and life of women in Britain. In practice this judgment was also applied in New Zealand. At the same time, abortions were not taken lightly; National Women's HMC passed a resolution in 1946 that terminations had to be carried out by the senior visiting surgeon or assistant visiting surgeon.[68]

In the early 1950s the hospital set up a 'termination committee', comprising two senior consultants; in the event of a difference of opinion they could co-opt a third senior consultant, and obtain further specialist advice if necessary.[69] The purpose of this committee was probably to provide legal protection for the gynaecologists performing abortions, and possibly to protect the consultant from being pressured by the patient or her GP to carry out the abortion. Yet therapeutic abortion was always a grey area. According to American historian Leslie Reagan, therapeutic abortion committees, which had been established there from the 1940s, provided a check on physicians' practices and therefore represented a 'new intervention in the relationship

Contraception, Sterilisation and Abortion

between physicians and patients and an erosion of physicians' freedom to make medical decisions'.[70]

John Taylor, who had joined National Women's staff in 1961 and who believed in a woman's right to abortion, later commented on how difficult it was for a woman to get an abortion in hospital at that time. He explained that in those days 'you just about had to have a psychiatric report to say that the woman was raving mad before you could consider that the termination was justified on grounds of mental health'. He went on to narrate his own personal experience of looking after a 22-year-old woman who had had an illegal abortion and eventually died, adding 'I'll never forget it.'[71]

As Taylor intimated, the number of therapeutic abortions performed in the 1960s was small. Fifty-eight cases of therapeutic abortion were carried out at National Women's from 1959 to 1967. The rate increased in the course of the 1960s – while eighteen had been performed between 1959 and 1963, there were 40 from 1964 to 1967. Almost all were performed by just three of the eighteen consultants at National Women's.[72] The HMC periodically discussed the constitution of the termination committee, commenting in 1968 on 'the great difficulties and diversities of opinion associated with this matter'.[73] Doctors could choose not to serve on the termination committee, however; for example, Green declined to be part of the committee after 1965.[74]

In 1966 the HMC decided to employ the services of a psychiatrist, particularly to help decide on termination cases, and appointed Dr Laurie Gluckman.[75] However, Gluckman did not feel well integrated into the hospital and soon complained about the small number of cases referred to him.[76] Yet in one case during his first year he did influence the course of events. In his case notes he described a pregnant woman at the clinic who had been deserted by her husband, had five children and worked as a barwoman:

> The reasons for termination were social. She had paid an abortionist £40 before I saw her, but when she told him she had informed me he refunded her money and refused to touch her. She had recently taken an overdose with suicidal intent. I explained to her the dangers in abortion, but she returned a few days later having douched herself several times daily with high pressure douches. She had several blackouts subsequent to or while douching, due to air or soap-water embolism. Try as I would, I could not make her cease such activity. I could not make a diagnosis of psychiatric disorder. Several obstetricians felt that interference was unwarranted. I took the view purely as a physician, she was substantially

endangering her life and termination was justified. This was more than an empty threat. She was ultimately terminated on these grounds.[77]

In her history of abortion in America, Reagan noted that psychiatrists were often leaders in the pro-abortion campaigns; as 'the newly liberal and socially activist wing of the medical profession in the post-war period, [they] responded sympathetically to the emotional distress of pregnant women'.[78] John Werry, professor of psychiatry at the University of Auckland, fits the bill. Vice-president of the Abortion Law Reform Association of New Zealand set up in 1971, he criticised the abortion service at National Women's in 1972. He complained that two gynaecologists were required to agree to the abortion, besides the referring doctor, even if the referring doctor was a psychiatrist. He believed that, since psychiatric factors were the major indication for therapeutic abortion, the certificate of a psychiatrist should be considered valid without scrutiny.[79]

Dr Pat Dunn, who had co-founded the Society for the Protection of the Unborn Child in 1970, responded that it was a professional matter and cautioned that they should be careful not to permit the development of the situation which had arisen in Britain and the USA where gynaecologists had given up their independence and had become technicians, performing operations on the say-so of a specialist in another discipline. For Dunn it was not just a matter of professional territory, however; he believed that 'only the obstetrician and the paediatrician perceive clearly that they have two patients under their care during pregnancy'.[80] The HMC responded to Werry that it was not inclined to change the current practice of 20 years' standing; with the law as it stood, they found it reassuring to have the support of a second consultant. They also denied that the majority of indications were psychiatric.[81]

Speaking to the Auckland University Women's Liberation Group, Werry declared that there was one abortion law for the rich and another for the poor. He said that those who had to go to public hospitals found legal abortions more difficult to procure than those who could afford to take advantage of the private hospital system.[82] In 1974 the Abortion Law Reform Association wrote to public hospitals throughout New Zealand to ascertain how requests for abortions were handled. They found the usual practice was for the application to be reviewed by a termination committee, consisting of two or three gynaecologists. The association believed that the Health Department should order public hospitals to discontinue the use of abortion committees, on the basis that these violated the rights of patients and doctors alike by preventing doctors from obtaining treatment for patients according to their judgement of needs.[83] This view was clearly influenced by a 1973 decision of the Supreme Court in America (*Doe v Bolton*) which had decreed the hospital therapeutic abortion committee system unconstitutional, violating the rights of women to health care and of physicians to practise.[84]

In 1974 a visiting lecturer to National Women's, Hugh McLaren, professor of obstetrics and gynaecology at Birmingham University, was reported in the *New Zealand Herald* as calling abortion 'mass slaughter of the next generation'. McLaren, a Presbyterian and member of SPUC in Britain, said the social clause in the 1967 abortion law in Britain had amounted to abortion on demand. He campaigned for abortion tribunals, consisting of an experienced social worker, a nurse and a doctor who would consider applications for abortions.[85] Herb Green suggested that a GP experienced in family planning should be added to the committee which determined abortions at National Women's.[86]

Some gynaecologists at National Women's were becoming more liberal in their views on abortion in the 1970s, along with the general public. According to the 1977 Report into Contraception, Sterilisation, and Abortion, between 1963 and 1969 National Women's Hospital had accepted 34 per cent of patients who had applied for abortions, whereas in the period 1970 to 1976 it accepted 50 per cent.[87] In 1973 Bonham said that there had been a seven-fold increase in two years in demands for abortion at the hospital (from five a month in 1971 to 35 a month in 1973), most of which were successful.[88] In 1974 the HMC noted a backlog of patients waiting for an interview for an abortion and asked consultants to see an additional case per week to clear the backlog.[89] Bonham pointed out that private hospitals were charging $300 for an abortion, which was why he favoured restricting abortions to public hospitals, so that 'monetary gain would not be made from patients' distress'.[90]

In 1973 tutor specialist Ron Jones wrote a report for the HMC on antenatal diagnosis of certain genetic and biochemical disorders. He suggested that 'with our more liberal views on termination of pregnancy it is reasonable to offer those mothers with a substantial risk of bearing a handicapped child the chance of having the pregnancy terminated if prenatal diagnosis of the condition is possible'.[91] Jones's report clearly upset some members of the committee, as indicated by Bonham's comment at the next meeting that it was unfortunate that his report could be interpreted as facilitating termination of pregnancy. Bonham said that the object of these tests was mainly to reassure patients about possible abnormalities and this could reduce the number of requests for terminations. With this in mind, the HMC passed a motion in favour of 'the setting up of a clinic to investigate the antenatal diagnosis of certain genetic and biochemical disorders'. Liggins agreed to organise the mechanics for obtaining amniotic fluid.[92] At the same time Bonham was negotiating with the new professor at the Department of Community Health, geneticist Arthur Veale, for a diagnostic service to screen mothers over the age of 35 routinely for Down's syndrome of the fetus.[93]

One member of staff who was undoubtedly upset by Jones's report was Bill Liley, who held firm views on fetal rights. He believed that the fetus was a 'young human, dynamic, plastic, resilient, in command of his own environment and destiny with a tenacious purpose'.[94] Another member of staff, Liley's wife Margaret, shared his views. In 1968 she wrote a book called *Modern Motherhood*. Reviewing the book, paediatrician and SPUC member Dr Neil Begg applauded her 'very perceptive' description of the growth, development and activities of the 'unborn child'.[95]

The social implications of viewing the fetus as a person led Liley to become founder president of SPUC in 1970. His 1983 *NZMJ* obituary declared that he communicated directly with the fetus using light and sound, and also that it grieved him that others seemed to devote so little effort and expense to these most important of all patients compared to what was spent elsewhere.[96] Discussing the rising tide of demands for abortion reform, Liley maintained that it was 'a bitter irony that just when the fetus achieves some medical status and importance there should be pressure to make him a social non-entity'.[97] Liley was not in the mould identified by historian Linda Gordon when writing about the anti-abortion lobby in America: 'Underlying all this discourse [about the fetus] was religiosity – most antiabortion advocates [were] not just churchgoers but involved in a personal relationship with God.'[98] Liley's motivation was humanistic rather than religious, although in 1975 he accepted an appointment as a non-Catholic member of the Pontifical Academy of Science, the scientific academy of the Vatican.[99]

As Liley became more involved in anti-abortion politics, certain developments at National Women's disturbed him. As historian Monica Casper noted, he became quite distressed that certain procedures he had developed to save fetal lives were subsequently used in abortion practices. Amniocentesis, a 'lifesaving diagnostic tool', was being 'misapplied to detect the handicapped unborn so that it could be destroyed'.[100] He and Margaret adopted a baby with Down's syndrome in 1976. He was also disturbed to find that techniques developed by him for transfusions were used in a solution for saline abortions. His perspective mirrored Ian Donald's in Scotland, who wrote, 'My own personal fears are that my [ultrasonic] researches into early intrauterine life may be misused towards its more accurate destruction.'[101] Liley wrote bitterly of the 1967 Abortion Act in Britain that it now accounted for the deaths of 140,000 babies a year and yet one pro-abortion group in New Zealand called the Act 'a great piece of humanitarian legislation'.[102]

In January 1973 the US Supreme Court announced its landmark decision (*Roe v Wade*) that a woman's constitutionally protected right to privacy included the right to abortion. The American 'pro-life' (anti-abortion) movement sprang into action following this ruling, with advocacy groups all over the country.[103] Three months after the ruling, the District Federal Court at Providence, Rhode Island, called Liley to give evidence on behalf of the Rhode Island Legislature, which was conducting a 'legislative finding of fact' resulting from the Supreme Court decision. The legislature was apparently one of 29 seeking to circumvent the decision.[104] Again in 1974 the US Supreme Court invited Liley to give evidence on whether abortion infringed the constitutional rights of the fetus. The committee interviewed him for two hours, together with another internationally recognised authority, the French geneticist Dr Jerome Lejeune, who had discovered the genetic cause of Down's syndrome and was a member of his local SPUC. The constitutional change being considered was one of several 'human life amendments' which would extend constitutional protection to human life from the moment of conception. Liley drew on the 'facts' uncovered from his research, which he said gave him no alternative but to regard the 'unborn child' as his patient with the same legal rights as any other age group.[105] Liley was thus used in the abortion wars in America to give the pro-life lobby scientific legitimacy. However, in 1975 the Supreme Court upheld the earlier rulings that, 'For the first trimester, the abortion decision and its implementation be left to the medical judgement of the pregnant woman's attending physician.'[106] These legal battles were to continue in America in the following decades: as Gordon noted, the leading right-to-life strategy from the 1970s to the 1990s was through the legal system.[107] Liley was not, however, directly involved after the mid-1970s.

Back in New Zealand, in March 1972 Liley chaired the first SPUC national conference in Wellington where it was decided to unite its 25 branches, with a combined membership of 20,000, into a national organisation. Liley was elected president. The society decided to focus on providing welfare assistance to women contemplating abortion. Liley thought SPUC's motto, like that of the Plunket Society, should be 'To help the Mothers and Save the Babies'. This goal of SPUC, Liley declared, 'disproved the idea that people opposed to abortion are a lot of moralists, completely out of touch with reality and taking good care that they don't have to deal with these problems'.[108] SPUC also sought to gain political support to oppose the liberalisation of abortion. In 1972 Liley told the Auckland branch of SPUC that more than 20 MPs and a number of aspirants had publicly declared support for their society.[109]

A decade later, in June 1983, Liley committed suicide.[110] While there were clearly multiple factors involved in this unfortunate happening, Casper later wrote that, 'It is both ironic and tragic that Liley, who had claimed such deep and abiding respect for life, would take his own.' She concluded that Liley's clinical work had had widespread significance in political debates in helping to imbue the fetus with 'autonomous personhood and constructed as worthy of protection and advocacy'.[111] Other tributes to Liley following his death stressed his activism relating to the rights of the fetus or the 'unborn child'.[112]

Others at National Women's held similar views to Liley. Gynaecologist Bill Faris had told the *New Zealand Herald* in 1973 that he believed the fetus had rights, 'and I believe no gynaecologist can act as judge and executioner'.[113] Associate Professor Herb Green was not, as Coney and Bunkle claimed in their 1987 *Metro* article, a member of SPUC.[114] However, he was opposed to abortion and published a three-part article in the *New Zealand Nursing Journal* in 1970 entitled 'The foetus began to cry'. In this series, he reviewed the social, ethical and legal issues relating to abortion and concluded that whether to abort the fetus or not was generally a social or ethical decision which should not be left to the medical profession. In his opinion, 'Not by the wildest stretch of the imagination can this be regarded as a medical problem. To put physicians into the position of deciding who shall live and who shall die, as has the UK Act, must and will ultimately be regarded as one of the supreme follies of this age of technology.' He referred to Liley's acclaimed research, and argued that, 'By permitting such research at National Women's Hospital and publicly acclaiming its chief architect, New Zealand has declared that the unborn foetus has the right to receive treatment in the interests of its life and health.' He concluded that social problems could not be cured by surgery and 'all the enthusiastic abortionists in the world can but scratch vainly at the surface of a problem of which the only solution is better standards of living'.[115] A colleague at the hospital aptly described him as a socially conservative socialist.[116]

Staff at National Women's became embroiled in a public dispute about a private abortion clinic, once again revealing divergent views. In 1974 the Auckland Medical Aid Trust set up the Auckland Medical Aid Centre to provide low-cost terminations for $80, operating as a day clinic with five doctors.[117] The following year the trust moved its services into a private hospital and by 1977 it performed most of New Zealand's 5842 abortions carried out that year.[118] Four months after the clinic had opened in 1974, police raided the premises with a search warrant and seized 500 files, suspecting it of performing illegal abortions, although the trust later successfully challenged their search warrant at the Court of Appeal. Herb Green wrote an affidavit critical of the clinic's standards, stating that 'the women did not get, or expect to get the best medical care because of the lack of staff training'. In particular he thought the staff were 'ignorant of the possibility of cardiac arrest, the risk of uterine perforation by the sharp dilators used and the risk of infection was not adequately allowed for'.[119] By contrast, fellow gynaecologist Tony Baird later published a report about the clinic concluding, 'It is apparent that there is no completely safe way to terminate a pregnancy, but vacuum aspiration under paracervical block, as practised at the Auckland Medical Aid Centre, carries a low complication rate. The practice at the Centre appears to be satisfactory by world standards.'[120]

Bonham also became involved, giving evidence at the 1975 trial of Australian Dr James Woolnough, one of the operating surgeons at the centre, who had been charged on twelve counts of procuring unlawful abortions. Bonham responded to a statement by Green disputing that pregnancy affected women's long-term mental health status. He thought this 'an incredible statement', and suggested that Green was 'pretty inexperienced in dealing with psychological matters'.[121] The Court of Appeal eventually acquitted Woolnough in 1976, upholding an earlier verdict that he had held an honest belief that there had been a danger to the physical or mental health of the twelve women involved. According to Werry, Bonham's evidence in favour of Woolnough was key to his acquittal. Evidence used against Woolnough claimed that he did not always personally assess patients, but Bonham stated that this also happened at National Women's where medical registrars would sometimes operate.[122]

Herb Green also clashed with medical superintendent Algar Warren in 1977 when he reported a case of septic abortion to the local medical officer of health. Warren thought this unethical, and referred the case to the Medical Council's Central Ethical Committee. In the event the committee upheld Green's actions as an appropriate way of dealing with infection.[123] There were clear personal divisions within National Women's over abortion.

Law Reform and the Epsom Day Hospital

From the late 1960s there was much public discussion of abortion law reform, particularly in light of Britain's 1967 Abortion Act that had legalised abortion there. While he was not opposed to abortion, Bonham did not believe a law change was necessary, as it currently allowed considerable flexibility.[124] In 1970 the Crown Solicitor affirmed that abortion in New Zealand was 'not a crime or unlawful if it is done in good faith for the preservation of the life of the mother or the physical or mental health of the mother'.[125] In 1971 Dr Brian Corkill, honorary secretary to the New Zealand Council of the RCOG, analysed 87 replies to a questionnaire sent to its members (a 93.5 per cent response rate): 70 per cent of respondents felt the law should be left unchanged, 'if interpreted liberally', although they believed it 'should be clarified specifically to include abortion for cases of suspected fetal abnormality'.[126] The broader medical profession supported a law change, however, according to the report of a survey which appeared in the *NZMJ* in 1971. Of the 1726 doctors interviewed in 1969–70, about 60 per cent favoured some reform and '80 per cent held views consistent with a revision of the statutes'.[127]

Abortion was also at the forefront of the feminist politics of the early 1970s, as feminists 'retheorized' its meaning.[128] They viewed abortion not as a health issue or a personal crisis but rather as fundamental to the right of women to control their own bodies and lives. The personal had become political and the right to abortion symbolised women's liberation.[129] In 1972 the press announced that the Women's Liberation Movement in Britain and America was teaching women how to help their friends have an abortion with a simple plastic suction instrument called menstrual abstraction. The do-it-yourself kits worked in the same way as the apparatus commonly used in hospital. Liggins warned women against using it, as the dangers were too great for those not properly trained in the method. Perforation of the womb and infection were two obvious problems, and there was a risk of death through air embolism.[130] Some New Zealand women flew to Australia for an abortion, where the law was more liberal. It was reported in 1975 that about 4000 New Zealand women flew to Australia annually for this purpose.[131]

In 1972 a new Labour government had been elected to office, under Prime Minister Norman Kirk, who was known to be supportive of modern social movements. However, he did not support the liberalisation of abortion, and indeed his wife became patron of SPUC.[132] However, Labour suggested a public investigation into abortion, and in 1975 Bill Rowling, who became Prime Minister when Kirk died in 1974, set up a commission to inquire into contraception, sterilisation and abortion, with Supreme Court Judge Duncan McMullin presiding. The commission held public hearings for 79 days and heard 317 submissions and 379 witnesses, and issued its report in 1977. It identified the status of the 'unborn child [as] the cornerstone of the abortion argument'.[133] According to a later analysis, in his discussion paper on 'The Status of the Unborn Child', McMullin 'drew principally' on Liley's submissions.[134] Yet in its report the commission tried to reflect the broad range of public views on the issue and recommended the establishment of an Abortion Supervisory Committee 'to accommodate mixed public feeling'.[135]

New legislation relating to abortion came in with the 1977 Contraception, Sterilisation, and Abortion Act and the 1977 Crimes Amendment Act. The latter included a clause specifying that abortion was permissible only when danger to the life or health of the mother could not be averted 'by any other means'; fetal abnormality was not included as a reason for abortion. This sparked heated and extensive public debates over the following months until amendments in July 1978 deleted the restrictive phrase and added possible fetal abnormality as a ground for abortion.[136] The extent of the debates can be gauged through the press. From December 1977 to May 1978, '245 news stories, eight editorials and "many hundreds" of letters to the editor' on abortion and related issues were published in the *Auckland Star* alone. The editor wrote, 'At one time, the newspaper received more than 100 letters a day on this topic alone.' In a submission following a complaint by SPUC of biased reporting in the *Star*, he stated that in some 40 years of journalism he had known no other controversial issue to be accorded more space or attention or 'to arouse such emotional, personalized and extreme responses'.[137] This continued following the 1978 amendment; the Women's National Abortion Action Campaign pressed for repeal of the law, and a petition for repeal signed by 318,000 people was presented to Parliament in August 1978.[138]

In its final form adopted in July 1978, the law permitted abortion to be performed for up to 20 weeks following conception to preserve the physical and/or mental health of the woman, and in cases of rape or incest, or if there was a substantial risk that the child, if born, would be seriously handicapped. The woman had to have the approval of two certifying consultants, one of whom had to be a practising obstetrician or gynaecologist, appointed by a central Abortion Supervisory Committee (ASC) and overseen by Parliament.

By 1980 there were 207 certifying consultants. That year 4786 women saw certifying consultants and 4223 abortions were authorised.[139] Liam Wright, a gynaecologist at National Women's Hospital, maintained that this showed that abortion on demand was now being practised in New Zealand.[140] Others disagreed. Feminists set up SOS, Sisters Overseas Service, to help women go to Australia for abortion where the laws were still more liberal.[141] Between 1977 and 1979, about 2500 did so (admittedly still less than the 4000 who had made the trip in 1975 prior to the law change).[142]

In 1980 Vivienne Boyd, NCW president who had taken over as ASC chair from Auckland magistrate Augusta Wallace the previous year,[143] resigned in protest when Parliament did not reappoint two members – Dr Bruce Grieve from National Women's Hospital, and Dr Heather Thomson of Invercargill. She interpreted this as evidence of SPUC influence on MPs. Grieve told the *New Zealand Herald* that his stance on abortion had always been 'middle of the road' and that the new appointees were known to be 'pro-life'. He thought the change would result in more abortions being done in Australia.[144]

The ASC had a difficult role to play. The new chair in 1980, Heather White, stated in her annual report that it aimed to reduce the number of abortions, but the following year she reported a 13 per cent increase.[145] Most were granted on psychological grounds. In 1981 this was the case in 75 per cent of all abortions; the corresponding figures for 1982 and 1983 were 91.3 per cent and 87 per cent respectively.[146] In 1986 White commented that critics varied from those who claimed that abortion had been liberalised in New Zealand to the point of 'abortion on request', to those who regarded the existing law as ill-contrived, restrictive and inconsiderate of women's rights to self-determination. The committee was aware that no legislation concerning abortion, or the constitution of membership of the committee to administer that legislation, would satisfy every section of opinion.[147]

In a commentary in the *NZMJ* Sarah Clarkson of the Department of Psychological Medicine at the University of Otago wrote about the dilemmas attached to modern abortion. She argued that the 1977 Act had 'placed firmly in the lap of the medical profession . . . the impossible task of becoming the arbiter of morals of New Zealand society'. She believed that the law required not a medical decision but a moral decision, and commented, 'Not surprisingly, medical practitioners are finding themselves unable to resolve a problem which has defeated the wisest philosophers throughout the history of mankind.' In her view, 'In the final analysis the morality of an act of abortion depended on the rights afforded the fetus.'[148]

The rights of the fetus formed the central focus of a new organisation set up in 1983 by a group of doctors who believed that 'human life begins at conception'. New Zealand Doctors for Life had 494 members by 1987. They referred to the 1949 Geneva Declaration and its reiteration of the Hippocratic Oath which decreed: 'I will maintain the utmost respect for human life from the time of conception; even under threat I will not use any medical knowledge contrary to the laws of humanity.'[149] The president, Invercargill doctor Norman MacLean, drew parallels between abortion and the Holocaust: the 'mental patients' who were killed in Nazi Germany, he said, 'were weak, defenceless, burdensome, and uneconomic; the unborn are weak, defenceless, burdensome, and uneconomic'.[150] Liam Wright supported MacLean, declaring, 'The only criteria for admission to society and its basic rights are that he/she be human and alive. Scientific work confirms commonsense and logic – humanity and life both begin at conception.'[151]

Meanwhile, National Women's had been asked by the Auckland Hospital Board to set up services in accordance with the 1977 Act. Premises for an abortion clinic were found at 5 Warborough Avenue, Epsom, occupying half of what had previously been St Margaret's Hospital. The new clinic, opened in 1978, was called the Epsom Day Hospital. It quickly became the largest abortion clinic in the country; 2304 abortions were performed there in 1985 by twelve consultants, increasing to almost 3000 the following year, with a further 300 at National Women's.[152] The hospital conducted first and second-trimester abortions; abortions beyond seventeen weeks, which would be due to gross fetal abnormality or a life-threatening situation to the woman, were passed over to National Women's.[153] The Epsom Day Hospital also had counselling staff, and the deputy head orderly became 'a "Father Figure" to distressed Patients, which [was] very much appreciated by both Nursing and Counselling Staff'.[154]

Broadsheet published an assessment of the attitudes of the operating surgeons at Epsom Day Hospital in 1979, as part of a nationwide survey of certifying consultants. These ranged from 'very liberal' (John Taylor) to 'very conservative' (Bill McIndoe). Bonham got a favourable mention as 'liberal, good with patients', while Tony Baird, who was the first clinical coordinator of the hospital, was said to be 'becoming more liberal. Sympathetic to older women.' Celia Liggins was also 'sympathetic to older women, particularly with contraceptive failure'. Not all comments were positive: one consultant was apparently 'conservative and women often upset by him', although it added that he was 'sympathetic to under 15 year olds and women with possible foetal abnormality'.[155]

Some National Women's doctors, like Green, Faris and Wright, chose not to be involved in the clinic, and others like Colin Mantell who felt pressured to become involved subsequently withdrew because they found it too stressful.[156] In 1985 the hospital's new medical superintendent Gabrielle Collison told a journalist that she found her views on abortion had become more conservative as a result of 'making friends of some very tiny babies, alive as a result of the techniques developed at the hospital'. But, the journalist noted, in a professional capacity she was also superintendent of Epsom Day Hospital.[157]

Anti-abortion activities continued following the 1977 Act. Parents of several girls attending Otumoetai College were 'up in arms' in 1979 about the showing of the anti-abortion film 'I'd Like Her Back', narrated by Bill Liley, as part of the school's health education programme. Twenty-four girls out of a class of 30 had walked out before the film ended. One girl was reported to have fainted. A sixteen-year-old said the film was 'pretty sickening' and 'enough to put her off pregnancy completely'.[158]

Like abortion clinics overseas, Epsom Day Hospital was a target for protests. John Taylor, who followed Baird as clinical director, found this particularly distressing when it was directed at his home, but he found consolation in the fact that 'we had very supportive neighbours and they used to be occasionally watering their garden in front and the hose used to be inadvertently directed towards the protest'.[159] In 1984 and again in 1987 the clinic was the object of arson attacks, the second of which caused $30,000 worth of damage.[160] As in America, some anti-abortionists were fanatical. In 1991 the Epsom Day Hospital closed and services were relocated to Green Lane Hospital, which it was hoped would give clients 'more privacy and security'. National Women's general manager Sue Belsham explained that the remote location had 'made clients clearly identifiable as consumers of the sensitive service, and vulnerable to harassment'.[161]

As noted, Bonham did not oppose abortion; indeed, he was one of the operating surgeons at the Epsom Day Hospital. Yet he did not see it as the optimal solution to the problem of unwanted pregnancies and continued to regard abortion as a failure of education in contraception. He thought the Abortion Supervisory Committee should lead an advertising campaign aimed at helping women avoid unwanted pregnancies. In 1979 Bonham surveyed a hundred women seeking abortions at the Epsom Day Hospital. Nearly half had taken no contraceptive measure, and only 20 per cent were using reliable methods. About 20 women had had a misunderstanding with their medical adviser, which he thought a contributing factor to their pregnancies (he related how 'one woman was told by her doctor she was a naughty girl for taking the pill because she was single'). He recommended that 'There should be more social support for these women, and more education in the use of contraception', as he declared that the survey had 'proved conclusively that half the terminations now being done could have been avoided'.[162]

The doctors of National Women's Hospital found themselves caught up in controversial social issues that had formerly been private matters. In the 1970s and 1980s, their work came under close scrutiny. Despite this, they continued to provide a service for women and to negotiate their way through the issues as best they could. The ways in which they did so reflected not one but many medical responses to the changing social environment.

CHAPTER 9

OBSTETRICS AND THE WINDS OF CHANGE, 1964–1980s

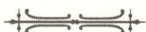

A FTER DENNIS BONHAM WAS APPOINTED PROFESSOR IN THE POSTGRADUATE School of Obstetrics and Gynaecology in 1964, those well beyond the hospital drew on his expertise. He became involved with the politics of maternity at a national level, being appointed to the Board of Health Maternity Services Committee in 1964 and consultant in maternity to the Health Department in 1967. His goals were to reduce New Zealand's maternal and perinatal mortality rates and to improve maternity services nationally.

Bonham took on this role in the midst of profound social changes. For some time he worked well with consumer groups: Parents' Centre and the NZFPA responded positively to his involvement. He was liberal in his views and was even on the side of the women's movement in the abortion debates. However, as the battle lines hardened and feminists became more radical, he found himself under attack. His involvement in the closure of small hospitals, and his opposition along with his colleagues to home births, eventually made him the enemy of the new women's health movement.

In 1979 the Maternity Services Committee produced a document, *Obstetrics and the Winds of Change*, which declared, 'Nowhere do the winds of change blow more strongly than across the field of obstetrics. We in the medical and nursing professions face a major challenge to meet the demands of a vocal minority, as well as the larger needs of the majority.'[1] This chapter focuses on the 'larger needs of the majority', or the involvement of doctors and nurses at National Women's Hospital in public debates relating to maternity services, including what kind of hospital was the best in which to have babies and what quality of care could be expected there. The following chapter will address the 'demands of a vocal minority' and the home birth movement.

Maternal Mortality Research Act 1968

One of Bonham's first actions in his attempt to reduce maternal mortality and improve maternity services in New Zealand was to bring to fruition, together with his deputy Herb Green, the 1968 Maternal Mortality Research Act. This was based on the British model, where 'confidential maternal mortality reports' had been published since 1957. Following closely its British counterpart, the structure established under the New Zealand Act involved appointing a number of medical practitioners as regional assessors and a maternal death assessment committee with seven members appointed by the Minister of Health. Bonham was appointed chairman. Doctors who had attended a woman during an illness or injury that contributed toward her death, and who thought that the death was a 'maternal' one, had to notify the District Medical Officer of Health within 24 hours of the woman's death. The medical officer then passed the information to the regional assessor. Bonham explained that arrangements would be made to ensure the anonymity of medical, midwifery and nursing staff involved with maternal deaths.[2] Similarly in Britain, the Chief Medical Officer Sir George Godber had written in the most recent *Confidential Report* (1966):

> This enquiry is a unique exercise in medicine in this country. It is a careful review of each maternal death in an attempt to ascertain whether additional or different action in accordance with the best current practice in obstetrics might have given the patient a better prospect of survival. The object of this enquiry by obstetricians, general practitioners, Medical Officers of Health and midwives, co-ordinated by the Ministry, is to seek the opportunities that remain for further advance, not to apportion blame to individuals or to particular parts of the services .... Superficial or sensational use of any of the material in this report would be a disservice to the mothers of the future.[3]

Godber also pointed out that these reports were strictly confidential, examined and analysed only by regional assessors, consultant advisers and a Ministry of Health doctor.[4] After his appointment as a New Zealand regional assessor in 1973, Ian Barrowclough, an obstetrician at National Women's Hospital, expressed his belief that the process would improve the safety and wellbeing of mothers and of obstetrical standards.[5]

The press had a different take on the confidential nature of the reports, believing they should be made public. The popular tabloid *New Zealand Truth* complained in 1973 that the committee's findings were 'top-secret'.[6] The *Sunday News* carried an article a few months later under the title, 'Why Did Your Mum Die?' This declared that a confidential Health Department report on maternal deaths in New Zealand, which the *Sunday News* had obtained, revealed an 'alarming situation', and that in nearly all maternal deaths there had been 'avoidable elements of unsatisfactory care'. Health Department officials were concerned that the *Sunday News* had a copy of the report but the journalist defended the leak on the grounds that it was 'of vital public interest'.[7]

Bonham declined to comment when approached, but Health Minister Bob Tizard wrote to the *Sunday News* explaining that the medical profession supported the 1968 Act on the understanding that the work and proceedings of the committee would be confidential, subject to the limited exceptions spelled out in the Act. In 1974 Bonham told Wellington's morning paper, the *Dominion*, that the research was a 'professional auditing system' similar to one operating in relation to perinatal deaths. Asked who decided what was a matter of public interest, Bonham replied that the public had to trust the committee and 'to have reasonably good faith that the profession will look after their interests . . . . If doctors felt relatives would be "on their backs" they might clam up.'[8]

Two years later the issue re-emerged in an article headed 'Pregnancy Deaths', after a report had been leaked to *The Week* by a doctor. Commenting on the confidential nature of the reports, the journalist advised, 'If doctors are serious in their desire to reduce the number of women who die in pregnancy then they must stop talking to themselves and start acknowledging their accountability to the community and the role to be played by a fully informed public.'[9] Two years later, in 1978, Bonham again stressed the importance of audit. Agreeing to appear on a TVNZ documentary, he told the Health Department that he believed it 'important for the public to know what is being done in this, one of the earliest forms of quality control in medicine that is being run in New Zealand'.[10] While Bonham viewed it as an exercise in auditing, public demand for transparency and accountability was indicative of a rising consumerism and suspicion of paternalistic medicine in the 1970s, a trend that was to accelerate in the following decade.

The Fate of Small Maternity Hospitals

Another public debate in which Bonham and some of his colleagues crossed swords with members of the public and other medical practitioners related to the status of small maternity hospitals vis-à-vis institutions like National Women's Hospital. As a member of the Maternity Services Committee and consultant to the Health Department on obstetrics, Bonham was asked by the department to assess maternity services throughout the country. This involved visiting, together with Dr Joan Mackay, director of Maternal and Child Welfare in the Department of Health, 160 hospitals during the period 1969–74. They published their report in 1976.[11]

When Bonham arrived at National Women's he had already been involved in a British survey of perinatal mortality, sponsored by the National Birthday Trust Fund and initiated by his boss, Professor William Nixon. The British Perinatal Mortality Survey consisted of an analysis of about 17,000 births and 7000 stillbirths and neonatal deaths in England, Wales and Scotland, over a three-month period in 1958. Just as Bonham was leaving Britain, on 6 December 1963, *The Times* reported an emergency informal meeting of the National Birthday Trust Fund to put forward 'a crash programme for sweeping reforms in maternity services', based on the findings of the survey's first report. This had shown that 200 of the 600 babies who died each week throughout the three-month period covered by the survey died of anoxia (lack of oxygen) before, during or after birth. *The Times* reported that about half these babies might have been saved if the mother had received proper antenatal care and been given access to adequate facilities at the time of the confinement. The solution, according to the report, was more hospital beds and more skilled staff.[12] In his biography of Nixon, obstetrician Geoffrey Chamberlain wrote that 'Bonham was attacked for exposing facts and antagonizing the general practitioners; soon afterwards, he went to New Zealand as Postgraduate Professor of Obstetrics at Auckland', implying some connection between the two events.[13]

British sociologist Ann Oakley wrote of the survey that it was almost certainly responsible for a substantially increased use of induction for post-term babies, and contributed to the invasion of obstetrics into the domain of normal delivery.[14] In her book Joan Donley referred to the belief that the aim of the survey was 'to nail down the coffin of home delivery'.[15] In Donley's view, therefore, Bonham had arrived in New Zealand with a marked agenda.

Bonham and Mackay's 1976 report expressly criticised small maternity hospitals run by single general practitioners with no specific obstetric training and no midwives present.[16] While they were impressed by the quality of some of the midwives in the smaller hospitals, they were distressed that some charge nurses were registered nurses without maternity training rather than registered midwives.[17] They declared that some of the smaller units provided 'no more protection for the patient than domiciliary confinement'.[18] The previous year Donald Aickin, professor of obstetrics and gynaecology in Christchurch, had also stated that there were 'still many relatively ill-equipped and inadequately staffed hospitals undertaking full obstetric care' and commented on the mistaken belief that such hospitals necessarily offered a more satisfactory environment for having a baby.[19]

Bonham and Mackay's report contributed to the shutting down of some smaller units; Donley said that general practitioners called the closures 'the Bonham squeeze', and she herself saw the closures as an attempt to 'consolidate O & G power'.[20] Between 1970 and 1984, 29 rural maternity hospitals, about one-third of such units, were shut down. In Auckland, the Salvation Army's Bethany Hospital closed in 1975; 1976 saw the closure of three small maternity units (the Devonport, Eastern Bays and Franklin hospitals);[21] and the Mater Misericordiae Maternity Unit was shut down in 1979. That year Prime Minister Robert Muldoon announced that private maternity hospitals were a thing of the past.[22] A decade later Auckland's St Helens was amalgamated with National Women's.

The same year that Bonham and Mackay published their report, another consultant from National Women's also became embroiled in the public debates about small hospitals. Bill Faris, who as well as working at National Women's had been medical superintendent of Auckland's St Helens Hospital from 1963 to 1972, was a member of the Auckland Hospital Board when the future of maternity services for Auckland came up for discussion. He proposed that 'in future within urban or metropolitan Auckland, no obstetric or maternity beds ever be developed unless there are accompanying facilities for adequate specialist anaesthesia, caesarean sections, and specialist paediatric consultation and care, preferably always in the environment of a general hospital'. This was defeated, Faris said, 'amidst emotional and anecdotal arguments that "our grandmothers had their babies at home [and that] specialists lived in ivory towers and did not know what the women themselves, the community, and general practitioners and midwives wanted".[23]

Another member of the hospital board, Mrs L. F. Miller, claimed that medical authorities were conducting an 'insidious indoctrination' of trainee doctors and nurses to make them believe that the only safe place for the delivery of babies was a large specialised obstetric hospital.[24] Faris countered this, declaring, 'It is a God-given right of every baby to be born where the circumstances are the very best', pointing out that things could go wrong in the space of a few minutes.[25] Faris wished every mother to be asked, 'does she prefer social convenience, or does the safety of her baby come first?' He argued that the lack of amenities at North Shore Maternity Unit should never be allowed to happen again; it serviced 100,000 people, but had no caesarean or paediatric facilities. National Women's was the only hospital in the area able to deal with caesarean sections and major neonatal problems. Middlemore Hospital in south Auckland, which had set up a maternity unit in 1961, had minimal neonatal services, and St Helens Hospital had no resident anaesthetist and its neonatal services were limited. According to Faris, transferring babies carried unacceptable risks, 'both in the short term and in subsequent brain damage and disability'. He stated that amongst those patients booking at National Women's Hospital, sixteen out of 1000 lost their babies, while the death rate was 97 per 1000 births for those (allegedly low-risk) patients – over 1000 in all – who each year in Auckland booked into hospitals without facilities and subsequently had to be transferred.[26]

Another local doctor, Albert Henderson, joined the fray. He had worked in India and declared that anyone who had practised in an underdeveloped country would challenge the necessity for such a high rate of interference in a healthy developed community.[27] Auckland Hospital Board chairman Dr Frank Rutter, himself a GP who delivered as many as 250 babies each year,[28] spoke on the concept of choice. He declared that many mothers were prepared to run a small calculated risk and have their babies at home or in a cottage hospital where they were better able to establish a close and emotional link with their newborn children. He added, 'If society placed an absolute value on human life cars would travel no faster than five miles an hour and beer and cigarettes would be banned.'[29]

In 1982 another Maternity Services Committee report advocated 'regionalisation' of maternity services within New Zealand, following an American model, with three levels of maternity hospitals in each region. These levels would be classified as level 1 (primary), level 2 (secondary) and level 3 (tertiary). For Auckland, National Women's would be categorised as level 3 and Middlemore and St Helen's Hospital would be upgraded to level 2 (later Waitakere and North Shore Hospitals were also upgraded to level 2).[30] Regionalisation was also being discussed in Britain at the time: a 1980s British obstetric textbook explained that the 'need to avoid excessive duplication of the costly equipment, high level technology, and specialised skills required for the care of tiny preterm and severely ill newborns made centralization [or regionalisation] necessary'.[31]

Donley viewed things differently. In 1986 she argued that regionalisation was a euphemism for the consolidation of specialist-controlled, high-technology care in a university/hospital complex. Regionalisation was, she declared, supported by the multinational drug companies that made huge profits from supplying the equipment and technology, and was a self-perpetuating system which guaranteed obstetricians and gynaecologists 'a monopoly of clinical material', that is, the women.[32] Some observers even suggested a personal motivation on the part of Bonham. In her history of maternity, Sue Kedgley quoted midwife Karen Guilliland stating: 'Bonham wanted everything centralised at one big hospital so he could control the lot.'[33]

Humanising Maternity Care in Hospital

In his 1964 inaugural lecture, Bonham stressed the importance of human relations in medicine. He took his cue from his mentor in London, William Nixon, whom he credited with initiating the drive for better human relations in obstetrics and gynaecology in Britain.[34] In fact, such concerns in obstetrics were being widely aired in Britain before Bonham's departure. In 1961 the Central Health Services Council's Standing Maternity and Midwifery Advisory Committee had published a report on 'Human Relations in Obstetrics' based on the inaugural lecture by Norman Morris, professor of obstetrics and gynaecology at London's Charing Cross Hospital Medical School and published in *The Lancet*.[35] Bonham's 1964 inaugural lecture reflected this trend when he stated, 'For the clinician, the time spent with the patient is one incident in a busy day, for the woman, her husband and family, it may be an awe-inspiring and alarming event or sequence. At all times we must provide an individual personal service for each patient and it is noteworthy that obstetrics is taking the lead in a field which covers all branches of medicine.'[36]

Obstetrics and the Winds of Change, 1964–1980s

In 1964 the Federation of New Zealand Parents' Centres appointed Bonham to its medical panel; the consumer activist and historian of Parents' Centre Mary Dobbie later described him as a 'benign' member of the panel.[37] The following year Bonham hosted a seminar on psycho-prophylaxis in childbirth at National Women's, where Mrs Valerie Leech, former teacher to Auckland Parents' Centre classes, was now charge physiotherapist. Leech ran regular refresher courses at National Women's for obstetric physiotherapists and the hospital provided overnight accommodation for out-of-town physiotherapists.[38] Like Nixon, Bonham supported natural childbirth.[39] He also felt strongly that babies should be breastfed and not bottle-fed; as paediatrician David Knight later said of Bonham, 'He wanted them breastfed, he wanted them with their mothers, he didn't want unnecessary interventions.'[40] In 1970 Bonham made the postgraduate school available to Parents' Centre for a two-day conference. Dobbie commented that Bonham approved of the high standard of physiotherapy in the Parents' Centre, and its encouragement of father participation in childbirth.[41]

By the 1970s the 'patient's perspective' was much more in the public consciousness than ever before, aided by the rise of the consumer movement and the new women's movement. A 1971 *NZMJ* editorial declared that reducing mortality in childbirth was now 'not enough'; it stated that women wished 'to enjoy their obstetrical adventure and have warm inner feelings of achievement' and that obstetricians needed to be aware of this.[42]

In their 1976 report, Bonham and Mackay included a section on human relations. They critiqued some of the smaller hospitals for being regimented and old-fashioned. In particular they specified rooming-in as an important aspect of modern maternity hospital care, but found that this was actively practised in just a few hospitals although it was more broadly available if the mother insisted. They reported that some of these hospitals 'resembled a factory routine which appeared designed to discourage the normal establishment of breast feeding'. Their report recommended a major educational programme to inform midwives about rooming-in, demand breastfeeding and modern concepts of infant management.[43]

A public perception that larger specialised hospitals like National Women's were more impersonal and streamlined than smaller ones was not necessarily borne out by evidence. In a 1977 undergraduate community health study comparing National Women's with a small maternity hospital in Te Puke, the researchers found that in the latter hospital only 33 per cent of mothers were breastfeeding their babies, because facilities did not allow for rooming-in, whereas all of those surveyed at National Women's were breastfeeding on demand.[44] Rooming-in at National Women's also allowed women to develop confidence in handling their new babies: one mother there told the researchers that when she went home after having a baby at another Auckland hospital, where there had been no rooming-in, she had been at a loss to know what to do with the baby.[45] Like Bonham and Mackay, some women found that smaller units did not necessarily provide a better birthing environment.

In a 1977 memorandum to National Women's HMC, Faris advised that they needed 'to make even greater efforts to counteract the oft-stated remark that large hospitals are "impersonal"; to that end much greater emphasis must be placed on personal care and friendly communication at all levels'.[46] The committee agreed, reaffirming its belief that the best outcome for patients lay in improving staffing and human relations at the larger hospitals rather than developing smaller hospitals.[47]

This message was reinforced during a visit in 1980 of Dr Ann Cartwright, the Auckland Savings Bank Visiting Professor for that year. Director of the Institute for Social Studies in Medical Care in London, she was well known for her critiques of medical intervention (particularly induction), and had conducted patient surveys on maternity in Britain. She told her Auckland audience that partnership between doctors and patients was important and that obstetricians should adopt a 'more scientific and self-critical attitude'.[48]

In 1977 a consumer group, Feminists for Life, took the initiative themselves and drafted a 'Maternity Patients' Bill of Rights', under the direction of Mrs Connie Purdue and in consultation with doctors, midwives, Parents' Centre, La Leche League and mothers. Purdue was the third daughter of Miriam Soljak, a pioneering New Zealand feminist and communist, and was herself active in the Labour Party, a member of the Auckland Hospital Board (1974–86) and inaugural president of the National Organisation of Women (1972–74).[49] She later recalled that Herb Green had helped to draw up the Bill of Rights.[50] The Bill, reproduced in the *New Zealand Listener*, stressed informed consent (with non-technical language provided for medical explanations), and the right of women to choose who should be present at the birth for emotional support, to refuse pain-relieving injections, to choose the labouring position, and not to decide about sterilisation during or immediately after the birth.[51] The Bill of Rights also included the mother's entitlement to have the baby with her in hospital at all times, to feed according to the baby's needs and not the hospital routines, to be visited by persons of her choice (including her other children) during all visiting hours, to have her ethnic and cultural attitudes respected, to have her medical records made available to a doctor of her choice, and finally to be treated with respect and courtesy and given emotional support by the staff.[52]

The document was sent to the Auckland Hospital Board, which forwarded it to National Women's for comment. Pat Dunn picked up on it and wrote an impassioned response, claiming that the Bill 'obviously misunderstood the nature of the professional relationship between doctor and patient, that this was a free association from which either party may withdraw and which implied mutual trust'. He believed the Bill would do little to enhance the rapport between patients and staff by framing them in opposition. While Dunn was among the more conservative members of the medical staff, there was a general agreement that a separate 'Bill of Rights' was not needed and that the statement, *Code of Rights and Obligations of Patients and Staff*, already issued by the board, covered the position adequately.[53]

Yet the issue did not go away. Two years later, in 1979, the Maternity Services Committee published its pamphlet, *Obstetrics and the Winds of Change*, as a guideline for obstetric hospital staff. The pamphlet explained why staff had to pay attention to this advice: 'How can we protect the lives and IQs of our future citizens and counter this move away from our hospitals? We can do so by making our hospitals more like homes, by abandoning our rigid attitudes, by listening to each patient's request, and by combining with each other to make her feel that she is the centre of the universe in her moment of triumph.'[54]

Recommendations listed in the pamphlet included allowing husbands and boyfriends into the delivery suites, even for complicated births, rethinking the attitude that professionals knew best, and being prepared to withhold sedation if a mother so wished. Soft lights, sweet music, warm baths, mirrors and cameras were to be encouraged, although the authors cautioned that, 'Cyanosis by candlelight could be a difficult diagnosis and suturing episiotomies [i.e. stitching the perineum following a cut to avoid tears] chaotic'. They also suggested improvements to décor, including carpets, armchairs, warm colours, gaily patterned wallpapers, curtains and pictures. Finally, conditions could be improved 'by not sheltering behind excuses of over-crowded conditions or overworked staff to prevent our providing tender loving care for our patients'. The document concluded, 'We live in times of rapid change and the voice of womanhood calls more loudly than ever before. Rights are being demanded and jealously guarded and we who look after women in their hour of need, ignore these rights at our peril.' The reward of paying attention would be 'deeper rapport with our patients'.[55]

Three months before the publication of this pamphlet, National Women's HMC passed a motion proposed by John Hutton and seconded by Herb Green, that a sub-committee be convened to examine recent press allegations about unsatisfactory care at their hospital.[56] Adverse publicity included an editorial in the *Auckland Star* in early 1979 which reported a swift and angry response to a suggestion from a mother-to-be that patients were treated as numbers. According to the editor, a certain professor called the comments a gross and unwarranted slur on the institution, an outburst which the editor said simply confirmed the institution's insensitivity.[57] Others rushed to defend the hospital, however. One woman, who had recently spent ten days there, declared she could not find anything to complain about: she had been treated as an individual and 'wanted for nothing'. She concluded, 'Frankly, it is the best hotel I've ever stayed in. Keep up the good work, National Women's.'[58]

In the wake of this publicity the HMC set up a sub-committee on the 'Care and Respect of Public Patients at National Women's Hospital'. The sub-committee conducted a series of interviews, inviting 20 clinic patients, ten postnatal patients, ten gynaecological patients and ten mothers of infants in the neonatal ward to participate. Criticisms related to the facilities, seeing different doctors at each clinic, inadequate explanations to patients by doctors, long waiting times in clinics and for blood tests, impersonal attention, the unavailability of doctors in obstetric and gynaecological wards, visiting hours, privacy, car parking and the food.[59] As a result the committee came up with suggestions which echoed the Maternity Services Committee pamphlet, relating to a more relaxed and homely environment for the mothers, their babies and their families.[60]

A Family Environment in Hospital

While most women opted for hospital childbirth from the 1950s, they constantly sought to make conditions there more comfortable. From that time, as part of their demand for 'quality experience' in childbirth, women campaigned for their husbands to be allowed to come with them into the maternity hospital. Auckland Hospital Board policy at that time did not permit this.[61] In his 1964 inaugural lecture Bonham declared that husbands should be allowed to be with their wives 'not only during the first stage but also at delivery'.[62] In

May that year Bonham persuaded the HMC to request the hospital board to delete the word 'very' from the ruling that 'husbands and other lay people be not allowed in the precincts of the Labour Ward suites except in very special circumstances and then only after permission'.[63] Two months later Bonham produced a memorandum suggesting that husbands might be present provided that both the mother and her husband desired it and that they had secured the agreement of the doctor or midwife in charge of the delivery. There were certain requirements for the husband: he had to have attended a course of antenatal instruction or been present at his wife's previous confinement; he had to realise he was there 'to support, encourage and comfort his wife at the head of the table and not as a spectator'; he had to be 'properly garbed in cap, gown, mask and overboots to conform with routine theatre technique'; and, finally, he had to agree to leave the delivery room immediately if asked.[64]

Not all members of the medical staff approved of the presence of fathers, even under these strict guidelines. Senior consultant Bruce Grieve thought the scheme might embarrass the delivery suite nurses because of the large number of cases handled in the delivery suite and also because the nurses would have to decide whether or not the husband could remain with his wife if no doctor were present. He advocated 'very strict control' and a trial which should not be publicised. The HMC agreed to Bonham's proposal on condition that it be marked 'Not for Publication'.[65] The Nursing Advisory Committee also discussed the proposal and agreed to a trial. The board chairman and the superintendent-in-chief responded that the hospital board adhered to its policy of no husbands, but advised that this could be 'overruled on clinical grounds'.[66]

The demand to allow men to accompany their wives into hospital for childbirth had its ideological roots in the writings of British gynaecologist Grantly Dick-Read who believed it to be an important cornerstone of future family relationships. As he advised in *Childbirth without Fear*, which ran into many editions and was widely read in New Zealand as elsewhere, obstetricians needed to understand that the father's presence at the birth enabled the husband and wife

> ... to be united in the most wonderful, awe-inspiring experience that can possibly fall to the lot of wedded human beings. There is no drama or playacting in the full recognition of the magnitude of this event to both of them. The first cry of the child is shared by both husband and wife in almost unbelievable ecstasy and relief from tension.[67]

He believed the father's presence created a 'marriage which is indestructible for all time', and advocated strongly that 'all husbands should make the pregnancy of their wives a heaven-sent opportunity for an association in marriage at the highest level'.[68] In other words, he believed that future marital happiness was enormously advanced by fathers' participation in childbirth.

Fathers were becoming more interested in being involved, as indicated by the success of mixed antenatal classes at National Women's from 1965; medical superintendent Algar Warren reported in 1966 that 'the two evening sessions . . . when husbands and wives come together have proved very popular'.[69] By the 1970s the programme consisted of six classes, held weekly, and parents were encouraged to complete these at least a month before the delivery date. Mothers attended physiotherapy for 45 minutes before each class, during which time their husbands (or parents or friends, who were also invited) were shown childbirth films. The classes themselves lasted an hour, and were held in the morning and in the evening (so husbands could attend). Topics included pregnancy, preparing for the baby, breastfeeding, labour, birth and the delivery suite, husbands helping in labour, and demonstrations of how to handle the new baby.[70]

In the late 1960s Bill Liley held lectures for men which he called 'Preparing for Fatherhood' and they also proved popular. He explained that questions ranged from why many pregnancies resulted in miscarriages, to whether or not it was desirable for the father to be present at the birth. Liley told his audience that there were several factors deciding the latter, including the views of the mother and the doctor, but that the most important requirement was that the father knew exactly what to expect by having attended an antenatal class. Verna Murray, principal nurse at National Women's from 1970 to 1983, thought that having the father present at the birth helped many women but that the man had to be 'the right type'. She recalled several having to be helped off the floor after they fainted during deliveries.[71] Liley too told his classes of one delivery where the mother required no stitches but the father did, after fainting and striking his head.[72] Such concerns contributed to the continued insistence that fathers remain seated during the birth. In 1979 tutor specialist Dr Andrew Mackintosh told the delivery suite staff: 'If husbands are present at delivery they must be placed on a stool on the mother's right, at the head of the table. They must not be standing or walking around the theatre please.'[73]

Not all doctors favoured fathers being present. In 1973 the local press published a statement by British psychiatrist Louise Eickhoff which elicited a heated response from Bill Liley's wife Margaret, physician in charge of antenatal and postnatal education at National Women's. Eickhoff claimed that the presence of a father at the birth was harmful to the baby, as it 'would be confused if it sensed its father's smell and vibrations before it could see him . . . . the father's scent and rhythms would recall for the child the traumatic experience of birth . . . [and] this makes an underlying pathological association which could ultimately land the child in my clinic'. Margaret Liley dismissed this as ridiculous, and commented that some women felt more secure in the presence of their husbands, adding that her husband was present at the birth of their five children (between 1955 and 1962). Bonham said that the majority view in New Zealand was now in favour of the husband being present at the birth.[74]

While most doctors were supportive of fathers being at the birth, some of the older ones continued to be reluctant. Bernie Kyle, who had joined National Women's staff in 1954, explained that he allowed men to be present under strict conditions such as keeping to the top end of the bed, firmly telling them, 'Don't come down here and have a peep show, and tell me my job.'[75] Another doctor, Pat Dunn, continued to be firmly opposed, explaining in 1973:

> From the point of view of the doctor, having the husband present leads to a second-rate service. I think that all professional people realise that they do a better job if somebody is not looking over their shoulder. Childbearing is a private function of the body and only the people who are really necessary, such as the doctor and the nurses, should be there. It is really partly a matter of professionalism and partly a matter of taste.[76]

He later expanded on his view of birth as a 'private function', explaining that there were certain bodily functions which were private: 'The reproductive and the excretory functions particularly. People realise that instinctively. It's like cleaning false teeth or putting on make-up . . . . From the point of view of aesthetics and personal integrity, the woman deserves more respect.'[77]

While Dunn was clearly old-fashioned, particularly in the permissive environment of the 1970s, some women responded well to him. He did not fit the feminist stereotype of a male obstetrician intent on controlling women's bodies and being dismissive of women and their needs. Indeed, one woman later wrote that she deliberately sought out Dunn because he was less judgemental than others. She declared, 'Dr Dunn had absolute regard for your dignity as a woman. He treated you like a queen.'[78] A further glimpse of his attitudes can be seen in a short piece he wrote in the *New Zealand Medical Journal* in 1979 advocating the left lateral position for women in childbirth (that is, lying on their side). He said that women preferred it and that doctors only had them on their backs ('dorsal position') out of laziness or so that they could 'stand aloof with hands joined like a high priest at a sacrificial altar'.[79] He had no time for such posturing. He regarded his own role as a kind of father-figure and therefore asexual; he did not see his presence as a male interfering with the woman's dignity. Dunn delivered 14,000 babies between 1960 and 1980.[80]

By 1983 Bonham felt able to observe that human relations were now better understood in New Zealand obstetric hospitals. Several hospitals allowed husbands to be present at caesarean births, particularly under epidural analgesia, and 'Despite our initial anxiety, this arrangement appears to work well.'[81] Historian Judith Leavitt called caesarean sections 'The Last Frontier' in denying fathers access to the birth room.[82] At National Women's attendance was at the discretion of the clinician, and this included caesarean sections. However, this came up in discussion at an HMC meeting in 1981 following an incident in the theatre when a husband had fainted and hurt himself. Discussing the case, the theatre supervisor explained that, 'Male staff never wear identification and with changing residents it is difficult to tell staff from relatives of patients.'[83] This had clearly been a case of mistaken identity, with the husband required to do more than he had bargained for.

The HMC minutes for the meeting which followed this incident show a variety of views on the subject. The medical superintendent pointed out that nurses could call the police if there was trouble with relatives in the theatre, although he expected the nurses to contact him first. Another doctor said he had no problem with the presence of relatives in theatre and at times found their presence helpful.[84] The hospital's solicitor, who was also consulted, related the story of a 'difficult' relative who had insisted on being present in the operating theatre while his wife was having a caesarean section, fearing she might be raped by one of the doctors. He said that Bonham accompanied the husband into the theatre and to his great delight found that the operating surgeon was a female registrar and the anaesthetist was also female, as were all the nurses.[85] This instance possibly reflected a growing public distrust of male doctors in the 1970s, or the conviction of some activists that men were excluded because they threatened the masculinity and superiority of the obstetrician over the mother, as expressed later in one anthropological study which starkly declared that 'male obstetricians assert sexual power over birthing women'.[86] Yet it was becoming more common for fathers even to attend caesarean sections by the mid-1980s, and gowns had become optional. Indeed, in 1981 the tutor specialist advised theatre staff to exercise their own discretion over this, declaring there was no compelling reason for 'clean husbands' to be gowned 'when there are lots of dirty doctors around'.[87] Creating an aseptic environment was no longer a consideration.

Some overseas studies in the 1980s continued to question whether husbands really did carry out their intended support role in the delivery suite. The French doctor and natural childbirth advocate Michel Odent thought that a particularly overprotective and possessive man could have a negative effect on labour. British feminist and childbirth educator Sheila Kitzinger also saw drawbacks with fathers being present. She pointed out that allowing husbands to be present, 'if they keep their place', deprived women from having other women present, giving them less choice.[88] A 1986 Scottish study concluded that husbands remained marginal figures in the birthroom: 'They were treated as children might be; given a "pretend" role in the birth (eg allowed to cut the cord) and referred to as if they were spoilt babies unaware of the real world of women's lives.' The authors concluded that these dismissive attitudes coexisted uneasily with ideas of father involvement and family togetherness.[89] In her study of fathers and childbirth in America, historian Judith Leavitt also found that 'significant numbers of fathers voiced feeling at sea, abandoned, out of control when they entered into their wives' labour and delivery rooms'.[90] A nurse in the National Women's delivery suite, Elizabeth Wood, reminisced about fathers' attendance in the 1980s, 'I only had one man pass out', but she added, 'Some men are not greatly helpful during labour. Somehow they either ignore the wife or they overdo it and we have to say, "Go away, leave her alone." Or say, "Excuse me, we are having a life-altering event here. We don't want to listen to the rugby thank you very much!"'[91]

Fathers were increasingly welcomed into neonatal wards as well. Neonatal paediatrician Simon Rowley, who worked at National Women's from 1984, commented that in the modern neonatal unit, 'you might see a father with his shirt off with his baby on his chest'. Admittedly he continued to see gender differences, explaining that 'the fathers seem to be more interested in the technical aspects of the baby's care, and the mother more interested in the pastoral aspects. So the father will come in and look at the monitors and the mothers will come in and look at the babies.'[92]

The story of the entry of men into hospital maternity wards was not a straightforward move towards acceptance and inclusion. Women pushed for it as part of the attempt to humanise childbirth. The desire to have male partners rather than female companions was related to the ascendancy of the modern nuclear family, a legacy of the popular psychology emanating from Dick-Read that future family relationships would be enormously improved by fathers' involvement from the beginning. Some men welcomed the involvement, others felt pressured; in the maternity hospital they remained second-class citizens.

The opening up of maternity hospitals to men was followed by entry for other family members. In 1977 Liley drew attention to a notice barring children from the delivery suite, something he found offensive: 'What I presume it is intended to proscribe is visiting by children. As the notices stand pregnant women would be forgiven for thinking they were coming to an abortorium.'[93] Glenda Stimpson, a midwife at National Women's from 1966 and supervisor of the delivery suite from 1976, explained that the notice was the result of an increasing number of children being brought into the delivery suite, sometimes for hours on end; in most cases they were not directly related to the labouring patient. These children, many of them toddlers, were noisy and obstructive as they ran up and down the corridors. Principal nurse Verna Murray backed her up, arguing that these infringements were inconsistent with the kind of atmosphere they wished to create for women in labour.[94]

Stimpson also pointed out that the presence of extended families was sometimes problematic. She gave one example of a sixteen-year-old woman who was well supported in labour by her mother and boyfriend, but after the delivery the woman's mother brought six other children into the theatre to visit their sister. In another instance, the labouring woman's grandfather and mother along with four children came to witness the birth. When the nurses suggested that the family leave just one member present, the grandfather objected. The third case was a thirteen-year-old girl in labour, whose ten-year-old brother and twelve-year-old sister insisted they be allowed to watch the birth as she was their sister.[95] Another midwife in the delivery suite, Val Dickens, later commented on the difficulty in managing extended families and that there were sometimes confrontations 'which is a terrible thing when a woman is trying to have a baby'.[96] In 1979 Liggins went to the HMC to ask permission for one of his patients to have her eight-year-old son present at the birth, only to be told that the decision should be based on his clinical judgement.[97]

In 1980 one of the hospital consultants, Liam Wright, received a letter from a patient complaining that there were too many visitors in the postnatal wards, which was disturbing to patients, especially at night. Other members of the HMC said they had received similar complaints. The HMC decided it would not take action unless a consensus was reached in the postnatal ward.[98] While no such consensus emerged, the discussions revealed that not only nurses but also some mothers had mixed feelings about a more relaxed environment in hospital.

In response to consumer demands, Liggins, in 1979, raised the possibility for some births occurring in motel-type accommodation that would have a family environment and be staffed by non-uniformed personnel. Staff opposed this when he first suggested it. However, a year later, when Mrs Connie Purdue made the same suggestion to the HMC after the *Winds of Change* document and the recommendations of the hospital's sub-committee relating to the hospital environment, they gave this proposal serious consideration. Such centres were known to be operating in Wellington and in Perth, Australia, and medical superintendent Ian Hutchison was asked to research these ventures.

Dr Stanley Reid of the King Edward Memorial Hospital for Women in Perth described the Perth Alternative Birth Centre (ABC), which had been functioning since 1979, as 'hardly . . . a roaring success'. He advised Auckland, 'If you wish to establish an ABC then you should not make your traditional delivery unit too attractive.' He explained that they accepted women having their first baby into their ABC but that about 50 per cent had to be transferred, mostly because they needed more assistance in labour and delivery than could be provided in the ABC.[99]

When National Women's HMC discussed the idea, some members dismissed it as 'emotional, idealistic and based purely on enthusiasm'. Others feared the ABC would be used by an elitist, articulate middle-class group only. Bonham declared he was delighted that women were questioning the birth service offered, allowing them to consider changes. The senior social worker at the hospital, Kate Harbutt, argued that ABCs were far from radical; she had three of her four children at home, and said this would provide another option. Nora Calvert, who had recently been appointed chaplain to the hospital by the Presbyterian Social Services Association,[100] also contributed to the debate. She compared the trend to the modern hospice movement, with people wanting to 'return life and death to the family'. The HMC remained less than enthusiastic, concluding that although there was a need for an ABC, it should be 'low in the list of the priorities for the use of available funds'.[101]

Four years later, however, the hospital got its ABC, in line with trends overseas; indeed, by the early 1980s America had over 150 ABCs.[102] Leavitt argued that these ABCs were the 'ultimate step in men's move through hospital spaces', a culmination of the movement 'to free fathers from the confines of the waiting rooms and admit them to labour rooms and then to delivery rooms'.[103] ABCs provided a family-centred environment in hospital and paved the way for other family members to attend. National Women's opened its ABC in 1984, with the daily press announcing, 'Women giving birth at National Women's Hospital can now have their baby in the home-like comfort of a birthing room. The room was completed a week ago with the arrival of a $6000 obstetric bed from Britain.... Other features are piped music (which is also available in the other labour rooms at National Women's), a telephone, a coffee table and tea and coffee facilities.'[104] A journalist for the *New Zealand Listener* enthused about the new 'pink room' at National Women's, with 'moire taffeta wallpaper, carpet, slimline venetians and gentle muzak'. This was a showcase room, the hospital's response, she said, to the pressure for low-tech birth.[105] Mothers could not book this room in advance, and the only requirement was that the birth was expected to be normal; as the manager of the delivery suite explained when Joan Donley inquired, the double bed could not be pushed through the door should a 'non-ambulant woman require delivery in a theatre'.[106]

A month after the 'pink room' opened, a delivery suite staff meeting recorded their belief that this facility should be available for all normal deliveries, and not solely 'to persuade those who wanted a home delivery to come to hospital'.[107] The hospital environment had most definitely changed since the 1950s; while the 'pink room' was a showcase, changing practices filtered down to affect other parts of the hospital as well.

Whanau Room

When National Women's opened in 1946 most Maori still lived in rural areas and did not give birth in hospital. However, by 1960, 90 per cent of Maori births occurred in a hospital, and by 1968 the percentage was 98.8, roughly equivalent to the non-Maori rate.[108] This trend coincided with the growing urbanisation of Maori, and with Auckland being the major destination.[109]

From the time of National Women's opening, Maori women gave birth there. In 2004, as part of her Master of Arts thesis in history, Christina Jeffery interviewed eighteen Maori women who gave birth there from the 1950s to the 1990s, and she found that for some, at least, it had been a positive experience. For instance, one of her interviewees who had a child in the old Cornwall hospital in the 1950s told her, 'It was nice there and the nurses were nice. I got to know them quite well. There were some Maori nurses, they were lovely, all of them, even the European ones were nice.'[110] Others commented on their delight in encountering other Maori women there, and Maori and Pacific Island women nursing and domestic staff.[111] For some Maori women, however, the hospital experience was less than satisfactory, with the main complaints being the lack of privacy and having to undress in front of male doctors.

Expectations held by Maori women and staff alike relating to birth experiences began to change in the 1970s and the 1980s in the light of broader social trends. The 1970s saw a heightened awareness of cultural sensitivity in the context of the international civil rights movement and local Maori activism. One result was the 1975 Treaty of Waitangi Act which allowed Maori complaints about breaches of the 1840 Treaty of Waitangi to be heard by a tribunal (which in 1985 was given retrospective powers to 1840). This was accompanied by a cultural resurgence, including the use of Te Reo (the Maori language) and an awareness of customs and practices, such as retaining the whenua (afterbirth or placenta) following childbirth so that it could be buried in a place special to the family. One woman, who first gave birth at National Women's in 1978, asked to keep the whenua and commented that there was a Maori nurse there who was 'probably educating her colleagues along the way', as it was not yet common practice.[112] Not all Maori women wanted to follow this custom, however. Jeffery recorded the negative response of another woman to obstetrician Colin Mantell (who was himself Maori) asking her if she wanted to take the whenua home in 1982.[113] In other ways, however, this woman appreciated a greater sensitivity amongst the staff. For instance, she commented that 'both the nurses and the doctors were always careful with blankets and things, making sure I was always covered when they were doing checks etc.'[114] Another interviewee, who gave birth there in 1980, commented on the hospital's willingness to allow visitors: 'I had crowds of visitors and no one ever said anything.'[115] The hospital was becoming more accommodating to different cultural demands.

In February 1988, at a time when Maori births comprised 12 per cent of all births in the Auckland region, a 'Whanau Room' was officially opened at National Women's for Maori mothers and their families. Medical superintendent Gabrielle Collison explained its objectives as being the 'sharing of resources, educating the young Maori mothers in traditional child care and in modern Pakeha care, changing of attitude within the health care system and bringing about environmental changes in the hospital'.[116] This development resulted from Collison's meetings with the Te Umere branch of the Maori Women's Welfare League, and the league provided resources for the room. The Maori Women's Welfare League itself dated back to 1951, set up in the context of Maori urbanisation, and it had a particular interest in the health and welfare of Maori women and children.[117] At the same time that the Whanau Room was established, two Maori community workers were appointed to work closely with Plunket nurses to provide 'a more effective support and health care service for young Maori women and their babies'.[118]

Feminising Childbirth Services

The goal of the new medical superintendent, Gabrielle Collison, appointed in 1984 as the hospital's first female incumbent, was to further feminise this institution to meet consumer demand. The same *Listener* article that reported favourably on the 'pink room' also commended the 'eminently sensible – and belated – move of having a woman medical superintendent for the country's major women's hospital'. The reporter described her as 'very feminine' and added, 'It's rather a local joke that she'll be best remembered for getting doors on the toilets [instead of curtains].'[119]

Like other areas of medicine, the profession of obstetrics and gynaecology was dominated by men, although by the 1970s and 1980s those in this specialty increasingly saw this as a problem. In her edited collection on New Zealand women doctors, Dr Rosy Fenwicke reminisced about her training at National Women's Hospital in 1980–81:

> At that time, there was no better place for a woman doctor wanting to advance her career in obstetrics and gynaecology (O&G). The largely male staff of consultants actively promoted women to train in the specialty. The teaching was inclusive and supportive and I especially remember the hugs and congratulations from senior staff when I passed the first part of my membership in O&G.[120]

In her contribution to the same collection, gynaecologist Hilary Liddell wrote:

> After I graduated I worked at NWH in Auckland as a house surgeon in the days when it was a powerhouse of male gynaecologists of international repute. It was a paternalistic, inflexible institution, but a hospital where the patients were put on a pedestal and the standard of care and continuity they received was exceptional.[121]

Liddell explained that Bonham worked to increase the number of women specialising in obstetrics and gynaecology. He recognised the obstacles to women choosing this path and introduced job-sharing to enable young women to combine families with their career. Liddell recalled that when she applied for the training scheme in 1978 Bonham was very encouraging and, in 'a typically far-sighted move', he arranged a job-sharing position for her and Lynda Batcheler, both of whom had young children.[122] Liddell also explained that Bonham later encouraged her to set up a recurrent miscarriage clinic at the hospital in 1987 after she had trained in London and worked in such a clinic there.[123] Bonham also established a part-time academic post in the mid-1980s for another young female gynaecologist with a family, Lesley McCowan. She later commented that he actively encouraged women into obstetrics and gynaecology.[124] Bonham's wife, Nancie, played her part; in 1968 she worked with Sandra Coney and others to set up the University of Auckland crèche, to enable new mothers to attend lectures.[125]

Dr John Werry, Foundation Professor of Psychiatry at the University of Auckland, reminisced about the early days of the Medical School in Auckland (opened in 1968). He explained that the number of women in the class rose each year to the point where it looked as if soon women would outnumber men. He said:

> At an HOD meeting in 1972, one of the professors expressed alarm at this as we all knew he said that women would go off and have children and never come back to medicine. He proposed that a quota should be put on women. He was joined by another head who said that because women matured earlier than men they presented better at interview but when they got into medical school they couldn't think especially scientifically. At that point Dennis [Bonham] exploded into one of his monumental and famous tantrums. Thumping the table he said

this is bloody nonsense, we have got to get far more women into medicine and into obstetrics in particular. Fortunately the idea [of quotas] then died an early death.[126]

In the 1960s and 1970s there were only a handful of women obstetricians and gynaecologists at National Women's. They included Jennifer Wilson, who started at National Women's but then moved to St Helens;[127] Margaret Liley, who was in charge of antenatal education from 1957 to 1984; and Florence Fraser, who started at National Women's in 1970. Two women paediatricians, Keitha Farmer and Pat Clarkson, joined the neonatal ward staff in 1970 and 1971 respectively. In 1976 Cecelia (Celia) Liggins joined the obstetrical staff.

English-born and trained, Celia Liggins was later described by fellow gynaecologist Lynda Batcheler as a 'very down-to-earth practical woman from Yorkshire', whom patients remembered with great fondness.[128] Celia had married Mont Liggins in 1956, and they held the distinction of becoming members of the RCOG at the same time: 'The examiners, who at first thought they were twins, said it was the first time they had admitted a husband and wife together.'[129] Celia ran a private obstetrics and gynaecology practice in Auckland from 1959, whilst bringing up four children and holding the fort during Mont's frequent absences overseas.[130] Five years after Celia joined the staff of National Women's in 1976, the HMC decided that it would be good to have a woman on the ethical committee which had been set up in the previous decade, and approached Celia.[131] She responded to the invitation to join the committee by saying that she would not do so 'as a member of a minority group'; however, she was persuaded to change her mind when Green and Howie proposed that she be appointed 'as a member of medical staff'.[132] Perhaps typical of many women of her generation, she felt it was important to be identified as a professional and not by her gender. The downside of this, according to the first male charge midwife at National Women's, Barry Twydle, who was appointed in 1982, was that patients could not be assured of more empathy by virtue of the obstetrician being a woman, although he did not say this with Celia in mind.[133] Midwife Val Dickens commented that Celia enjoyed an excellent rapport with patients, midwives and doctors alike.[134]

The goal of humanising National Women's Hospital, to which Bonham declared a commitment from the time he took up the chair in 1964, became more urgent in response to growing consumer demands for 'quality childbirth' over the next two decades. By the 1980s new family-centred spaces had been created within the hospital walls. This was partly a reaction to the negative public image of highly technological hospitals as against the smaller maternity units which some obstetricians did not consider a safe option for women in childbirth. It was also in response to a smaller but very vocal feminist campaign to opt out of hospital births altogether. The 1979 *Maternal Mortality Newsletter* warned that 'Women rejecting conventional care may become an increasing problem'; in response it recommended a 'flexible approach' to services.[135] However, a flexible approach was not enough to satisfy those rejecting conventional care, who became vocal and politicised during the following decade, a topic which forms the central theme of chapter 10.

CHAPTER 10

FEMINISTS, MIDWIVES AND NATIONAL WOMEN'S HOSPITAL

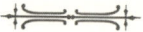

RADICAL FEMINISTS OF THE 1970S AND 1980S VIEWED SCIENCE AS patriarchal and medical technology as tools developed by men to control women and their bodies.[1] These feminists believed that men had no place in childbirth (except perhaps as husbands or partners providing support) and questioned the motives of male obstetricians. They were supported in this by midwives, who were fighting their own battles with the medical profession and became increasingly politicised during these decades.[2] National Women's Hospital, with its Postgraduate School of Obstetrics and Gynaecology, was perceived as a powerhouse of patriarchal male medicine and research on women's bodies. Its head, Professor Dennis Bonham, was described by feminist activist and independent midwife Joan Donley as 'the emperor [who] moulds the thinking of obstetrics and gynaecology in New Zealand'.[3] He was an emperor whom Donley and her colleagues sought to dethrone. A government inquiry in the late 1980s, ostensibly about a particular research programme led by Associate Professor Herb Green but effectively into the conduct of National Women's Hospital, presented them with this opportunity and considerably advanced the interests of feminists and domiciliary midwives at the expense of obstetricians and gynaecologists.

Bonham and the Women's Health Movement

Bonham saw opportunities in the new women's health movement. He claimed in 1980 to be 'delighted to find women questioning the birth service offered'.[4] He thought obstetricians and women should work together to improve women's health services. When Sandra Coney interviewed him about Green's research in 1986, he sought her help to lobby for an increase in the time allowed in the medical school undergraduate curriculum for obstetrics and gynaecology, which he said had been eroded over the years.[5]

Another of Bonham's initiatives from the early 1970s was an invitation to Coney to address medical students on 'Women in the New Society'. She delivered her first talk in 1973. She spoke at Bonham's request on other occasions, but later explained that she was eventually dropped after one visit when she decided to 'say what she thought instead of being lightweight and humorous'. She heard that Bonham found her 'too militant'.[6] In the late 1970s she was asked to speak on a panel together with someone from the Council for the Single Mother and Her Child, and later told the Cartwright Inquiry, 'Instead of just talking to the students we decided we would do a dramatised presentation of one of my colleagues' experience at National Women's Hospital, and Professor Bonham was present and became hysterical about what we were saying and shouted at us that it was lies.'[7] Nevertheless, her connection with National Women's continued, and she was still speaking by invitation at the hospital in 1987.[8]

While Bonham encouraged women in medicine, as discussed in the previous chapter, and attempted to draw in or work with feminists, from a feminist perspective there was little room for compromise or negotiation. The women's health movement questioned men's motives for involvement in women's health. Former women's groups had campaigned for free hospital care in childbirth and believed that pain relief in childbirth was a woman's right; the new feminists dismissed these women as having been duped by men (and 'honorary men', the women gynaecologists).

Feminist Views of Obstetricians

Many feminists believed that the introduction of men into the world of childbirth had been detrimental to women's interests and had been imposed on them against their will. Local feminist views can be gauged from the Auckland-based magazine *Broadsheet*, which was established in 1972 and edited by Coney until 1986. In 1974 it featured an article on childbirth, including an account of an International Childbirth Conference in Connecticut, USA, in 1973, attended by over a hundred feminists. The article quoted one speaker on the decline of obstetrical care with the advent of the male obstetrician:

> The male obstetrician, confident of his superiority over women and at the stroke of a jealous hand changed childbirth from a natural process to a barbarous event. Refusing to stoop in front of a woman he put her beneath him, prone on a delivery table. Male egos could be swabbed and satisfied with women flat on their backs and male control over women was complete with women strapped to a table with their legs spread wide apart in stirrups. Helpless and vulnerable women were forced into a position that was directly opposite to that which would allow quick and safe labour and delivery.... Doctors are known to plunge their fists into the vagina occasionally to check for dilation when women are experiencing contraction – an act that is calculated to intensify pain and increase humiliation.[9]

Thus she portrayed childbirth in the hands of a male obstetrician as a form of rape.

A few years later, Sandra Coney gave her own views on men's entry into obstetrics, which she believed was a result of 'womb envy':

> ... 'womb envy' explains man's determined, and largely successful, attempt to control who gives birth, and to whom, and how and where this will take place.... In alienating woman from her creative abilities during birth man has created the space for himself to step into the spotlight. In fostering her passivity, in keeping her ignorant, in isolating her from her familiar support systems, in promoting the view that birth is dangerous and unnatural he brainwashes and coerces her into powerlessness so that he can take over, do it his way and gain for himself the false emotional satisfaction that comes from believing that he is doing the birth.... The inert unconscious woman, hidden behind sterile theatre guards, allows the man to come the nearest he can to really giving birth – he can 'take' the baby – symbolically he can birth himself.[10]

Coney's co-activist Phillida Bunkle viewed obstetricians as misogynistic. She reminisced about her experience of total powerlessness at the birth of her first child in 1975. She said, 'As the doctor bullied and yelled and threatened, it became apparent that this was *his* theatre and *his* drama.' She recounted the glee with which he inserted stitches following an episiotomy without anaesthetics, his face 'alive with pleasure . . . . My flesh would no longer defy his power.' She added that, since then, she had listened to hundreds of women who had been abused by the medical system.[11]

Not surprisingly these feminists rejected obstetricians and hospitals in favour of midwives and home births. Midwives were natural allies, as consumer activist Judi Strid explained in *Broadsheet* in 1987, quoting a member of the UK Association of Radical Midwives: 'To be a midwife is to be with women – sharing their travail and their suffering, their joys and their delights.' Strid believed the medical profession's preoccupation with technology was simply a sophisticated strategy to undermine midwives, but she added that, throughout history and 'herstory', midwives had shown great determination to protect their position of supporting women in childbirth.[12] According to Joan Donley, the only 'real midwives' were those practising in the domiciliary field.[13]

Home Births and Joan Donley

By the 1970s home birth in New Zealand appeared to be a thing of the past. Bonham and Mackay's 1976 report announced that domiciliary midwifery, which was still funded through the maternity benefit, had 'almost disappeared'. In 1970 there were only 87 home births (comprising just 0.13 per cent of all births), and in the year following the 1971 Nurses Act, which made it illegal for midwives to provide maternity care unless a medical practitioner undertook responsibility for the woman in childbirth, there were only 24 such deliveries nationwide.[14] In the 1970s some doctors were prepared to support midwives delivering babies at home, and the number of home deliveries actually increased after 1972, as Coney reported in 1977. She wrote, 'Women must be seeing what's radically wrong with present maternity care to decide to ignore the scare tactics of doctors who tell horror stories about childbirth or even tell their patients it's illegal to have a baby at home.'[15] In 1979, 289 out of 52,279 births were known to have occurred at home (0.6 per cent of all births).[16]

There were only three home-birth midwives in Auckland at the time and, according to Coney, they found it difficult to keep up with demand.[17] One of these was Vera Ellis-Crowther. She had been a firm advocate for the availability of pain relief for women in childbirth back in the 1930s, but was later converted to the natural childbirth movement. By the time she retired in 1976 at the age of 79 she had delivered over a thousand babies at home.[18] The other two domiciliary midwives in Auckland were Carolyn Young and Joan Donley, who took over Ellis-Crowther's practice following her retirement.

Joan Donley was to receive an OBE for services to midwifery in 1989 and an honorary Master's degree in midwifery at the Auckland Institute of Technology in 1997.[19] Born in Canada in 1916, Donley (née Carey) had trained as a nurse and worked in a small hospital on the British Columbia coast where she delivered the babies of Indian women and loggers' wives.[20] She married in 1941, and the following year gave birth to the first of her five children. In 1964 she and her husband immigrated to New Zealand but divorced in 1970. She gained her New Zealand maternity certificate at National Women's Hospital and in 1971 did a midwifery course at St Helens and worked for two years at Waitakere Hospital. In 1974 she delivered her first baby at home, her granddaughter. Later (in 1979) Donley delivered her co-worker Carolyn Young's first baby at home.[21]

The practice and politics of midwifery became the major focus of Donley's life until she died, aged 89, in 2005.[22] 'It's your tea party', she told her mothers, 'I'm just here to help pour the tea.'[23] In her 1993 biography of Donley (as one of 21 'notable women in New Zealand health'), Patricia Sargison wrote, 'This dynamic grandmother continues to blaze trails in the fight against what she calls the "modern medical megalomaniac" which neglects to ask, "Whose body is it? Whose baby is it?"'[24] Donley herself argued in *Broadsheet* in 1985 that having a baby at home was a 'feminist and a political act', and that home birth was a 'challenge to the white, male-controlled obstetrics and gynaecology (O&G) which is trying to gain a complete monopoly of childbirth in New Zealand'.[25] One commentator, who called her 'our birthing matriarch', referred to her campaigning spirit and explained how she 'always talked about how on day three or four after the birth, she would talk to women and make them aware of the political issues'.[26] The 1997 National Homebirth Conference report described her as a 'homebirth midwife and political activist extraordinaire'.[27]

Home birth associations were set up in Christchurch in 1976 and Auckland in 1978. Donley explained that the founders of Auckland's association, Barbara Macfarlane and Deryn Cooper, were motivated by their 'anger at the powerlessness of women being forced into the medical model'. Cooper (who had a home birth in 1978) was a lecturer in psychology at the University of Auckland, and Macfarlane (who had two home births by 1980) was a law graduate. Both, according to Donley, saw home birth as a 'focus of women-power'.[28] As Rea Daellenbach later noted in her doctoral thesis on home-birth associations in New Zealand, activists sought to represent home birth as a right, a responsible decision and empowering for women.[29] Advocacy for home birth was often accompanied by promotion of breast-feeding, bed-sharing and non-immunisation.[30] Daellenbach also found that the activists tended to be white women; few Maori were involved in these emerging networks before the 1990s.[31]

Home birth was given a considerable boost in 1977 when TVNZ screened a 57-minute documentary produced by Parents' Centre president Helen Brew and R. D. Laing, a Scottish psychiatrist and well-known critic of modern psychiatry. Brew met Laing at a conference in London, and several years later, when Laing was visiting New Zealand to give the Vice-Chancellor's lectures at Victoria University of Wellington, Brew proposed to him that they make a film together. Brew had opposed hospital births since the 1950s; she had had her first two babies in the 'inhumane regime' of a hospital and her next three at home. She believed that a good birth experience would help to bring about a 'world of emotionally mature and loving human beings'.[32]

Brew and Laing recorded more than a dozen births around Wellington and the Hutt valley. They interviewed the women and Laing provided the commentary. The documentary won the Feltex award for best documentary for 1977 and the Best TV Film at the 1978 Melbourne Festival. Press reports claimed that it 'caused a row' about delivery methods in some New Zealand hospitals, fostered an interest in home birth, and sparked discussions and changes in several other countries.[33] Mrs Diony Young, director of the International Childbirth Education Association, recounted seeing the film at 'two very big childbirth conferences' in the United States.[34]

In his commentary Laing questioned how Western medical systems handled childbirth, which he categorised as 'one of the disaster areas of our culture'.[35] He argued that the conditions under which babies were born often led to the presentation of insanity later in life. He spoke of 'umbilical shock', the moment of cord-cutting when 'a few seconds can make a profound difference for the rest of one's life'. He claimed to remember his own birth, which he described as 'a body blow, a searing pain, a complete total organismic reflex'.[36] One of Laing's biographers said of the film that its reverberations lasted well into the 1980s, when Laing's preoccupation had become not only the 'process of medical birth but the therapeutic process of rebirthing'.[37]

Home births were also the subject of a lively debate at a seminar at Green Lane Hospital in 1976. National Women's paediatrician Jack Matthews argued that if all high-risk pregnant women were given the advantage of well-equipped, well-staffed hospitals, there would be fewer perinatal deaths. Dr Jill Calverley, a general practitioner from Kumeu and mother of two, responded that stillbirths and neonatal deaths were 'a form of natural selection and [she] felt mothers were philosophical about this'. In keeping with the psychology relating to the natural childbirth movement, she argued that juvenile delinquency was 'due to poor mother/child relationships which were initiated by the humiliating, terrifying experiences [for women] in hospital'.[38] Interviewed by Coney for *Broadsheet*, Calverley stated that she had no 'strong feeling' on hospital versus home births but that, 'If people are very interested in infant and maternal mortality and saving as many mothers and babies as possible – then yes, you must have your maternity hospitals. If women as a whole are prepared to accept a slightly higher maternal and foetal mortality, and perhaps enjoy a higher quality of childbirth, I'd say have home births as well.'[39]

In 1977 Colin Mantell was appointed professor of obstetrics and gynaecology at the University of Auckland. His inaugural lecture in 1978 was entitled 'Where should babies be born?' Not surprisingly, he argued the case for hospital births. Vanya Hogg, the 'Midweek for Women' columnist for the *Auckland Star*, described the lecture: 'Pacing the carpet square round the lectern in his beautiful imported shoes, Dr Mantell looked every inch a successful professional man.' He claimed to be an advocate for babies rather than mothers, and stated that labour and delivery were times of great risk to the baby. Labour, he said, was unpredictable: 'We should beware of the rose-tinted nostalgic view of hypothetical societies, young, robust and strong, glorying in the experience of delivering painlessly, simply, safely – for most [it] is simply not true.' Hogg noted that he was 'watched approvingly by the doyen of National Women's, Professor Denis [sic] Bonham'. She also noted that Auckland had 38 home-birth doctors at that time, and on the apparent risks quoted one doctor who said, 'The real nub and hinge of the whole matter, is what level of risk are we prepared to accept to enjoy the advantages.'[40]

In an interview with Jenny Wheeler of the *New Zealand Woman's Weekly*, Mantell reiterated that childbirth was unpredictable; he explained how a third of the problems came from normal pregnancies and claimed that the stage had been reached where the prospects for babies of very sick mothers could be better than the prospects for babies from unmonitored normal pregnancies. He added that the majority of women preferred to have their babies in hospital, but that these women were often forgotten in the debates.[41]

Another contributor to the debate was obstetrician Charles Jockel, who wrote to the *NZMJ* in 1979 in response, he said, to Margaret Crozier of the Values Party who 'blandly states that 40 percent of confinements could be handled in the home – presumably the "normal ones". I wish with my 30 years of obstetric experience I could forecast the 40 percent "normal ones". I shudder at memories of manual removals, PPH's, pulmonary emboli, inadequately repaired perineums, in a sagging bed in a poorly lit small room.'[42] National Women's principal nurse, Verna Murray, who had been nursing for 40 years when she retired in 1983, also supported hospital births, explaining that she had seen too many cases of home birth 'going wrong'.[43] So did Penelope Dunkley, a member of the national executive of the New Zealand Nurses Association and charge nurse of the neonatal unit at National Women's Hospital, who declared in 1979 that the hospital was the safest place to have a baby.[44]

Those supporting home births included Dr Victor McGeorge, an Auckland general practitioner and psychotherapist (and one-time president of the New Zealand Association of Psychotherapists) who had been delivering babies at home since 1942. He stressed the importance of bonding: 'If it fails to establish itself [in the first 24 hours] a vicious interaction may occur instead, with crime, depression, drug dependency and delinquency as its results.' He described those who chose home birth not as protesters but rather as concerned and responsible parents.[45]

In 1980 the first National Conference of Home Birth Associations was held in Auckland, with 150 attendees who formed a national incorporated Home Birth Association.[46] A panel discussion entitled 'What is the future of home birth in NZ?' included as speakers Drs Andrew Mackintosh and Tony Baird from National Women's and Sister Patricia Clark, supervisor of Auckland St Helens antenatal and outpatients' clinics. Opposing them on the panel were general practitioner Dr Ron Grieve, psychologist Dr Geoffrey Bridgman (the research officer for the Auckland branch of the New Zealand Home Birth Association whose wife Deryn Cooper was one of the association's founders), and Linda Daly-Peoples. Daly-Peoples, an Auckland lawyer, had previously published an article in *Broadsheet*, in which she described women as 'victims of discrimination in every conceivable area of their lives', and hospitalised childbirth as a 'major technique in the suppression of women, reinforcing their dependence in a male power structure'.[47] For her, the personal was political: the 'driving force' behind her involvement in the women's movement was, she said, the 'horrible' experience of giving birth to her first child in hospital; she had her second baby at home.⁴⁸ Donley summarised the debate, describing Mackintosh and Baird as 'conciliatory'. Mackintosh urged domiciliary midwives to collaborate with the hospital board and to book women into hospital in case they later needed to transfer them. Baird assured them that obstetricians were not their enemies, despite the impression given by some of the speakers. Donley was not convinced; nor was Daly-Peoples, who declared that until the twentieth century the human race had survived without being born in hospital and that it was time to reaffirm their faith in women and in the human race.⁴⁹

The Second Asia-Oceania Congress on Perinatology was held in Auckland in 1982. The guest speaker was Richard Beard from St Mary's Hospital, London, who had been obstetrics adviser to the British House of Commons Select Committee on Perinatal Mortality, which produced a report in 1980 advocating 100 per cent hospital delivery with electronic monitoring of every labour. During the congress the press reported Beard describing home birth as 'Russian roulette'.⁵⁰ Health Minister Aussie Malcolm, who opened the congress, also opposed home birth. According to Donley, however, he simply regurgitated the so-called dangers fed him by experts.⁵¹

Bonham's 1982 blueprint for the future of obstetrics in New Zealand, *Whither Obstetrics?*, recommended that all first-time mothers, all mothers over the age of 30, and any with a medical problem in their background should be classified as high risk and channelled into specialist care and delivery at a regional base obstetric hospital. There was no place for home delivery or home-birth midwives in his plan. Parents' Centre was apparently so upset by this report that it dismissed Bonham as one of its advisers.⁵²

Not all home-birth midwives were totally dismissive of Bonham, however. Sian Burgess, who was an Auckland domiciliary midwife from the time she arrived in New Zealand in 1979, later related an occasion around 1980 when Bonham asked to meet with a group of home-birth midwives. She said that when women whom the midwives transferred to hospital ended up under Bonham's care he would question them about their preferences. According to Burgess,

> ... he was a good communicator, he was a good listener and he would ask women what it was that had interested them in giving birth at home, was there something about the system that was different. He would ask them specifically about their care and he was one of the few doctors who would ask to view their records

because we kept, all my records are in there, about 2,000 women and he would look at maternity records.... [Bonham] was incredibly supportive of us, so I was ... really impressed with Bonham.[53]

It is clear from Burgess's account and others that Bonham valued professionalism, whether in midwives or doctors.[54]

In the 1980s domiciliary midwives became even more politicised by what they saw as a further attempt to squeeze them out of practice. In 1979 midwife education moved out of the hospital setting into technical institutes and became a postgraduate nursing diploma.[55] Whereas women prior to this date could undertake a course in midwifery following a maternity nursing programme, now they had to become a general nurse first. Domiciliary midwives saw themselves as separate and distinct from nurses, and together with consumers formed the Coalition for Maternity Action in 1980. A further amendment to the Nurses Bill in 1983 proposed that all midwives who were not trained nurses should work in a hospital, which further incensed these midwives and led them to form the Save the Midwife Association. Deryn Cooper thought the Bill was 'designed to demote the age-old profession of midwifery, subjugating the midwife to a role of assistant to the obstetrician and removing her as a practitioner in her own right'.[56] The association achieved a concession allowing direct-entry midwives already working as domiciliary midwives to continue to do so.[57]

Joan Donley wrote to the *Auckland Star* in 1983 that the real issues in the debate over home birth were obvious: it was a 'power struggle between obstetricians–hospital boards, with their huge investment in architecture and technology aggravated by a falling birth rate, and women who are trying to regain control over their bodies'.[58] She said of a 1984 review by Bonham and senior National Women's Hospital midwife Jan Clifton, that it displayed the 'contempt for consumers prevalent among powerful health professionals'. She also complained that the review accused the Home Birth Association of seeking confrontation rather than negotiation.[59] Yet confrontation was certainly on Donley's agenda: she conceived her 1986 history in terms of a political 'battle' for the home-birth option, explaining that she was marshalling information to be used when 'planning strategies, [and to aid] recognition of the traps and ambushes', and described obstetricians as 'generals in the war against normal childbirth'.[60] She might have found Mackintosh and Baird 'conciliatory' in the 1980 debate, but she was in no mood for conciliation herself.

The New Labour Government and Feminism

In 1984 a new Labour government was elected to office. Responding positively to the burgeoning women's movement, the government set up a Ministry of Women's Affairs in 1985 and appointed Ann Hercus as its first Minister. A midwifery journal quoted Hercus as declaring that at a United Nations World Conference for Women, the WHO set out a gendered vision for health by 2000, a choice between one that was 'sane, humane and ecological (SHE)' and a 'hyper-expansionist (HE) scenario, standing for unconstrained technological development'.[61]

The Board of Health had disbanded the Maternity Services Committee in 1983, before Labour's election. Bonham appeared to be puzzled by this development, which had occurred without consultation. He declared: 'This is something else I protest about. Perhaps I should just continue to grow orchids and stop worrying about the health of New Zealand women and children!'[62]

The Maternity Services Committee was replaced by a new body called the Women's Health Committee, a clear response to the new women's movement. Thanking Donley in March 1985 for a letter outlining her work with midwives and home birth, Labour MP Helen Clark wrote, 'We will have to watch very carefully to see that that committee does not become a vehicle for anti-midwife and anti-home birth advocates.'[63]

Donley believed this was indeed the case. She expressed her views in the newsletter of the New Zealand Women's Health Network, set up following the 1977 United Women's Convention. She complained that the Women's Health Committee included two 'MALE O&G SPECIALISTS', writing in capitals to emphasise her indignation and outrage. These were Colin Mantell and Richard Seddon, whom she declared had not been supportive of women's issues in the past. She wrote that the Ministry of Women's Affairs had promised a home-birth option, but wanted to know how Labour proposed to implement this policy 'when the power to make the changes has been placed back into the hands of those who developed the maternity services in their own interest in the first place'. The following issue of the network's newsletter contained a draft letter to the new committee describing it as a 'sell-out' and requesting that it not insult them further by suggesting that it represented the interests of women.[64]

A Health Benefits Review conducted in 1986 pointed to the growing influence of the small but vocal home-birth movement. The review noted that, although there were fewer than 40 midwives claiming the domiciliary midwifery benefit and that home birth represented less than 1 per cent of all New Zealand births, it had been the subject of many submissions. The review stated, 'The ability of pressure groups in this area to make some headway against the medical establishment demonstrates their growing influence.'[65]

The mid-1980s saw a strong and growing feminist movement ready to take on the medical profession, aided by a Labour government which was fighting its own battles with the medical profession.[66] The feminists' opportunity arose when a local magazine, *Metro*, published an article in June 1987 by Sandra Coney and Phillida Bunkle on a medical scandal at National Women's Hospital. Readily accepted by the public, the government and some members of the medical profession, this was described by one local medical journal as a 'bombshell'.[67]

The 'Unfortunate Experiment' at National Women's Hospital

Coney and Bunkle's article, 'An Unfortunate Experiment at National Women's', resulted in Labour's Health Minister Michael Bassett hastily announcing a government inquiry. Silvia Cartwright, a district court judge (and later, from 2001 to 2005, New Zealand's Governor-General), was appointed to lead the inquiry and issued her report in July 1988. The article and the subsequent inquiry argued that Herb Green had divided his patients who presented at National Women's Hospital with a positive Papanicolaou ('Pap') cervical smear (a test for carcinoma *in situ* or CIS, which could lead to cervical cancer) into two groups, one treated conventionally and the other subject to medical experimentation, leading in the latter group to cervical cancer and, in some cases, death.[68]

There were never two such groups of patients at National Women's. The basis for the two-group theory was an article published by some of Green's colleagues at the hospital in 1984.[69] The authors of this article retrospectively divided patients who had come to National Women with CIS into two groups, and demonstrated from the records that those who had continued to have a positive smear over time were more likely to develop cervical cancer than those whose smear had reverted to normal. The authors stated clearly that these outcomes were regardless of treatment. The main author, Dr Bill McIndoe, confirmed to Coney that treatment did not enter their study, and the statistician involved in the study also affirmed that there had never been two groups who were differentially treated.[70] What the *Metro* article and subsequent inquiry had picked up on was an internal dispute between practitioners at the hospital about the appropriate treatment for CIS, and they significantly misinterpreted a crucial medical paper.[71]

Green was among a generation of doctors who, like British professor of social medicine Thomas McKeown, had grown sceptical of modern medical intervention.[72] Specifically, in relation to positive cervical smears Green questioned the need for radical responses such as hysterectomy or cone biopsy, responses which had emerged initially in America in the 1950s following the discovery of the Pap smear test but founded on no evidence.[73] Judge Cartwright later held, 'I have come to believe that Dr Green was in fact trying to prove a personal belief.'[74] This was far from the case. There was a substantial international literature questioning an aggressive approach to CIS and an increasing realisation that most smears (up to 95 per cent) would revert to normal over time and would not develop into cervical cancer (this was before the discovery of the Papillomavirus, which helped to explain the disease further). In 1977, for example, the Australian gynaecologist Malcolm Coppleson argued that 'many thinking gynaecologists' questioned the 'true indispensability' of cone biopsies and hysterectomies for CIS 'in the light of the increasing numbers of follow-up studies reporting excellent results from minimal interference in patients with abnormal smears and pathology'.[75] Moreover, there was an increasing awareness that cell changes occurred so slowly that intervention was possible if it was indicated during careful monitoring.[76] Subsequent studies have reaffirmed that approach.[77]

The medical tendency to over-react in relation to positive Pap smears had been picked up in the feminist literature in Britain and America before the inquiry, with one writer commenting: 'Only in a male dominated society could doctors have such a disregard for a woman's physical integrity.'[78] As British feminist medical sociologist Tina Posner was to write a few years after the inquiry, in 1991: 'The "medical dilemma" [in relation to CIS] was . . . to know when to treat the abnormality and when to leave it alone because no harm would result from doing so, whereas intervention could lead to a variety of unintended negative consequences.'[79] The irony of Green being effectively on the side of the feminists in his approach to CIS was lost at the time.

The important point, however, was that Green's research was based on an analysis of the data relating to all women with CIS at National Women's over an extended period treated by any of the 20 or so consultants at the hospital. He did not, as was later alleged, 'choose' or 'recruit' women for a study.[80]

Indeed, he treated his own patients on a case-by-case basis and was more forthcoming in explaining options to them than were many of his colleagues, as Bonham noted at the inquiry.[81]

Following the inquiry, the president of the RCOG asserted that Green 'undoubtedly had a profound effect on reducing the degree and number of unnecessary interventions' and that 'many thousands of women would be grateful for that'.[82] Nevertheless, the myth that Green had engaged in unscrupulous research, dividing his patients into two groups for the purpose of experimentation, persisted. In a speech to the 1990 General Scientific Meeting of the Royal Australasian College of Surgeons, Liggins commented how the 'famous' 1984 article was 'misinterpreted by the authors of the *Metro* article and by the judge. Once rolling, such minor matters became irrelevant to the course of the judicial inquiry which allowed its brief to expand to encompass every possible area of medical practice (fees excepted) about which there was public concern.'[83]

Green himself had retired in January 1982 and, as Liggins suggested, the details of his so-called experiments became sidelined as attention focused on modern medical politics. Cartwright concluded in her report, purportedly about a past medical experiment, that current National Women's staff were 'extraordinarily insensitive' and that there was a 'pervading atmosphere of defensiveness and even arrogance, [which] does not bode well for the future care of patients at National Women's Hospital'.[84]

In setting up the inquiry Bassett had stated the importance of having an 'all-women Inquiry', suggesting that the emphasis was on the relationship between women and their male gynaecologists rather than on establishing whether there had been any medical wrong-doing at National Women's. In its submission to the inquiry, the Ministry of Women's Affairs viewed the situation through a feminist lens, lamenting, 'Women are the major consumers of health care but our reproductive health is dependent on the attitude and skills of men who dominate medicine, in policy-making and practice.'[85]

Coney too explained that their intention had been 'to broaden the inquiry beyond the specific events at National Women's Hospital into a general critique of the practice of medicine, observance of patients' rights and the treatment of women within the health care system'.[86] They succeeded. In 1988 *Broadsheet* hailed the Cartwright Report as a feminist victory.[87] Cartwright herself later told *North & South* magazine: 'Because I had a Family Court background and was a feminist, I conducted that inquiry as a feminist and as a lawyer.'[88] In 1989 an article announcing that Cartwright had been given a presentation by a local feminist group, the Auckland Women's Health Council, included a photograph of her with Coney, Bunkle and an ex-patient Clare Matheson. The article opened with the words: 'Four women who took on the might of the medical profession'.[89]

Health Minister David Caygill, who had succeeded Bassett in August 1987, pronounced after the release of the Cartwright Report that 'future confidence in doctors would be largely dependent on the way they responded to the report. If they can respond in the same forward looking response that I can discern in the report, we can avoid a repetition of what has happened.'[90] In this way he contributed to a climate in which it was extremely difficult for doctors to question the findings of the report; as journalist Jan Corbett put it, 'for doctors to speak out in that climate would have made them look foolish, defensive and chauvinistic'.[91]

Following the inquiry, Fertility Action called for a 'fresh start' with new personnel at National Women's Hospital.[92] The New Zealand Medical Association (NZMA, successor to the NZBMA) requested an investigation into the conduct of doctors involved in cervical cancer research at National Women's Hospital. This further muddled the issue, as the inquiry had been about the treatment of pre-cancer and not cancer. However, importantly the NZMA hoped that such an investigation would help to restore public confidence in the profession.[93] Coney complained the following year that, 'Some of the doctors who publicly displayed disbelief and defiance [at the inquiry] are still stalking the corridors at National Women's.'[94]

Bonham retired as head of school in February 1989 after pressure from the NZMA and Fertility Action.[95] The Auckland Women's Health Council warned the Chancellor of the University of Auckland that bestowing emeritus status on Bonham would be an endorsement of his conduct, would distress many women and would be 'an insensitive step on the part of the University'.[96] He was denied emeritus status. Colin Mantell took over the headship of the Department of Obstetrics and Gynaecology following Bonham's retirement. Donley wrote to him, pointing out that the Cartwright Report had highlighted the arrogance of the medical profession, and asserting that women should play a major role in the decision-making process relating to their bodies and interests. She suggested that Mantell approach British obstetrician Wendy Savage as a possible replacement for Bonham, as in doing so, 'your Department would be demonstrating, both nationally and internationally, that the criticisms and recommendations of the Cartwright Report are being taken seriously and that there IS a will to confront and resolve old habits and attitudes'.[97]

Mantell received letters from others such as the Maternity Action Alliance. They told him that an appointment made from within New Zealand would be detrimental to women's health as it would perpetuate the teaching of Bonham and Green. They too supported Savage, on the grounds that she had proved not to be threatened by the reallocation of power to women and had experience in challenging medical authority.[98] Karen Guilliland, chair of the midwives' section of the New Zealand Nurses Association, wrote that women would trust Savage, which was necessary for them to regain their faith in health providers. She thought Savage would provide a role model for doctors, midwives and nurses, and restore the morale of New Zealand's maternal and child health services.[99]

Wendy Savage was a controversial figure. She had been suspended as senior lecturer and honorary consultant in obstetrics and gynaecology at the London Hospital after allegations of incompetence in 1985 but was exonerated and reinstated following a public inquiry.[100] She had previously spent three years in New Zealand in the 1970s, at Cook Hospital, Gisborne, where she had set up a family planning clinic.[101] She unsuccessfully applied for the chair in obstetrics and gynaecology at Wellington in 1983.[102] She was not appointed to Auckland, though the successful candidate was a woman from outside New Zealand, Dr Gillian Turner from Bristol. Back in Britain, Wendy Savage lamented that there had been 'remarkably little interest' in the Cartwright Inquiry in British obstetric and gynaecological circles, which she said, 'irritates the hell out of me because the issues apply equally to women here'.[103]

In July 1990 the Medical Council of New Zealand fined Bonham for disgraceful conduct for his part in the 'unfortunate experiment'.[104] During the Medical Council's deliberations, Bonham's counsel produced letters of support from 33 patients and 51 doctors, including Professors Sir John Scott, Sir Graham Liggins and Colin Mantell, Associate Professor Ross Howie, and the Dean of the Auckland Medical School Derek North.[105] Four of Auckland's female gynaecologists, Lesley McCowan, Hilary Liddell, Cindy Farquhar and Lynda Batcheler, wrote to the editor of the *NZMJ* declaring their support for Bonham. They were concerned that the negative publicity overshadowed his major contributions to obstetric practice in New Zealand.[106] Despite his long and distinguished career, Bonham's obituary in the local daily press declared that he was 'best remembered for his part in what became known as "the Unfortunate Experiment at National Women's Hospital" which led to charges of disgraceful conduct'.[107]

Following the inquiry, Bonham was summarily dismissed from the Maternal Mortality Research Committee, which he had led since its inception in 1969. The committee itself was disbanded in 1991, following an unsuccessful manslaughter charge against an anaesthetist. As Karen Guilliland and Sally Pairman explained in their 2010 history of the New Zealand College of Midwives, 'Following the manslaughter case, specialists refused to undertake analysis of cases fearing that their reports, obtainable under the Crimes Act, could be used to prosecute their colleagues and that they would also be required to account for their assessments in a court of law.'[108] When the committee was re-established in 2006, confidentiality legislation gave protection to the committee's processes as they were classified as quality-assurance activities and therefore not subject to the Official Information Act. As noted earlier, Bonham had believed that the previous committee's engagement in audit made it one of New Zealand's earliest forms of quality control in medicine.[109] In a period of profound public distrust of doctors, this view had counted for little.

Midwives and the 1990 Nurses Amendment Act

Interviewed for *Time* magazine in mid-1990, Helen Clark, Health Minister from January 1989 until November 1990 and a future Prime Minister, commented that the Cartwright Inquiry had politicised women's health and, discussing outcomes, she referred specifically to the Nurses Amendment Act 1990, which was due to come into force on 28 August 1990. She explained to *Time* that this legislation effectively made midwives equal to doctors in maternity care. In granting midwives the right to deliver babies without a doctor's involvement, it reversed the 1971 Nurses Act. But it went further, entitling midwives to provide antenatal care and to hold access agreements with area health boards in order to attend their clients during labour and birth in hospital facilities. It also entitled them to prescribe medicines and order laboratory diagnostic services that were commonly used during pregnancy and childbirth. Clark described this as 'an important move in curbing over-intervention in childbirth and encouraging a questioning of the medical model'. Donley, who was also consulted for the article, explained that the Cartwright Inquiry had changed the climate because it 'undermined the status and credibility of the obstetricians and gynaecologists', which made it easier for this legislation to happen.[110]

In her PhD on maternity services in New Zealand in the 1990s, Sally Abel noted that Helen Clark had been responsible for the 1990 Nurses Amendment Act, and that to some extent she had been influenced by Donley who wrote regularly on the issue to Clark as her local MP. Yet the proposal also appealed to Clark generally. Her commitment to strengthening the public health and health promotion orientation of the health system was evident in her introduction of the Health Charter and the Smoke Free Environments Act 1990. Also, as Minister of Labour she was proposing pay equity legislation to redress gender differentials in pay – and pay equity was to become an important component of the 1990 Nurses Amendment Act.[111]

At the same time, midwives were busy establishing their own professional organisation. A 1988 meeting of the Midwives and Obstetric Nurses Special Interest Section of the New Zealand Nurses Association, set up in 1972, decided to disband the section and establish a New Zealand College of Midwives, because they believed that the Nurses Association was undermining midwifery. The New Zealand College of Midwives (NZCOM) was officially formed in April 1989.[112] The college claimed to be different from most professional bodies in that it included consumer representation: 'Midwifery is intertwined with women and we are unable to separate ourselves from them – neither do we wish to! It is the women who define our practice and who give us our direction.'[113] New Zealand was not alone in this development. In Australia, a National Midwives Association had been formed in 1977. In 1983 it voted to split from the Royal Australian Nursing Federation and its nursing ties, and in 1987 formally became the Australian College of Midwives.[114]

On 18 August 1990, ten days before the Nurses Amendment Act was passed, Helen Clark opened the 1990 NZCOM National Conference. She explained that she had become interested in maternity services in two respects: first, how women's occupations were valued and the status they were accorded, and secondly, the way in which the treatment model had come to dominate the health service.[115] She explained that as Minister of Health she had the opportunity to do something about the injustice encompassed by the loss of autonomy for midwifery. In looking at options, she found that she had 'surprising allies' in the form of Treasury, which could also see strong arguments against an 'anti-competitive' monopoly of childbirth services by medical practitioners.[116] Citing this speech, historian Philippa Mein Smith noted how the 1990 Act fitted into the neoliberal political climate initiated by the fourth Labour government; she explained, 'Significantly, the Nurses Amendment Act 1990 suited both feminist and economic rationalist agendas.'[117]

In her speech to the midwives, Clark explained how the Nurses Amendment Bill introduced to Parliament in November 1989 had attracted 96 submissions, which were generally supportive. However, some submissions had questioned whether the safety of the mother and the child could be guaranteed by the change in the law. Others expressed reservations about the adequacy of midwifery training and accountability. She stated, 'While these concerns would merit serious attention if they were well based, it is my judgement that they are not.'[118] Clark also revealed that she strongly supported the home-birth option.[119] *North & South* magazine later reported, 'Clark says she changed the law to promote home births, which she viewed as more cost-effective than hospital ones.'[120] She also favoured direct-entry midwifery as a means of encouraging women who would not otherwise be attracted to the nursing profession to consider midwifery training.[121] Parents' Centre wrote to Clark congratulating her on the passage of the 1990 Nurses Amendment Bill.[122] Midwives became autonomous practitioners, and Otago Polytechnic and the Auckland Institute of Technology set up direct-entry midwifery programmes.

Abel pointed out that concerns about the 'safety' of midwifery practice and the call for 'team work' were to be ongoing features of the medical profession's responses to midwifery autonomy in the 1990s. The terms 'safety' and 'team work' had considerable rhetorical value, she wrote, but from the perspective of midwives the terminology 'masked the hidden agenda of medical control of the birth process'.[123]

While the Bill was before Parliament, an article in the *Listener* explored the difference between midwives and doctors, between 'natural' and 'technological' births. Amongst others, the article quoted Nelson domiciliary midwife Bronwen Pelvin:

> Giving birth, says Pelvin, can be an empowering experience which will affect a woman for the rest of her life: give her a minute to roll up her sleeves and she'll climb that mountain or become the first woman prime minister. But a woman who has been 'delivered', whose baby has been mastered by obstetric technology, so often comes out of it feeling like a victim 'violated in the worst way'. And a woman who does not have a good birth experience, says [local GP, Diana] Nash, 'will not mother easily'.[124]

Such pronouncements could lead to high expectations for women in childbirth which might easily come crashing down if problems occurred, apparently with dire consequences for the mothers. In her history of motherhood in New Zealand, Sue Kedgley quoted Donley explaining that if a woman had a drugged birth and could not hold her baby straight away, 'her innate mothering skills are suppressed'. Kedgley also quoted Judi Strid's view that this could 'profoundly influence a woman's relationship with her partner and child'.[125] While some feminists accused doctors of scare tactics when persuading women to give birth in hospital, they were not averse to using scare tactics themselves.

In October 1988 Coney was invited to speak at the Auckland Medical School about 'The Unfortunate Experiment: Implications for the Profession'.[126] In 1989 the university's Postgraduate Medical Committee invited Dr Ann Oakley as the 1989 ASB Visiting Professor. Oakley was a British feminist and author of many books and articles on women's health. The Dean of Medicine Derek North responded to the University Council sub-committee on the Cartwright Report (the Ryburn Committee) that this visit had been planned some months before the Cartwright Report and not in response to it.[127] These invitations show the university and the postgraduate school's willingness to continue to engage with these self-critical issues.

The public image of obstetricians and gynaecologists had been dealt a severe blow. A 1993 *North & South* article on childbirth referred to the 1984 piece by Carroll du Chateau (at that time Carroll Wall) in *Metro*, entitled 'The Glamorous Gynaecologists', where she had marvelled at the high-tech procedures which had taken over conception, pregnancy, birth and infancy (see chapters 6 and 7). The journalist wrote, 'Nine years on, du Chateau winces at the memory and says how much things have changed for the better . . . . Obstetricians and gynaecologists are today members of a battered and defensive profession. They are most certainly not gods. They are no longer glamorous.'[128] *North & South* pointed out that another article, by Coney and Bunkle, had been an important catalyst for the change of climate, and that the Cartwright Inquiry which followed had made it politically acceptable to question the medical establishment. Among its many repercussions, the journalist said, it gave impetus to the home-birth movement's calls to allow midwives to practise without a doctor's supervision.[129] For National Women's Hospital it was the end of an era.

CHAPTER 11

A HOSPITAL IN TROUBLE, 1990–2004

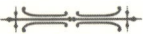

A 1993 AUCKLAND AREA HEALTH BOARD SURVEY FOUND THAT NATIONAL Women's Hospital had a poor public profile and was generally seen as a hospital where staff were under stress and the facilities run down.[1] Two years later, Jeffrey Robinson, professor of obstetrics and gynaecology at the University of Adelaide, was invited to lead a review of the hospital and provided a frank assessment of the problems it faced. He and his review team declared, 'Unfortunately, all is not well within National Women's Hospital.' This report too noted the dilapidated facilities for patients and staff. But it also commented on low staff morale and considered that communication problems had been compounded by a lack of trust between different professional groups and by rivalries between subgroups and individuals within groups. The review team thought this had led to a culture which fostered 'fear, anxiety and stress'.[2]

The major challenges of the 1990s were dealing with the aftermath of the Cartwright Inquiry and restoring public confidence in the hospital's services, teaching and research, in a climate of staff shortages, new management structures and legislative changes to maternity services. The academic side of the hospital, the reputation of which suffered a blow from the Cartwright Inquiry, gradually regained some of its former international status, but it was an uphill struggle. Another setback came at the end of the decade with a new judicial inquiry, this time in the newborn unit. This chapter focuses on various stakeholders, including mothers, nursing staff, midwives, GPs, consultants and academics, as they negotiated through the quagmires of the 1990s.

Management and Resource Problems of the Early 1990s

In 1989 the position of medical superintendent of National Women's Hospital was disestablished, making Gabrielle Collison redundant, and Sue Belsham was appointed general manager, in line with modern market-orientated trends in public sector and hospital management.[3] Belsham explained at the time that the 'changes were long overdue and reflected a new determination to recognise the consumer'.[4] However, she did not remain in the post for long, and by the time of Robinson's review in 1995, the hospital had had seven general managers.

Several factors influenced the functioning of National Women's in the early 1990s. One was a dramatic increase in the number of births as a result of the closing of Auckland's St Helens Hospital in June 1990. In 1989 there had been 5341 births at National Women's and 3618 at St Helens; in 1991 there were almost 9000 deliveries at National Women's.[5] The hospital struggled to cope with this expansion.

As part of the amalgamation of St Helens with National Women's, Anne Nightingale, principal nurse at St Helens from 1973 and recipient of a CBE for her services in 1988,[6] was appointed manager of maternity and neonatal services at National Women's, a post she held until 1995. She described National Women's as a 'sick hospital' when she arrived in 1990 and 'in deep gloom' following the Cartwright Inquiry.[7] She had expected other staff from St Helens to come with her, and some did. However, one midwife at National Women's told a reporter in 1990 that they were 'absolutely desperate for staff to the point of being unsafe', regretting that the staff who were expected to transfer from St Helens had not done so.[8] An article in the *New Zealand Nursing Journal* later that year also referred to a 'dire shortage' of midwives at National Women's.[9] The staffing crisis had in fact preceded the closing of St Helens. In March 1990, a *New Zealand Listener* article on maternity services claimed that the shortages had already led to one tragic result: 'a baby died in the hospital recently because staff were too busy to notice a foetal monitor showing that the baby was in distress. The parents were left alone for 84 minutes.'[10]

Despite the construction of two new delivery suites in 1990, the hospital was overcrowded, which, along with the run-down conditions, increased the pressure on nurses and midwives. The problem was exacerbated by an outbreak of methicillin-resistant staphylococcus aureus 'superbug' in 1990, which saw one postnatal ward closed temporarily.[11] Before the new delivery suites were ready, the overcrowding had reached crisis point. An obstetrician told the press that babies had been delivered in hallways because women arrived late in labour and the delivery suite was full. Two other doctors confirmed the corridor births.[12] A press report in October 1990 related how one pregnant woman was informed there was 'no room at the inn' when she rang National Women's to book in for the birth of her child. She turned up anyway, and found eleven others in labour but only three midwives and one doctor on duty.[13]

Physical conditions which received considerable publicity in the early 1990s included unclean toilets and cockroach infestations, with one report claiming that cockroaches were driving mothers away. It noted that these insects had been found on beds and in babies' cribs, in bathrooms, and in kitchens where babies' bottles were stored, with one patient finding 'up to 20 cockroaches crawling on the floor of her ward'.[14] Cockroaches became a symbol in the media for the hospital's malaise. Yet another report declared that cockroaches were not the worst problem facing patients. One mother, a former nurse, discharged herself twelve hours after giving birth because she felt neglected and because, she said, provisions for babies were non-existent. The article cited Nightingale who said that babies' supplies had been cut in a bid to help mothers to adapt to the outside world; the hospital was encouraging mothers to be thrifty by using toilet paper or the ends of nappies to clean their babies. She denied there had been cost-cutting measures and said staff were teaching mothers good habits. Recognising the publicity as a further attempt to defame the hospital, Nightingale pronounced that National Women's had been 'bashed enough' in the wake of the Cartwright Inquiry.[15] Concerns about the 'squalid' conditions at the hospital continued to be given publicity well into the 1990s.[16] One woman giving birth there in 1996 remembered the midwives looking 'frazzled, just too many women and too much to do'.[17]

One solution to the staff shortages was the recruitment of nurses and midwives from overseas. Nightingale had drawn attention to the lack of locally trained midwives as early as 1988, attributing it to the lack of an effective midwifery training course once nursing education had moved from the wards to tertiary institutions after 1979. In her eyes this accounted for the fact that up to 85 per cent of midwives in New Zealand hospitals were trained overseas.[18] By the mid-1990s National Women's was 'forced to take its search for midwives to

England and Australia'. The hospital was apparently short of 38 midwives, but had only managed to recruit eighteen locally.[19] Two National Women's representatives, Sandra Budd and Nicky King, visited the UK and offered jobs to 30 midwives.[20] The following year, the *New Zealand Herald* declared, 'all around are the voices of British midwives who are plugging the gaps'.[21]

Consumer Demands
'Choice' for consumers was a buzz word of the early 1990s. This had been a powerful rallying point for the New Zealand College of Midwives since its formation in 1989 and for those who advocated home births. They argued that women had the right to choose home births and independent midwives. National Women's invoked the same rhetoric as it sought to meet consumer demands. Describing the two new delivery units in 1990, *New Zealand General Practice* magazine declared that they 'incorporate[d] society's changed attitude toward birth and the expectations by the users of maternity services that they have choice in the care they receive'. General Manager Sue Belsham stressed that the units (with eleven and twelve beds respectively) were the result of consultation with women as users. The magazine described the units as 'family-centred', including rooms large enough for the father and children to spend time comfortably with the mother and baby. They also had access to outdoor spaces, while other facilities included an en suite and spa bath, with medical equipment hidden from view, creating a 'homely, low-tech non-threatening environment ... which can spring into high-tech quickly with a minimum of fuss'.[22]

Ironically, creating a more relaxed and less institutionalised environment did not suit all women who used the facility. In 1991, 'the irate mother of a 12-day-old baby claims her confinement at National Women's Hospital was ruined by the noise of unruly pre-schoolers dumped on other mums in the ward by dads who slouched all day in the TV room'. The mother said: 'The TV room is where a lot of mothers go to feed their babies. But often the room was full of men stretched out on the chairs, who didn't even bother to get up and give you their seat.'[23]

Mothers' complaints about noisy visitors, which had come to the staff's notice in the 1980s, continued into the 1990s. One woman complained about a group of relatives coming to see a Fijian woman and her baby, carrying large boxes. She thought they were presents, but found, 'after some sort of ceremony, they opened the boxes which contained food, and had a big feast, right there in the room', with food spread out on the beds. Nightingale responded, 'We allow people to do what is culturally appropriate when a new child is born. Other women may not agree with it, but we won't stand in the way of what they think is culturally correct.'[24]

One mother went so far as to organise a petition relating to conditions at National Women's. This was sparked by concerns about security at the hospital following the kidnapping of a baby who was fortunately returned safely. The organiser, Mrs Stewart, scolded, 'The present conditions are unacceptable, and it has been that way for far too long. A lot of people feel very sternly about the issue.'[25] Mrs Connolly, who helped to organise the petition, stated that the ease with which they collected a thousand signatures demonstrated widespread dissatisfaction with services at National Women's.[26] What eventually became a 5000-signature petition was sent to the Auckland Area Health Board in July 1991 and criticised the 'flexible visiting hours, the lack of security, and relaxed eating rules'. Nightingale responded that she would be reluctant to return to the stricter visiting hours of ten years earlier.[27] And, indeed, the relaxed atmosphere at least in the delivery suite did suit some women. One of Christina Jeffery's interviewees, who gave birth at National Women's in 1995, described her birth experience:

> The delivery was like a Kodak moment, a real epiphany really. I had my twin sister there and she was giving me wonderful foot massages, and [her husband] was there too. So my two favourite people in the world were there and encouraging me to push. My parents were behind me, and this whole team of people. My other sisters were there as well, so it was a real family experience. And the Kodak moment was when they were both telling me to push and the glee on their faces when they could see the head coming out, they both were looking very happy. It was definitely a very positive experience.[28]

One innovation which came directly out of the Cartwright Report was the appointment to the hospital of a patient advocate. Judge Cartwright had concluded 'with some regret' that she could not 'leave the encouragement of new habits and practices to the medical profession alone', and recommended the appointment of 'an independent and powerful advocate for the patient'.[29] She thus portrayed the relationship between doctors and their patients as adversarial, with the patient requiring strong support to counteract a powerful medical profession.

Lynda Williams was appointed patient advocate to National Women's and Green Lane Hospital in August 1989. Williams had four children (her last child was born at home in 1984, and she later commented, 'Giving birth at home is undoubtedly one of the most empowering experiences of a woman's life').[30] Williams had worked in private practice as a childbirth educator for ten years and was also employed as coordinator of Fertility Action.[31] On her appointment she told the press that, from her own childbirth experiences, 'she knew what it was like to feel helpless and powerless and not have the support needed to make choices'.[32]

Williams was patient advocate at National Women's for the next two and a half years, and her later comments about her experiences suggested her relationship with other staff had been adversarial. She complained about being 'constantly undermined'. She found charge nurses, midwives, senior consultants and junior doctors equally culpable, explaining that none of them would give her time to explain the problem before launching a personal attack on the person for whom she was advocating. She added that 'there were a few encounters with medical staff that tested every ounce of control and restraint I had as they made their unbelievably sexist and patronising attitudes towards women patently clear'.[33]

Williams might have found a hostile environment within the hospital but she also complained that women weren't allowed to stay long enough. In 1995, writing about early discharge, she cited one woman who left two days after her baby was born. She pointed out that mothers who remained in hospital had access to 24-hour midwifery care: 'If something happens to the baby in the middle of the night . . . there's always someone there while the woman is adjusting to something new and feeling vulnerable.' Sandra Coney also believed that early discharge increased the risk of feeding problems being overlooked.[34] Williams was still expressing concern about this three years later.[35]

Concerns about exploiting women in a teaching hospital, which had been highlighted in the course of the Cartwright Inquiry, also led to a new approach to teaching medical students. Dr Helen Roberts introduced Gynaecology Teaching Associates (GTAs) in 1992. She trained women volunteers to instruct medical students to perform gynaecological examinations. Recruited primarily through the Family Planning Association, GTAs were mostly health professionals and educators.[36]

Consumer activists continued to be disgruntled with National Women's, however. Robinson's 1995 review cited Coney's address on 'Quality in health care: A consumer perspective' to a Health Quality Management Conference in 1994. She told the conference that consumer groups felt excluded from National Women's, with little opportunity to contribute to the formulation of policy or the functioning of clinical areas. She also believed that women were not given enough information.[37] Following the 1995 review, the hospital opened a Women's Health Information Centre 'to give women and their families easy access to free information about issues and services in women's health'. Sandra Budd, then manager of Maternity Services, thought this 'a major step forward in empowering women to take charge of their own health'.[38]

Consumer activist Judi Strid was appointed to run the centre. Strid had been the consumer representative on the working party that established the College of Midwives and a member of the Auckland Maternity Services Consumer Council, set up in 1990 to 'enhance the consumer lobby' in maternity services.[39] Strid also represented the Auckland Women's Health Council at the 1992 Maternity Benefits Tribunal, established to determine pay rates for midwives and general practitioners for maternity services. Submissions to this tribunal had shown just how active consumer groups continued to be in the politics of maternity. These included Parents' Centre New Zealand (Inc.), fourteen local Parents' Centre branches, Maternity Action (Tauranga), Patients' Rights Advocacy Waikato Inc., Federation of Women's Health Councils (Auckland), The Health Alternatives for Women (Inc.) (Christchurch), Women's Electoral Lobby (Waikato) Inc., Auckland Women's Health Council, Women's Health Special Interest Group (Birkenhead, Auckland) and the Auckland Maternity Services Consumer Council.[40] Most of their submissions strongly endorsed the right of women to choose their childbirth practitioner.[41]

National Women's Hospital and Independent Midwives

In their 1994 address to the New Zealand College of Midwives, Karen Guilliland and Sally Pairman (at that time past and current presidents of the college) claimed that a partnership between midwives and women had been forged out of the climate created by the Cartwright Inquiry. The partnership, they said, was a political one, with midwifery having 'responsibilities as an emancipatory change agent', which required it to identify as a feminist profession.[42] The college was firmly rooted in feminism. Guilliland and Pairman dedicated their 2010 history of the college to Joan Donley as its 'official founder'; they held that without her 'amazing insight, conviction and energy' it would never have come into existence.[43] Throughout their history they portrayed women and midwives as partners fighting for women's interests against a predominantly male obstetrical profession. As Guilliland had told a journalist in 1993, it was not just about the choice of providers: 'It's a bigger picture than doctors versus midwives. It's the containment of women's rights. It's to do with the control of women's bodies by doctors. Midwifery is a partnership which helps women to make their own decisions.'[44]

A 1990 *New Zealand Listener* article explored the tensions in maternity hospitals between doctors and midwives. The article cited John Hutton, professor of obstetrics and gynaecology at Wellington Women's Hospital from 1983 (before that he had worked for a time at National Women's in Auckland), who claimed that 'the lack of trust and communication' between midwives and medical staff had almost reached crisis point. He blamed the midwives, referring to a 'small cabal of at least five Wellington Women's Hospital midwives' whose philosophy, he said, 'embraces not only radical feminism but misology [a distrust of logical debate]'. At National Women's, GP-obstetrician Diana Nash related how she encountered a great deal of hostility and tension between doctors and midwives, with new doctors given 'a horrible time' by midwives. By contrast, Lynda Williams, also interviewed, said that she had seen midwives who questioned medical decisions being 'eaten alive by very forceful, intimidating doctors'. Obstetrician Denys Court was adamant that this 'adversarial system of childbirth with all its animosity' was not helping the patient.[45]

The article did not specify whether the midwives referred to were hospital-based or 'independent' (self-employed), but there did appear to be particular tensions with the new independent midwives. The 1990 Nurses Amendment Act brought a new kind of midwife into the hospital setting. That year there were around 50 independent midwives working in New Zealand, who attended about a thousand births. Three years later there were 350 handling 11,000 births, and by 1995 there were over 500 independent midwives.[46] Gaining access agreements to deliver babies in hospital, these midwives could offer women a choice of birth place. Robinson's 1995 review noted that 118 independent midwives had access agreements with National Women's Hospital.[47]

Despite being given the choice of home or hospital, most women continued to opt for a hospital birth. Home births made up just 2 per cent of all births in 1990 and remained around that level in the following years.[48] Midwives came with their clients into hospital, sometimes causing tensions with medical staff and hospital midwives. In 1993 National Women's obstetrician Tony Baird commented on the 'division and distress in hospitals' caused by independent midwives: 'Hardly a day goes by when someone doesn't complain to me about a private midwife sweeping in and being rude to the ward staff. They behave in the same manner they criticise doctors for.'[49] A few years later he expressed his belief that medical practitioners were undermined and undervalued by midwives and not the reverse: 'Each week this month one of them [resident staff] has come to me upset, in two instances in tears because of the way they have been treated by midwives.'[50] Gillian Turner, a British obstetrician who was professor of obstetrics and gynaecology at Auckland from 1993 to 1999, later referred to 'the fearsome vehement single-minded feminist group of independent midwives'.[51]

In their history, Guilliland and Pairman commented on tensions between independent midwives and hospital midwives following the 1990 Act. They wrote that some independent midwives treated hospital midwives 'with disdain and disrespect making their workplace a place of continual tension'.[52] Yet Guilliland said of hospital midwives who trusted doctors that they were 'astonishingly naive and display[ed] oppressed group behaviour', adding her belief that failing to 'confront the issue [of midwives' "struggle" against doctors] is to deny women's struggle for autonomy'.[53] Hospital midwives were thus betraying the cause of feminism.

Hospital midwives on the other hand complained about the attitudes and pay rates of independent midwives. In 1994 one midwife from National Women's Delivery Unit 2 wrote an impassioned letter to general manager Sheryl Smail, asking her how she would feel if 'a new person moved into the office next door to you, her salary per hour was six times yours and you were asked to assist her in her role because there were aspects of the job she was not skilled to do'. This, she said, was how she and her colleagues felt.[54] Midwives from this unit had written a submission to the 1992 Maternity Benefits Tribunal complaining about the pay inequality between hospital and independent midwives, contrasting their $15 per hour to provide care at all levels with the $140 per hour paid to independent midwives as caregivers for normal obstetric patients.[55] Robinson's 1995 review commented on the poor relationships between hospital and independent midwives, with the former 'often feel[ing] side-lined and under-valued'. He described them as a 'disempowered workforce with low energy levels and increasing patient numbers, remunerated differently from their colleagues'.[56] A 2001 article on New Zealand midwifery also noted that hospital midwives felt like 'second-class midwives compared to their [independent] colleagues'.[57]

The tensions between hospital-based and independent midwives were mirrored by tensions between obstetricians and independent midwives. Obstetricians were not slow to point out that intervention rates had not gone down following the 1990 Act, which had been one of the selling points of the independent midwifery system. National Women's Hospital began publishing annual clinical reports in 1992, and in 1994 initiated a system whereby an 'expert' was invited to review the statistics. The first reviewer was James King, an obstetrician at the Mater Women's Hospital in Brisbane and Queensland director of the Perinatal Database. He noted that 7 per cent of the births at National Women's were booked under independent midwives, and that only 64 per cent of those had spontaneous deliveries, 14 per cent had caesarean sections and 19 per cent forceps. He found these high rates of caesarean section and forceps surprising for a group of women who should have been carefully screened: 'These results are way way higher than the Australian Birth Centres statistics so they are of concern.' He also looked at the outcomes for the 'domino' midwives (an acronym for 'domiciliary midwife in and out') whom National Women's employed from 1993 to look after women from the antenatal to postnatal periods. King reported, 'although only a small number at 207 births they have a 12% incidence of forceps and 15% c-section so if the role of midwives is being increased to address the high intervention rate – he would question whether this is actually being achieved'.[58] He noted that the rate of inductions by private obstetricians was 27 per cent, by public teams 20 per cent and by independent midwives 20 per cent. Again he was surprised at the high rate for independent midwives' clients since they should have been in the low-risk category.[59] Peter Stone, who came to National Women's to head the Maternal Fetal Unit in 1998, also later commented that the expected reduction in intervention following the 1990 Act had not occurred; rather the intervention rates 'inexorably climbed' in the 1990s.[60] Caesarean section rates did indeed increase from 15 per cent in 1992 to 23.7 per cent in 2000.[61]

There was a feeling amongst obstetricians that midwives were not referring women with problems to specialists early enough. A 1994 article in *Consumer* magazine questioned whether midwives knew when to transfer cases. It also noted that while the 1990 law had provided for 'radical change', no national database had been established to monitor results. There were no records of how many births involved an independent midwife, or what the intervention rates were for each group. The article added, 'More importantly, we do not know what effect different birthing practices have had on the safety of childbirth.'[62]

Anne Nightingale later commented on the 'violent swing' following Cartwright from 'professional control' to 'patients' rights', which meant that structures for patient safety were not necessarily in place. As manager of maternity and neonatal services she sought to review the access contract system for outside practitioners (doctors and midwives) to enter the hospital and to set up protocols for handover, to protect staff as well as patients.[63]

The press picked up on disputes between doctors and midwives in the mid-1990s. A 1995 article in the *New Zealand Herald* was dramatically headed: 'Babies dying for need of proper care says doctor'. Dr Allan Sutherland, a member of the Medical Practitioners Disciplinary Committee and a GP who had delivered more than 3000 babies, claimed knowledge from his work on that committee that babies were dying or being injured through lack of proper medical care during birth.[64] He was backed by Baird, then president of the Royal New Zealand College of Obstetricians and Gynaecologists,[65] who said that he was called out at least once a day when he was on duty to take over a case which had needlessly become dangerous. Referring to the attitudes of some 'natural birth lobbyists', he said, 'We are tired of being called the bad guys when all we really care about is the mothers and the babies.'[66]

Guilliland responded that the advent of independent midwives had not led to poorer maternity standards. She referred to the National Women's annual clinical reports of 1992 and 1993 as 'quite clearly illustrating the continued decline in baby deaths'.[67] She invoked the Cartwright Report and claimed, 'Midwives and women throughout the world, including New Zealand, are challenging the medical profession's claims to absolute truth.' At the same time she believed that 'many' doctors were responding positively to independent midwives and were 'working collaboratively with midwives and women in an effort to improve maternity care'.[68]

While Guilliland saw women and midwives as having common interests, not all women supported independent midwives. In February 1997 the *Sunday News* published an article entitled 'Home births under scrutiny'. This stated that six women who had given birth to brain-damaged or dead babies after deliveries by independent midwives were asking questions. One mother, herself a trained nurse, blamed her 'bad delivery' on an independent midwife and launched a 'baby safety campaign'. She was joined by several women who had similarly given birth to brain-damaged or dead babies in the past three years after deliveries by independent midwives.[69]

There was further adverse publicity for independent midwives in October 1997 when Robyn Stent, appointed as the first Health and Disability Commissioner in 1994, published details of a baby who had died at Hutt Hospital in 1996 under the care of an independent midwife.[70] Stent concluded that the midwife had failed to provide reasonable care and skill, and Hutt obstetrician Dr Howard Clentworth said it was an 'example of lack of consultation which was typical of some midwives'.[71] The Nursing Council eventually removed this midwife from the College of Midwives Register, but Stent had published her findings before the Nursing Council had investigated the case. The College of Midwives severely criticised her for this, and described it as a 'trial by media'.[72] Certainly it received a lot of media attention. A *New Zealand Herald* article declared, 'Maternity system puts mothers and babies at risk'.[73] Sandra Coney also stressed the need for accountability in an article entitled 'Nurses need to be as accountable as doctors'.[74]

Following the widespread publicity around this case, Guilliland leapt into damage control: in a press release she reassured women that, 'Babies have never been safer in New Zealand's history. Women choosing a known midwife are even safer.'[75] She rightly reminded women that most births were normal. Midwives had by this time become central to maternity services following changes in the funding structure, which had resulted in many GPs exiting from childbirth services.

GPs and Section 51

One unforeseen outcome of the 1990 Nurses Amendment Act was its apparent impact on the maternity services budget. The Act set the rate of pay for prolonged attendance at birth (after one and a half hours) for midwives and doctors at $139.60 per hour. This boosted midwives' salaries in particular as, unlike doctors, they tended to stay with the mother throughout the birth, so that according to a 1993 *North & South* article, the five top-earning midwives earned an average of $203,862 during a ten-month period, which it noted was considerably more than the prime minister. This article pointed out that Helen Clark was concerned about the sums claimed by midwives, and had said this was not what she expected when she promoted the Act. Government spending on primary maternity care had risen from $47.5 million in 1989-90 to $90 million in 1994.[76]

In an edited volume on health care in New Zealand in the 1990s, Dunedin GP obstetrician Glenn Blanchette also reviewed the different patterns of attendance by midwives and doctors, and came up with the following calculation: 'In contrast to the average GP claim of $600 for up to 1.5 hours in complicated cases, midwives are often with a woman in labour for eight to twenty-four hours and midwifery claims ranged from $2,000 to $3,000 for normal cases.' Like the *North & South* article, he blamed this for the doubling of the government's maternity benefit expenditure from 1990 to 1994.[77]

Guilliland disputed that midwives were responsible for a budget blow-out in maternity services and looked forward to the day when almost all babies were delivered by midwives. 'We'd be like GPs are today', she enthused to *North & South*.[78] However, shared care between GP and midwife seemed to be the preferred choice for many women. *Consumer* pointed out in 1994 that most of the estimated 11,000 women then using an independent midwife were also cared for by their doctor; having a GP and midwife was 'still the most common choice made by New Zealand women'.[79]

In the context of the general cost-cutting budgets of the 1990s for social services under a neoliberal National government elected in 1990, policy-makers looked at options to reduce the cost of maternity care. Section 51 of the 1996 Health and Disability Services Act contained a new schedule for payment of maternity benefits.[80] This placed all providers in competition for the one set of fees by way of the concept of a 'lead maternity carer', chosen by women amongst the available providers. Blanchette maintained that the change had predictable results. For a GP who had to subcontract a midwife (as they were unable to provide all the requirements of section 51 themselves), there was no cheap option and most gave up.[81] The number of independent midwives continued to grow: by 1997, there were about 600 of them.[82]

In 1997 Parents' Centre conducted a survey on maternity services, and found that 91 per cent of its 168 respondents were dissatisfied with the 'lead maternity carer' scheme, and would have preferred to have both a midwife and a GP.[83] Guilliland questioned how representative this was, given that only 168 out of the 8000 members of Parents' Centre responded. She commented, 'Parents Centre has been a naïve partner in the political campaign to undermine women's trust in the normal process of birth, and the midwifery services that attend them.'[84] Nevertheless, the *New Zealand Listener* concluded in 1999 that the so-called 'choice' offered by the 1996 changes had been illusory, as having a doctor in the role of lead carer was no longer a choice for most women. At that time fewer than a hundred New Zealand doctors were available for maternity care.[85] The number continued to decline. By 2004 there were between 30 and 40 GPs practising obstetrics in New Zealand, and in 2005 when GP-obstetrician William Ferguson resigned as maternity spokesperson for the Royal College of General Practitioners and opted out of providing maternity care 'in despair', the *New Zealand Herald* declared this would leave just fourteen obstetrician-GPs in New Zealand.[86] At National Women's there were a hundred GP 'access holders' in 1996 and just nineteen in 2000.[87]

What's the Buzz? Building Staff Morale

The 1995 Robinson Review acknowledged the problems that had beset National Women's and praised it for continuing to function: 'the clinical commitment of the nursing, midwifery, medical and technical staff . . ., despite low morale and low trust between professional groups, have continued to demonstrate a high professional commitment to patients' care'.[88] Nevertheless, the review recommended better leadership and improved lines of communication, and advised appointing a new general manager as soon as possible.[89]

The attempt to revitalise the hospital was dubbed 'Project 95'.[90] Dennis Pickup, the acting manager of the hospital and chief executive officer of the Auckland Central Crown Health Enterprise, seconded Dr Nigel Murray from the New Zealand Army, where he had been assistant director of Medical Services, for six months, to implement the changes. Murray's restructuring included appointing a new general manager, Gary Henry, who stayed in the post for the next five years. He appeared to be a popular choice with staff, dubbed 'Henry the Eighth' because he was the hospital's eighth manager in seven years.[91] Henry came to the hospital after eleven years at Melbourne's Royal Women's Hospital, where he had been the first non-medical CEO. According to the Royal Women's Hospital historian, under his influence the hospital had been open to new ideas, making the 1980s 'the most creative decade in the hospital's history'.[92]

Other changes occurred in the hospital, and a new newsletter, initially called *Project 95* and then *What's the Buzz*, kept staff informed. Murray appointed Sandra Budd, a nurse and midwife who had worked at National Women's for fourteen years, principally in the neonatal service, as manager of maternity services.[93] She replaced Anne Nightingale as acting manager in 1995, and became manager in 1996, a post she held until 2001 when she was head-hunted by the Women's and Children's Hospital, South Australia. Neil Pattison was appointed clinical head of maternal fetal medicine (later succeeded by Peter Stone), and Carolynn Whiteman was appointed manager of newborn services. During her time as manager of maternity services Sandra Budd led reviews of both consumers and staff; in 1996 she interviewed 175 medical, midwifery, clerical, ancillary and other hospital staff, aiming to improve communication.[94] That year Marjet Pot, a consumer advocate with a background in the Home Birth Association, was appointed Maternity Access Rights Co-ordinator to improve relations between hospital and independent midwives.[95] The following year, Professor Robinson was invited back to lead yet another review, this time of the obstetric and gynaecological staffing.[96] In 1997 the hospital employed a research company to undertake 'a major customer focused market research survey'.[97] In 1996 gynaecology services returned to the hospital from Green Lane where they had been relocated following the Cartwright Report. In 1997 the hospital also appointed a Maori Health Manager, Aroha Harris, who had written a report in 1994 on health services for 'Maori consumers' based on 161 interviews and which included a section on childbirth.[98] Two years later the hospital established a separate Maori midwives team to provide midwifery care to Maori and Pacific Island women.[99]

One initiative of the late 1990s was the construction of a new private wing, the Cornwall Suite. Described as 'a silver-spoon birth service', this was set up in response to consumer demand, and in competition with a private midwife facility called Birthcare that had been established in 1987.[100] The Cornwall Suite proved 'immensely popular' with women.[101] This short-lived venture ended prior to the hospital's move to Auckland City Hospital in 2004, and was not replicated at the new site, where all rooms had en suites.[102] Meanwhile, Birthcare secured a contract with the Auckland District Health Board to provide postnatal facilities to women and babies born at National Women's and also established birthing facilities for women who chose to give birth there.

The Academic Unit at National Women's Hospital
Recommendation 24 of the 1995 review was that National Women's Hospital 'should seek to regain and maintain its pre-eminence in research'. The reviewers noted that their 'attention was particularly drawn to the absence of strong academic presence in gynaecology and midwifery', a state of affairs they attributed to the Cartwright Report. They also commented on 'the absence of any records by which the review team could assess the overall research output of the hospital'.[103]

The Postgraduate School of Obstetrics and Gynaecology had been set up as part of National Women's Hospital with the appointment of the first postgraduate professor in 1951. The salary of the postgraduate chair was funded through a trust fund (the Obstetrics and Gynaecology Endowment Fund), from the fundraising orchestrated by Doris Gordon. Thus, when Auckland's Medical School was established in 1968, the Postgraduate School was funded separately and remained autonomous, with the professor reporting directly to the Auckland University Council through the Vice-Chancellor and not to the dean of the School of Medicine.[104] This created an anomaly for the Medical School, which had its own Department of Obstetrics and Gynaecology for undergraduate teaching.

From the time the medical school opened, Associate Dean David Cole, who was in charge of postgraduate studies, believed there was no reason 'other than sentimental' to maintain the postgraduate school in its present form.[105] The university reviewed the situation in 1973, and again in 1976, following the appointment of Cole as dean of medicine in 1974. The university and the school agreed in 1976 that 'the teaching unit should be named the Department of Obstetrics and Gynaecology (incorporating the Postgraduate School of Obstetrics and Gynaecology)'. Colin Mantell was appointed to a chair in obstetrics and gynaecology with special responsibility for undergraduate teaching. Dennis Bonham continued as head of the newly created department in his role as the senior professor.[106] However, tensions between the Postgraduate School and the School of Medicine continued. In 1979 senior staff at the Postgraduate School told the Vice-Chancellor that they were 'saddened by the continual pressure' from the Dean to 'submerge' the school into the School of Medicine.[107] In 1987 Bonham again complained to the University Registrar that the Dean appeared to be conducting a campaign to destroy the Postgraduate School.[108]

Following the Cartwright Report, Cole told the University Registrar that the Postgraduate School should now be disbanded as an entity, adding, 'I think the death knell for this Department has been the Inquiry, but it was in recent times a contrivance perpetuated largely by Dennis Bonham . . . . [the] Postgraduate School is an anachronism.'[109] Cole got his way and the school was disbanded, with its functions absorbed into the Department of Obstetrics and Gynaecology University Academic Unit. The postgraduate chair was kept and was advertised following Bonham's retirement in January 1989. However, it took four years to fill the post. Dr Gillian Turner, consultant senior lecturer obstetrician and gynaecologist at the University of Bristol since 1973, was appointed to the chair in 1992 and took up her post in March 1993. The following year she became head of department when Mantell, who had replaced Bonham as head in 1989, moved to Middlemore Hospital. Turner remained until 1999, when she returned to England.[110]

The demise of the Postgraduate School which had attained such a high international standing was the end of an era for National Women's Hospital. In an attempt to salvage its academic reputation in obstetrics and gynaecology, the university rebranded the academic side of the hospital in 1989, approving the establishment of a new Research Centre in Reproductive Medicine in the Department of Obstetrics and Gynaecology. The centre was administered by Mont Liggins as director, assisted by Professor John France as associate director, a management committee, and a board of trustees. The chair of the trust was John Hood, CEO of Fletcher Building and later Vice-Chancellor of the University of Auckland.[111] The Academic Unit attained some international recognition when senior lecturer Cynthia (Cindy) Farquhar, who was developing tertiary services in reproductive endocrinology, was appointed Cochrane Collaboration Coordinator in Menstrual Disorders. As the hospital's 1996 *Annual Report* recorded, this occurred with the support of National Women's Hospital, which provided funding.[112]

New appointments occurred in two other areas in the 1990s, in 'maternal fetal medicine' and neonatology, completing the post-1950 move to acknowledge the medical needs of the fetus and newborn baby as well as the mother.[113] Maternal fetal medicine was the new label for dealing with pregnant women who had complicated medical problems, such as diabetes and recurrent miscarriage. A special maternal fetal department was set up in 1993.[114] In 1998 the university established a new chair in maternal fetal medicine, with Peter Stone as founding professor and clinical director of maternal fetal medicine. In 1999 the department proudly reported, 'unlike our neighbouring maternity hospitals in the Auckland region, we have not had a maternal death at National Women's Hospital in the last 6 years. This is due to the high level of vigilance and expertise provided by the multidisciplinary Maternal Fetal Medicine service consisting of obstetricians, physicians, midwives and anaesthetists.'[115]

Another area of development was neonatology, which, like maternal fetal medicine, was part of an international trend. In 1997 Jane Harding, a former Rhodes Scholar who had been senior medical officer at National Women's since 1989, was appointed professor of neonatology, the first such appointment in New Zealand. Her personal chair was in 'recognition of her eminence in the profession and her achievements in both clinical medicine and pure research'.[116] Harding spent half her time on research, and the other half as a paediatrician in National Women's neonatal intensive care unit.

In 2001, in a further attempt to restore Auckland's international standing in reproductive health and medicine, the University of Auckland established a new research institute for the study of the fetus and the newborn, named after one of National Women's pre-eminent researchers, Sir Graham Liggins. At the official opening of the Liggins Institute in 2002 the director, Professor Peter (later Sir Peter) Gluckman, announced, 'Sir Graham has been our mentor, friend and inspiration and we plan to continue the pioneering traditions he has set for New Zealand medical science.'[117] The Queen, Prime Minister Helen Clark and a hundred invited guests attended the opening, welcomed by the Chancellor of the University of Auckland, John Graham, the Vice-Chancellor Dr John Hood, and Peter Gluckman.[118] In 2003 the university reported that the institute was 'rapidly becoming known for . . . groundbreaking research . . . . The institute has four groups of scientists investigating critical questions surrounding: pregnancy and labour, the foetus and newborn; the brain and behaviour; and growth, development and ageing.'[119]

When Peter Stone took over from John France in 2001 as head of the Division of Obstetrics and Gynaecology in the Faculty of Medical and Health Sciences, he observed that the University Department of Obstetrics and Gynaecology was inextricably linked with the hospital service. Stone worked collaboratively with the new hospital manager 'for common goals to enhance National Women's Hospital and its important position as the Centre of Excellence in Women's Health locally, regionally and nationally'.[120] In so doing he was seeking to dispel the negative association between patient care and research, a legacy of the late-twentieth-century climate which had given rise to the Cartwright Inquiry. Liley would have seen the seeds of the separation between clinical care and research being sown much earlier, however, in 1960 when the professor was no longer the director of the hospital, as discussed in chapter 3.

NICU and the Cull Report
In the 1990s the hospital had two units for newborn babies with medical problems: the Neonatal Intensive Care Unit (NICU) with sixteen cots, and the Special Care Babies Unit (SCBU) with 48 cots, making it the largest of its

kind in Australasia.¹²¹ By this time more premature babies than ever were surviving. Interviewed in 1997, neonatal paediatrician Tania Gunn said that when she first started in this field in the 1970s, critics said, 'Babies under 1,500g, forget them all!' Then it was babies under 1000, then 750, until by 1997 babies of 500–600 g or under were considered viable.¹²² A report at the end of the decade noted that in 1974, 60 per cent of babies with birth weights of 1001–1500 g (approximately 31 weeks' gestation) survived, whereas by 1999 more than 95 per cent survived. In the weight range of 501–1000 g, the survival rate had improved from 10 to 80 per cent.¹²³

During this period some commentators claimed that paediatricians were 'playing God' when they intervened to save babies who would otherwise die and argued that nature should be left to take its course.¹²⁴ There was nothing new in this: as noted in chapter 5 the Plunket Society had been accused of this in the 1920s when it set out to rescue premature babies. Yet the long-term health risks for extremely small babies surviving in the 1990s were still unknown. An article in the *New Zealand Woman's Weekly* in 1997 noted, 'Critics point out about one in five premature babies with a very low birth weight (under 1500g) is significantly disabled. There's a risk of cerebral palsy, loss of vision and hearing, low intelligence and other difficulties that may not become apparent until the child reaches school age.'¹²⁵ According to a 1999 report, National Women's records confirmed that the incidence of serious adverse outcomes for premature babies in terms of neurological functioning was around 20 per cent.¹²⁶ However, it was not the long-term health outcome for preterm babies that came into the public eye in the late 1990s, but rather a method used to treat them at the hospital.

The scandal which rocked National Women's at the end of the 1990s once again affected its public profile. The *Sunday Star-Times* commented that it revived the spectre of Cartwright; here again was 'a new treatment introduced without consent which had devastating results'.¹²⁷ The treatment referred to was chest physiotherapy provided for preterm babies in National Women's neonatal unit. Physiotherapists had started using this treatment in 1985, following overseas practices.¹²⁸ The treatment consisted of tapping the baby's chest with a soft latex face mask to clear chest secretions. From 1993 the hospital also trained nurses in the technique so that it would be available on a 24-hour basis.¹²⁹

Between September 1992 and June 1993 three newborn premature babies developed an unusual brain lesion. Such lesions also affected a further ten babies born between September 1993 and September 1994. Noticing there was a cluster of babies with brain lesions in their unit in February 1994, doctors began a case control study to identify the cause, and also contacted colleagues in Birmingham, England, following a literature search which revealed a cluster of similar brain-damaged neonates at Birmingham Maternity Hospital.[130] In December 1994 they decided the most likely link was with the chest physiotherapy being practised. They stopped the treatment immediately, and informed the parents of the affected babies.[131] Of the thirteen babies affected (with birth weights between 675 and 1100 g), five had died. The hospital issued a press release in February 1995 and alerted all other neonatal units in Australia and New Zealand.[132]

When informing the parents, staff indicated that they would be eligible for ACC for medical mishap, as the brain lesion was a serious and rare complication of medical treatment.[133] Applications to the Accident Compensation Corporation were successful. However, the ACC Medical Misadventure Advisory Committee determined that the injury sustained by two babies after receiving chest physiotherapy constituted medical error. It referred the matter to the Director-General of Health, who ordered an inquiry. The members of the inquiry team were Helen Cull QC; Dr Philip Weston, neonatologist at Waikato Hospital; and Jan Adams, Waikato's director of nursing.

The report, released in July 1999, vindicated the actions of National Women's staff. It declared that the steps taken to research and publicise the results of the link between chest physiotherapy treatment and the brain lesion were 'timely and appropriate'. It concluded that the hospital staff deserved 'commendation for their openness in acknowledging the tragic occurrence within their unit, to alert others of the potential consequences'.[134] The report made a number of recommendations, considered relevant for all neonatal units in New Zealand. The recommendations involved improvements in communication, consent processes and peer review. The Ministry of Health set up a working party to develop guidelines.[135]

The same month the report appeared, Sandra Coney announced in *The Lancet* that 'parents of damaged infants want greater accountability and compensation for the families'.[136] One of the parents of a baby who had developed cerebral palsy laid complaints against three paediatricians, ten nurses and six physiotherapists, and he was subsequently joined by others. The Medical Council, the Nursing Council and the Board of Physiotherapists heard the complaints respectively. Gary Henry, the hospital's general manager, expressed surprise at the actions of the parents, 'in the light of last year's Government inquiry which concluded that no individual was to blame for anything that had happened'.[137] The respective disciplinary bodies did not uphold the charges of malpractice, but not before the incident had received considerable media exposure.[138]

In 2002 an article in a British paediatric journal, describing the inquiry and critiquing neonatal chest physiotherapy, elicited a heated response from paediatricians within Britain, who lamented that scapegoating health professionals by media and politicians was fashionable.[139] Certainly what happened in Auckland was not unique. Two years before the Cull Report, a scandal which had broken out in England also received extensive adverse media exposure. It too was in a neonatal unit, in North Hampshire Hospital, Basingstoke. The story broke with a newspaper report in 1997 declaring, '43 premature babies, many only a few hours old, died or suffered permanent brain damage after being used as "guinea pigs" in a radical hospital experiment'. The campaign, headed by one set of parents, led to a government inquiry. The original article did not mention that the 32 babies in the control side of the trial suffered similarly, and this was not picked up by the press. It took a decade before allegations against hospital staff were dropped, by which time they had suffered severe demoralisation.[140] The 1980s and 1990s saw public trust of health professionals at an all-time low, in New Zealand as elsewhere, aided by the press.

National Women's came under fire yet again in March 2002 when the *New Zealand Herald* published an article headed 'Baby research breached ethics'.[141] The article stated that a pioneering study on cooling the heads of potentially brain-damaged newborns to limit injury had breached ethical guidelines. The controlled trial, carried out in 1996–97 by 'medal-winning researcher' Professor Peter Gluckman, paediatrician Associate Professor Tania Gunn and her son Dr Alistair Gunn, who was also a paediatrician, was written up in the journal *Pediatrics*.[142] It compared ten babies kept in the normal temperature range with twelve in whom minimal or mild hypothermia was induced for up to 72 hours through the use of a 'cooling cap'. The cap, which fastened under the baby's chin like a bonnet, circulated cold water through tubes next to the head, with the aim of preventing cerebral palsy and other complications of asphyxia. A North Health ethics committee had approved the trial, but the report in *Pediatrics* showed that the babies and the water were cooled below the approved temperature. The *Herald* article reported the MRCNZ's chief executive, Dr Bruce Scoggins, saying, 'Although it was not possible to establish precisely how the breach occurred, the evidence would appear to indicate that omitting to submit the amendment to the committee until November 1997 was an inadvertent error by Dr Tania Gunn.'[143] Gunn herself had died in 1999.

The 2002 *Herald* article also reported that the Auckland study had led to an international trial. The trial featured in the *Herald* two years later when it boasted: 'A head-cooling cap developed in Auckland is expected to save the lives of thousands of brain-damaged babies worldwide, after a successful international trial proved its effectiveness.' This article reported that a four-year trial at 28 hospitals in four countries had found that a quarter of lightly brain-damaged babies were saved by the cap, and that the rate of cerebral palsy and other movement disabilities among those who survived was cut from 28 to 11 per cent. Gluckman, who led the US$5–7 million (NZ$8–11 million) trial, told the reporter, 'This is the first time ever that people have shown that brain damage can be reversed in newborn babies.... Worldwide, the cap could save thousands of newborn babies every year.'[144] Taken together, the two *Herald* pieces demonstrate how perceptions of National Women's see-sawed between accusations of breaching ethics and praise for its ground-breaking international research.

National Women's Hospital Closes
By the time of Robinson's 1995 review, National Women's days as a stand-alone unit were numbered: the review referred explicitly to the 'plan to rebuild National Women's Hospital at the Auckland Hospital [Grafton] site'.[145] This was in part owing to the disarray at the hospital following the Cartwright Inquiry, but was also in line with international trends to reintegrate women's health into mainstream medicine. For instance, four years after National Women's was moved, Melbourne's Royal Women's Hospital was relocated in 2008 to Melbourne Hospital, a large general hospital.[146]

The planned move was part of a bigger project by the Auckland District Health Board, hailed as 'the largest health redevelopment in New Zealand's history'. This involved a building project costing in excess of $420 million, concentrated within a new high-tech acute hospital in Grafton, the site of the existing Auckland Hospital, and centralising many of Auckland's medical services. The decision to move National Women's to the Grafton site was announced in 1999, apparently after 'five years of open discussion and planning with doctors and professional groups, public meetings and surveys'.[147] The Auckland District Health Board described opposition to the move in 2003 as 'a storm in an infant-sized teacup', declaring that 'the move will bring unwell mothers and babies closer to specialist care'.[148] Liggins had told a reporter in 1995 that his department had always believed that National Women's should be housed within (and not alongside) a general hospital.[149]

The hospital moved to the new site in October 2004, over 40 years after it shifted to the purpose-built women's hospital in One Tree Hill.[150] National Women's Hospital was no more, but the relevant unit at Auckland City Hospital was named 'National Women's Health'. A year later, Kay Hyman, clinical services general manager, reported that the National Women's Health facilities on the ninth and tenth floors of the new building had been greatly appreciated by women and staff alike.[151] Outpatient services at the Green Lane Clinical Centre campus moved to improved facilities in the early part of 2005, completing the integration of women's health with general medicine.

One woman gynaecologist, Hilary Liddell, reflected in an interview in 2005 on the history of National Women's Hospital that the move to Auckland City Hospital had diminished women-centred services. She thought it sad that a hospital set up as a result of women's fundraising should be taken away from them:

> There may be theoretical advantages of having it within a big public hospital, but I don't think enough was done to preserve the entity of a women's hospital, and I've worked in a lot of big hospitals where the woman focus has been very downplayed by stronger disciplines of medicine that are more male dominated. And I think there are huge risks of the service being not allocated its proper share of resources because it's part of now a big set-up, and I think it's dominated by paediatrics, and it's dominated by anaesthetics, and not enough by gynaecology and obstetrics.[152]

Cindy Farquhar, a successor to Bonham as postgraduate professor of obstetrics and gynaecology from 2002, also reflected on National Women's as a stand-alone hospital. She recalled the problems they had when gynaecological services were transferred to Green Lane Hospital in 1990, a less woman-centred institution:

> I can remember going to see a woman in the acute ward who was having a miscarriage and needed to go to theatre. She was covered in blood and there was blood on

the sheets and the orderly came to get her and he exposed her legs, and he didn't realise, you know, whereas the orderlies at National Women's had been fantastic about privacy and personal issues and all that sort of thing. We actually had to train the Green Lane orderlies about things like miscarriage and things like that.[153]

A separate women's hospital was something that women had lobbied for and achieved around the middle of the twentieth century. Women's health in the post-Second World War era had attained a privileged status. By the end of the century it would lose that privileged status, ironically in part at least as a result of activism by another wave of women's organisations.

CONCLUSION

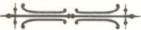

As New Zealand's largest women's hospital, National Women's touched the lives of many New Zealanders during the second half of the twentieth century, including those at the giving and receiving ends of its services. A large number of New Zealand women passed through National Women's at some point in their lives. Some attended its gynaecology, infertility or other clinics, but the most common experience for women was to give birth there – by the 1990s around 10,000 women a year were having their babies at the hospital. Some babies ended up in the neonatal care units, extending the relationship which their parents had built up with the hospital, sometimes for several months. Those who encountered National Women's in the course of their working lives included doctors (as obstetricians and gynaecologists, paediatricians, anaesthetists, general practitioners, pathologists, psychiatrists, radiologists, registrars and house surgeons), midwives, nurses, nurse aides, physiotherapists, laboratory technicians, tradesmen, hospital administrators, secretaries and receptionists, social workers, domestic staff and many others. All these participants in the hospital's history have stories to tell. Dr Jenny Carlyon's interviews for this project revealed multiple narratives, both tragic and heart-warming, as well as giving a first-hand account of the everyday life of the hospital.

Conclusion

This history draws on those accounts in order to understand social relations in the hospital and beyond, as well as the reception of new medical practices and the environment in which they occurred. I have focused in particular on the public image of the hospital, both celebratory and contested, high points and low, in order to place this institution in its wider national and international context. Interviews supplemented the vast array of printed sources, which included the daily press, women's magazines, and feminist and other writings on the hospital. Heroic medical achievements as well as battles fought between different sectors have always been subjects of widespread popular interest and are never far from public consciousness. Unpublished sources, such as the hospital's own meetings, and the records from the Department of Health and consumer organisations such as Parents' Centre also provided insights into the motivations and strategies of various interest groups. The focus of this history then was on the interactions between, and the respective influence and power of, the different sectors and stakeholders, particularly doctors, midwives, nurses, patients, activist groups, the government's health agencies and hospital boards. Personalities, new technologies, social movements – specifically the consumer and women's movements – and changing health-care systems, were all important contributors to the hospital's changing fortunes.

Women and their Organisations

This history has challenged some views of women's place in modern childbirth services which emerged from the 1970s and became accepted largely as orthodox. In her 1997 PhD thesis on New Zealand's maternity services, Sally Abel drew on the French philosopher Michel Foucault's notion of 'biopower' to argue that for much of the twentieth century, 'through its control of childbirth practices the medical profession was instrumental in effecting the governance of women as a population'. Only in the late 1980s, she argued, did the 'dissenting counter-conduct' of politicised consumers and midwives begin to disrupt the dominance of prevailing medical ideologies and practices.[1] Contrary to this interpretation I have argued that throughout the twentieth century maternity services were the result of interactions and negotiations between various interest groups, including women. Through researching the records of women's organisations prior to the 1950s, such as the National Council of Women and the Society for the Protection of Women and Children, I came to question the view that women were forced into hospital to give birth against their better judgement. Indeed, organised women's groups played a major role in persuading the government to provide free hospital care for women in childbirth in 1938, and to found National Women's Hospital with its Postgraduate School of Obstetrics and Gynaecology in 1946.

Consumer involvement in National Women's began as soon as the hospital opened, and was formalised through the Parents' Centre movement from the early 1950s. Once in hospital, women did not passively accept hospital regimes and routines but constantly lobbied to change conditions to suit their needs. While some women described feeling lonely and disempowered in hospital, others appreciated the two-week stay there after giving birth, which was provided free of charge in New Zealand from 1939. Some welcomed and even demanded pain relief and other interventions. At an organisational level, women frequently carried out consumer surveys and lobbied for changes. In the 1950s women as consumers did not adhere to what feminists later called the 'natural' alliance between women and midwives, but rather sided with the doctors, whilst the nurses and midwives bore the brunt of their criticisms. When Parents' Centre representatives reported that they had engaged in a 'very frank and thorough exchange of views, opinions and information' with National Women's obstetricians in 1958,[2] it would be condescending to them to suggest that they were mere victims of the medical profession, as some feminists would later assert.

Women's ideas and allegiances changed over time but their confidence in expressing their views and making their demands known did not. Some women lobbied to create a more family-friendly environment in hospital. National Women's Hospital in the 1980s was a very different place from the 1950s. The trend to provide what women wanted was epitomised in the hospital's showpiece birthing suite known as the 'pink room', but services throughout the hospital had by this time become less regimented and formal, reflecting not only the activities of lobby groups but also broader societal changes. Other alliances of women, emerging from the new women's health movement, rejected hospitals altogether in favour of home births in the 1980s. Home birth remained a minority activity, but nevertheless its advocates became a powerful lobby group, contributing to the passage of the 1990 Nurses Amendment Act, which gave midwives the power to practise autonomously. Consumer organisations had advocated for the right to choose midwives as their caregivers at birth. Yet by the mid-1990s another shift had occurred, with Parents' Centre lamenting the withdrawal of general practitioners from childbirth services and their replacement by midwives.

Conclusion

This history has attempted to explain and contextualise these shifting alliances, contending that throughout the period under consideration, women were far from being passive victims of the medical profession. Their voices were ever-present and comprise an important part of the hospital's narrative and that of New Zealand's maternity services. Funding restraints, owing to different government policies and strategies, were also important, however. While women had persuaded the government to provide fourteen days' free care in hospital at childbirth in the context of the classic welfare state in the 1930s, by the 1990s they were permitted only a few days of such care under a neoliberal regime. Women's reproductive capacity for the nation, it appears, was no longer valued as it had been in the 1930s, although equally importantly, medical and social ideas surrounding childbirth had also changed.

Nurses and Midwives

The 2004 issue of the *New Zealand College of Midwives Journal*, marking one hundred years of midwifery registration in New Zealand, included a guest editorial by historian Pamela Wood, in which she gently reminded midwives of the importance of 'sound historical knowledge' and 'facing the possibility that current beliefs [about their history] might be mythical'. These myths included a romanticised view of a 'golden age of non-interventionist midwifery' and the subsequent disempowerment of midwives by doctors. The truth was, she said, more complex.[3] Another contributor to that same issue, midwife Jane Stojanovic, took a different stance. Stojanovic drew on her recently completed Master's thesis on hospital childbirth in the 1950s and 1960s, based on interviews with four mothers, but located in a broader history which spanned centuries. She claimed that, as a result of medicalisation and hospitalisation of childbirth, midwives 'lost the experiential knowledge of birth that had been handed down for centuries from woman to woman'.[4]

Stojanovic wrote about the process of 'nursification' of midwifery in a hospital context, which she depicted as a negative development, causing midwives to become powerless and invisible, forced to work according to hospital rules, dictated to by doctors. Her interpretation echoed that of Elaine Papps and Mark Olssen in their 1997 history, which told a story of disempowerment of midwives by doctors and nurses, aided by the state.[5] Similarly, in her 1986 history of midwifery Joan Donley had asserted that most New Zealand midwives had become a 'nurse-midwife, a hybrid, a medically-oriented handmaiden, while the real midwife is an endangered species'.[6]

Such views were part of a political movement which emerged in the 1980s when home-birth midwives led by Donley allied themselves with feminists, stressing the feminist roots of their profession and the partnership with women which had been lost as a result of oppression by doctors and nurses. History, or what midwives often called 'herstory', was a tool for explaining the roots of that oppression. Midwives began to distance themselves from nursing, contrasting the biomedical and illness focus of nursing and its deference to doctors and medicine, with midwifery's focus on health and wellness, and pointing to what they saw as its traditional autonomy from nursing. In 1989 midwives separated from nurses to form their own College of Midwives.

This history does not engage with childbirth practices, romanticised or otherwise, before hospital births became the norm. However, it does challenge the view that hospital midwives were disempowered. Records from National Women's Hospital suggest that midwives were highly valued members of the professional team. Far from being the handmaidens to doctors, they effectively ran the wards. Their prior nurse training and 'indoctrination' or integration into modern obstetrical science did not diminish them.[7] For instance, when Verna Murray, who had done her midwifery training at Auckland's St Helens Hospital in 1950, was appointed matron at National Women's Hospital in 1970, she told the press that it was a 'terrific honour to be matron of this hospital which has a world-wide reputation as one of the leading obstetric hospitals'. She certainly did not feel invisible or disempowered. The reporter noted that Murray had charge of 181 obstetric and 74 gynaecological beds, together with premature and isolation units.[8] Her intellectual and professional base was the hospital and she was proud of her contributions to modern hospitalised birth. The political movement for midwifery autonomy and direct-entry midwifery training is an important part of the story of New Zealand's maternity services, including National Women's. However, this should not belittle the contributions and standing of those hospital midwives who had commanded great respect from other health professionals, including senior doctors, since the hospital opened.

Doctors

National Women's Hospital academic medical staff were members of an international community of researchers, a 'two-way traffic', as Sir Douglas Robb proudly called it in 1966.[9] Sir William Liley and Sir Graham Liggins in particular put New Zealand on the international map, and the manner in which this small nation achieved such status is an important part of the hospital's history. Serendipity played a part in their research accomplishments, but the hospital also provided a fertile environment for research. While Liggins encouraged young researchers, he was not involved in large research teams; he was, in the words of his biographers, a 'self-taught clinical and laboratory researcher'.[10] Yet his trial into corticosteroids now features on the logo of the Oxford-based Cochrane Collaboration. The logo shows that the original trial results achieved by Liggins and Ross Howie were almost identical to those that would be seen in the integration of a series of trials by meta-analysis. As Liggins' biographers rightly pointed out, 'Today it might also be seen as a beautiful example of translational research.'[11] 'Translational research' is a modern concept which signifies a gold standard for medical research encompassing all the steps involved in translating laboratory research into effective clinical practice.[12]

It was not, however, all plain sailing for doctors who worked, taught and researched at National Women's. When Auckland's *Metro* magazine published its feature article on 'The Glamorous Gynaecologists' in 1984, this was already the end of an era.[13] Ironically, obstetrics and gynaecology was probably the first branch of medicine to be acutely aware of the importance of good patient relations. Doctors were well aware of the criticism that some women felt dehumanised in the bureaucratic and technological settings of a hospital. In their study of childbirth services in Britain, Jo Garcia, Robert Kilpatrick and Martin Richards noted, 'Interestingly, one of the first places within medicine where these concerns surfaced was obstetrics; and by the early 1960s they had become sufficiently serious for the Ministry of Health to issue a policy statement entitled *Human Relationships in Obstetrics*.'[14]

In the 1950s Harvey Carey was well known for his good relations with women's consumer groups such as Parents' Centre, and Dennis Bonham maintained that rapport until the 1980s. Following the rise of the women's movement of the 1970s and 1980s, not just in New Zealand but throughout the Western world, obstetricians and gynaecologists became arguably the most beleaguered branch of the medical profession. Negative representations can be found in the feminist publication *Broadsheet*; for instance, consumer activist Judi Strid wrote in 1987, 'The medical professions are totally dependent on women's bodies for providing the clinical material they need to maintain their high-income professional practices and also for the training of their successors.'[15] In a similar vein, feminist perspectives were provided in a book entitled

Women, Health and Reproduction edited by Dr Helen Roberts in 1981. At that time Dr Roberts was a senior researcher at Ilkley College, West Yorkshire, but soon after she was based at National Women's Hospital. In her chapter in this volume, medical sociologist Pauline Bart wrote, 'Basically every gynaecologist doesn't like women, otherwise he couldn't work with them. The fact is that he is the god, king, they do what he tells them, which is what he would always want women to do, because every man wants his women subservient to him.'[16] Another contributor to the book, Gail Young, who had qualified in medicine at Edinburgh in 1973, took a less critical stance, suggesting there might be reasons for doctors to choose the specialty of obstetrics and gynaecology other than gaining power over women or financial considerations:

> Many doctors see obstetrics and gynaecology as attractive because they deal with a younger, healthier population, because they demand a mixture of practical and academic skills, because patients in obstetrics are often happy, and there is wide scope for preventive work and for analysis of the results of treatment policies, and therefore areas for improvement are easily pinpointed.

Nevertheless, when she added that 'a few obstetrician/gynaecologists have a genuine interest in, and concern for women', she appeared to be suggesting that the majority did not harbour such concerns.[17]

Certainly the public image of doctors changed over the period covered by this book. They enjoyed a high social status immediately following the Second World War and even into the 1980s as the harbingers of dramatic medical developments. Yet by this time they were also increasingly subject to public distrust. Nowhere is this story of the changing public image of doctors better illustrated than through the history of National Women's Hospital. This distrust culminated in the Cartwright Inquiry, during which the public was more than ready to accept that the medical profession had placed research above concern for patients.

This history has questioned the existence of an inclusive entity called 'the medical profession'. It has sometimes been argued that doctors supported ever-increasing medical technology until forced to modify their views by the burgeoning women's movement, but doctors did not necessarily support medical interventions. For instance, Harvey Carey was among those male doctors in the 1950s who favoured 'natural childbirth' as an alternative to providing pain relief in childbirth. The natural childbirth movement itself has sometimes been presented as a consumer-based movement which rejected medical intervention. For instance, British childbirth activist Sheila Kitzinger wrote of the movement that, 'Some critics still see it as a group of self-centred women, wrapped up in their own emotions, who scorn medical knowledge and are prepared to put their babies at risk as a result.'[18] However, historically the movement, emerging from the work of Grantly Dick-Read and others, reflected a direct concern about the health of the newborn baby, particularly its psychological health. This explains why psychotherapists and psychiatrists, such as R. D. Laing, were drawn to it. Others, like Carey, were drawn to natural childbirth primarily out of concern for the physical wellbeing of the baby. Whether relating to psychological or physical health, the natural childbirth movement presaged another important strand in the history of National Women's over the period of this study, the increasing attention paid not only to mothers but also to the newborn baby and the fetus.

When National Women's Hospital opened in 1946 it contained a premature nursery, but the hospital's medical committee commented on the ready acceptance of deaths among the newborn compared to any other age group. By the 1990s the hospital provided 64 beds in its special care units, catering for around 1500 babies a year and making it the largest unit of its kind in Australasia.[19] Following Liley's ground-breaking work in the 1960s and other technological developments, medical attention had increasingly extended beyond the baby to the fetus as well. Acknowledging the importance of the fetus as a patient culminated in the establishment of a chair in Maternal Fetal Medicine in 1998.

Through its research activities, National Women's contributed internationally to the care of the newborn baby and the fetus and to the evolution of their status as patients in their own right. While this evolution was related to technological and medical developments, it had significant social implications. To some, the rights of the newborn and the fetus were pitted against the rights of women. This created tensions and moral dilemmas, again with no single perspective amongst the medical profession. What is clear is that obstetricians and gynaecologists by the very nature of their work were drawn into social issues well beyond the practice of medicine.

This history grapples with the ironies and ambiguities of the past: on the one hand, medical advances were celebrated (infertile couples could have babies, more mothers and babies survived); on the other, in the context of new social movements, the motivations of those responsible for the advances were questioned. Consumer groups had allied with doctors in the 1950s to improve services in National Women's Hospital. By the late twentieth century the Cartwright and Cull inquiries were indicative of a change not in medical practice but in the social relations of medicine, specifically a distrust of the medical profession as guardians of health. Such misgivings were fuelled by the feminist movement and by territorial disputes between doctors and midwives as well as a media receptive to scandal. Meanwhile, mothers and their partners continued to take advice and choose the best services they could within existing constraints. The history of National Women's Hospital provides a lens through which to view the history of reproductive health services at a national and international level during the second half of the twentieth century. The rise and fall of this hospital as a stand-alone unit reflected broader social, political and medical trends.

NOTES

INTRODUCTION

1. 'The New National Women's Hospital, Auckland', *New Zealand Medical Journal (NZMJ)*, vol. 63, April 1964, pp. 241–2; 'Official Opening of National Women's Hospital Souvenir Issue', *Health and Service*, vol. 18, 4, 1964, p. 21; reprinted in Robb's memoirs: George Douglas Robb, *Medical Odyssey*, Collins, Auckland, 1967, p. 81.
2. Robin Carrell, 'Essay Review: Trial by Media', *Notes and Records of the Royal Society*, 12 July 2012, p. 1, doi:10.1098/rsnr.2012.0028.
3. *Sunday Star*, 12 April 1992.
4. *New Zealand Herald (NZH)*, 26 December 1992.
5. *NZH*, 14 May 2005.
6. Linda Bryder, *A History of the 'Unfortunate Experiment' at National Women's Hospital*, Auckland University Press, Auckland, 2009; reprinted as Linda Bryder, *Women's Bodies and Medical Science: An Inquiry into Cervical Cancer*, Palgrave Macmillan, London, 2010.
7. Diana Wichtel, 'Delivering with Style', *New Zealand Listener*, 21 September 1985, p. 14.
8. Judith Walzer Leavitt, *Brought to Bed: Childbearing in America, 1750 to 1950*, Oxford University Press, New York, 1986, p. 3.
9. Ibid., pp. 4, 5.
10. Jo Murphy-Lawless, *Reading Birth and Death: A History of Obstetric Thinking*, Cork University Press, Cork, 1998, p. 22.
11. Cited by Judy Barrett Litoff, 'Midwives and History', in Rima D. Apple (ed.), *Women, Health, and Medicine in America: A Historical Handbook*, Garland, New York, 1990, p. 446; Barbara Ehrenreich and Deirdre English, *Witches, Midwives and Nurses: A History of Women Healers*, Glass Mountain Pamphlets, Oyster Bay, New York, 1973.
12. Ann Oakley, *The Captured Womb: A History of the Medical Care of Pregnant Women*, Basil Blackwell, Oxford, 1984, pp. 2, 250; see also Ann Oakley, 'The Medicalized Trap of Motherhood', *New Society*, vol. 34, 18 December 1975, pp. 639–41; and Ann Oakley, *Women Confined: Towards a Sociology of Childbirth*, Schocken Books, New York, 1980, where she 'speculates[s] about the ways in which women's treatment as mothers is associated with their oppression as women': Introduction, p. 1.
13. Oakley, *The Captured Womb*, p. 274.
14. Ibid., pp. 254–5.
15. Marjorie Tew, *Safer Childbirth?: A Critical History of Maternity Care*, Free Association Books, London, 2nd edn, 1998, p. 10.
16. Ibid., pp. 7, 20.
17. Ibid., p. 20.
18. Joan Donley, *Save the Midwife*, New Women's Press, Auckland, 1986; Elaine Papps and Mark Olssen, *Doctoring Childbirth and Regulating Midwifery in New Zealand: A Foucauldian Perspective*, Dunmore Press, Palmerston North, 1997.
19. Joan Donley to Silvia Cartwright, 8 December 1987; reply from Cartwright, 17 December 1987, Joan Donley Papers, MSS & Archives 2007/15, item 9/1/A/1 pt. 2, University of Auckland Library, Special Collections (UOASC).
20. 'Obituary: Joan Donley', *NZH*, 17 December 2005.
21. Joan Donley, *Birthrites: Natural vs Unnatural Childbirth in New Zealand*, Full Court Press, Auckland, in association with New Zealand College of Midwives, Christchurch, 1998, p. 11.
22. Donley, *Save the Midwife*, p. 117. The

school's logo was intended to show that it was a training centre for the whole country and not just Auckland; the hospital's logo by contrast did not include the map but rather the local landmark, One Tree Hill.

23 Wendy Mitchinson, *Giving Birth in Canada, 1900–1950*, University of Toronto Press, Toronto, 2002, p. 302; Wendy Mitchinson, 'Agency, Diversity, and Constraints: Women and Their Physicians, Canada, 1850–1950', in The Feminist Health Care Ethics Research Network, co-ordinator Susan Sherwin, *The Politics of Women's Health: Exploring Agency and Autonomy*, Temple University Press, Philadelphia, 1998, pp. 122–49.

24 Mitchinson, *Giving Birth in Canada*, p. 159.

25 Janet Greenlees and Linda Bryder (eds), *Western Maternity and Medicine, 1880–1980*, Pickering Chatto UK, London, 2013.

26 Sara Dubow, *Ourselves Unborn: A History of the Fetus in Modern America*, Oxford University Press, Oxford, 2011, p. 5.

27 G. S. Dawes, 'Chairman's Closing Remarks', in G. E. W. Wolstenholme and Maeve O'Connor (eds), *Foetal Autonomy: A Ciba Foundation Symposium*, J. & A. Churchill, London, 1969, p. 316.

28 'The Abortion Doctors: A Nationwide Survey of Certifying Consultants under the CS & A Act', *Broadsheet*, vol. 68, April 1979, p. 21.

1: CHILDBIRTH SERVICES IN NEW ZEALAND, 1900–1939

1 Report of Committee of Inquiry into Maternity Services, *Appendices to the Journals of the House of Representatives (AJHR)*, H-31A, 1938, pp. 1–112.

2 See Keith Sinclair, *A History of New Zealand*, Penguin, Auckland, revised edn, 2000, p. 195.

3 For further discussion of this literature, see Linda Bryder, *A Voice for Mothers: The Plunket Society and Infant Welfare 1907–2000*, Auckland University Press, Auckland, 2003, p. 2.

4 *New Zealand Parliamentary Debates (NZPD)*, vol. 131, 1904, p. 481.

5 *NZPD*, vol. 140, 1907, p. 852.

6 *NZPD*, vol. 131, 1904, p. 110; see also Philippa Mein Smith, *Maternity in Dispute: New Zealand, 1920–1939*, Historical Publications Branch, Department of Internal Affairs, Wellington, 1986, p. 17.

7 Duncan MacGregor, Department of Public Health Annual Report, *AJHR*, H-22, 1906, p. 3. England and Wales also passed a Midwives Act in 1901: see Joan Mottram, 'State Control in Local Context: Public Health and Midwife Regulation in Manchester, 1900–1914', in Hilary Marland and Anne Marie Rafferty (eds), *Midwives, Society and Childbirth: Debates and Controversies in the Modern Period*, Routledge, London, 1997, p. 134.

8 J. A. Rodgers, '"A good nurse . . . a good woman": Duty and Obedience in Early New Zealand Nursing', in Roger Openshaw and David McKenzie (eds), *Re-interpreting the Educational Past: Essays in the History of New Zealand Education*, New Zealand Council for Educational Research, Wellington, 1987, pp. 54–63.

9 Confinement cost £1 10s 0d per week in 1917 and £5 5s 0d by 1935. Nurse attendance for home delivery was £1 in 1917 and £2 by 1935, and if a doctor attended at delivery an extra 10s was charged. Income limits were £4 in 1917 and £5 per week in 1935: see Department of Health, *The Expectant Mother and Baby's First Month*, Government Printer, Wellington, 1935, p. 2.

10 This was still the case in 1937: see Transcripts of Committee of Inquiry into Maternity Services, comment by Dr Thomas Paget during evidence given by Dr Siedeberg McKinnon, 21 May 1937, MS 78, Auckland Museum Archives (AMA).

11 On this service, see Elizabeth Peretz, 'A Maternity Service for England and

Wales: Local Authority Maternity Care in the Inter-War Period in Oxfordshire and Tottenham', in Jo Garcia, Robert Kilpatrick and Martin Richards (eds), *The Politics of Maternity Care: Services for Childbearing Women in Twentieth-Century Britain*, Oxford University Press, Oxford, 1990, pp. 30–46; and Nicky Leap and Billie Hunter, *The Midwife's Tale: An Oral History from Handywoman to Professional Midwife*, Scarlet Press, London, 1993, pp. 55, 201–2.

12 Report of Committee of Inquiry into Maternity Services, *AJHR*, pp. 73–74.

13 Ibid., p. 90. In Britain, too, there had been dissenting voices to a midwifery-based service. Specifically, a consultant-based maternity service was proposed by the president of the British College of Obstetricians and Gynaecologists, William Blair-Bell, professor of obstetrics and gynaecology at the University of Liverpool and co-founder of the college: see A. Susan Williams, *Women and Childbirth in the Twentieth Century: A History of the National Birthday Trust Fund 1928–93*, Sutton Publishing, Stroud, 1997, p. 53; and John Peel, *William Blair-Bell – Father and Founder*, Royal College of Obstetricians and Gynaecologists (RCOG), London, 1986.

14 New Zealand Obstetrical Society (NZOS) minutes, 13 September 1929 (Minute books held by Professor R. W. Jones).

15 NZOS minutes, 16 March 1933; see also J. B. Dawson, 'New Zealand Obstetrical Society Section: Doctor and Midwife, Colleagues or Rivals', *NZMJ*, vol. 32, 1933, p. 23. For differences between 'midwives' and 'maternity nurses', see p. 21 and chapter 4, p. 71.

16 NZOS minutes, 20 March 1934.

17 Dawson, 'New Zealand Obstetrical Society Section', pp. 20–23.

18 Henry Jellett, *The Causes and Prevention of Maternal Mortality*, Churchill's Empire Series, J. & A. Churchill, London, 1929, p. 15.

19 T. F. Corkill, 'The Trend of Obstetric Practice in New Zealand', *NZMJ*, vol. 32, 1933, pp. 42–52.

20 On these women, see also Philippa Mein Smith, 'Hutchinson, Amy May', *Dictionary of New Zealand Biography. Te Ara – the Encyclopedia of New Zealand*, updated 30 October 2012, http://www.TeAra.govt.nz/en/biographies/4h40/hutchinson-amy-may; Margaret Lovell-Smith, 'Kent-Johnston, Agnes Gilmour', *Dictionary of New Zealand Biography. Te Ara – the Encyclopedia of New Zealand*, updated 30 October 2012, http://www.TeAra.govt.nz/en/biographies/5k8/kent-johnston-agnes-gilmour; Hilary Stace, 'Fraser, Janet', *Dictionary of New Zealand Biography. Te Ara – the Encyclopedia of New Zealand*, updated 30 October 2012, http://www.TeAra.govt.nz/en/biographies/4f21/fraser-janet.

21 Mrs McGuire, Onehunga Labour Party, Evidence to Committee of Inquiry into Maternity Services, 7 September 1937, MS 78, AMA.

22 Mein Smith, *Maternity in Dispute*, p. 1.

23 Hester Maclean, 'Report: Nurses Registration Act, Midwives Act, Maternity Hospitals and Private Hospitals', *AJHR*, H-31, 1918, p. 9; *AJHR*, H-31, 1919, p. 11.

24 Jellett, *Causes and Prevention of Maternal Mortality*, p. 201.

25 New Zealand Society for the Protection of Women and Children (NZSPWC) minutes, 19 August 1936, p. 73, MS 1144/7, AMA.

26 Report of Committee of Inquiry into Maternity Services, *AJHR*, p. 76.

27 T. L. Paget, *Maternal Welfare. Report of the Inspector of Private and Maternity Hospitals, 1930–31*, *AJHR*, H-31, 1931, p. 29 (by 1934 there were five St Helens hospitals still in existence); on the unlicensed homes, see NZSPWC minutes, 12 February 1939, MS 1144/7, AMA.

28 See Dorothy Page, *The National Council of Women: A Centennial History*, Auckland University Press with Bridget Williams Books and National Council of Women, Wellington, 1996.

29 National Council of Women (NCW), Auckland Branch minutes, 22 June 1936, NCW MS 879, 32, AMA, my emphasis.

30 Leavitt, *Brought to Bed*, p. 194.
31 Mitchinson, *Giving Birth in Canada*, p. 179.
32 Jane Lewis, 'Mothers and Maternity Policies in the Twentieth Century', in Garcia et al. (eds), *The Politics of Maternity Care*, p. 20; Jane Lewis, '"Motherhood Issues" in the Late Nineteenth and Twentieth Centuries', in Katherine Arnup, Andrée Lévesque and Ruth Roach Pierson with the assistance of Margaret Brennan (eds), *Delivering Motherhood: Maternal Ideologies and Practices in the 19th and 20th Centuries*, Routledge, London, 1990, pp. 11–12. Despite outlining these conditions and campaigns, Lewis still argued that, 'The move to hospital birth was dictated more by professional developments and the changing status of obstetrics as a specialty than by women's campaigns, although the latter were invoked to legitimize the change': '"Motherhood Issues"', p. 12.
33 Alison Clarke, *Born to a Changing World: Childbirth in Nineteenth-century New Zealand*, Bridget Williams Books, Wellington, 2012, p. 172.
34 *NZPD*, vol. 128, 1904, pp. 70–71, 80.
35 Department of Health, 'Maternal Mortality in New Zealand: Report of Special Committee set up by Board of Health to Consider and Report on the Question of the Deaths of Mothers in Connection with Childbirth', (Chairman, C. J. Parr), *AJHR*, H-31B, 1921, p. 1.
36 Ibid., p. 6.
37 Lewis, 'Mothers and Maternity Policies', pp. 15–16.
38 Leavitt, *Brought to Bed*, p. 176.
39 Dr Siedeberg McKinnon, Evidence to Committee of Inquiry into Maternity Services, 21 May 1937, MS 78, AMA.
40 Leavitt, *Brought to Bed*, p. 117.
41 Clarke, *Born to a Changing World*, pp. 54–56.
42 Williams, *Women and Childbirth in the Twentieth Century*, p. 126.
43 Donald Caton, *What a Blessing She Had Chloroform: The Medical and Social Response to the Pain of Childbirth from 1800 to the Present*, Yale University Press, New Haven, 1999, p. 141. See also Jacqueline H. Wolf, *Deliver Me From Pain: Anesthesia and Birth in America*, Johns Hopkins University Press, Baltimore, 2009, pp. 44–47.
44 Jennifer Beinart, 'Obstetric Analgesia and the Control of Childbirth in Twentieth-Century Britain', in Garcia et al. (eds), *The Politics of Maternity Care*, p. 120.
45 Irvine S. L. Loudon, 'Childbirth', in W. F. Bynum and Roy Porter (eds), *Companion Encyclopedia of the History of Medicine*, vol. 2, Routledge, London, 1993, p. 1064; Hilary Marland, 'Childbirth and Maternity', in Roger Cooter and John Pickstone (eds), *Companion to Medicine in the Twentieth Century*, Routledge, London, 2003, p. 566; Irvine Loudon, *Death in Childbirth: An International Study of Maternal Care and Maternal Mortality, 1800–1950*, Oxford University Press, Oxford, 1992, p. 348; Williams, *Women and Childbirth in the Twentieth Century*, p. 128; nor did twilight sleep take off in Canada, see Mitchinson, *Giving Birth in Canada*, p. 218.
46 Doris Gordon, Evidence to Committee of Inquiry into Maternity Services, 13 September 1937, MS 78, AMA.
47 Ibid.
48 Beinart, 'Obstetric Analgesia', in Garcia et al. (eds), *The Politics of Maternity Care*, pp. 120–1.
49 NCW, Auckland Branch minutes, 24 July 1933, 30 October 1933, NCW MS 879, 31, AMA; see also NZOS minutes, correspondence from NCW, 11 September 1935, *NZMJ*, vol. 34, 1935.
50 NCW, Auckland Branch, Report of Social Welfare Committee, 11 October 1933, NCW MS 879, AMA (my emphasis).
51 NCW, Auckland Branch minutes, 24 July 1933, NCW MS 879, 31, AMA.
52 Caton, *What a Blessing She Had Chloroform*, p. 157.
53 Beinart, 'Obstetric Analgesia', in Garcia et al. (eds), *The Politics of Maternity Care*, pp. 123–4; Caton, *What a Blessing She Had Chloroform*, p. 162.
54 Vera Crowther, 'Maternity and the

Working Woman', *Woman To-day*, October 1937, pp. 150–1; Vera Crowther, 'Correspondence: Maternity and the Working Woman', *Woman To-day*, January 1938, p. 240. This correspondence is also discussed in Eve Ebbett, *Victoria's Daughter: New Zealand Women of the Thirties*, A. H. & A. W. Reed, Wellington, 1981, pp. 114–15. On Crowther, see also *Broadsheet*, September 1976, pp. 16–17, 25.

55 Raewyn Dalziel, *Focus on the Family: The Auckland Home and Family Society, 1893–1993*, The Home and Family Society, Auckland, 1993.

56 NZSPWC minutes, 19 August 1936, p. 73, MS 1144/7, AMA.

57 Ibid.

58 Department of Health, 'Report of the Committee of Inquiry into the Various Aspects of the Problem of Abortion in New Zealand', *AJHR*, H-31A, 1937, p. 9.

59 NZSPWC, Minutes of Executive, 9 November 1936, visit paid to St Helens Hospital, 22 October 1936 by Mrs Moore, Mrs Bates, Agnes Preston Chambers and Amy Hutchinson, MS 1144/7, AMA.

60 Nellie Molesworth, NZSPWC, Evidence to Committee of Inquiry into Maternity Services, 6 September 1937, MS 78, AMA.

61 Janet Fraser, Evidence to Committee of Inquiry into Maternity Services, 1 September 1937, H 131/139/15 9402, Archives New Zealand, Wellington (ANZW).

62 Nellie Molesworth, NZSPWC, Evidence to Committee of Inquiry into Maternity Services, 6 September 1937, MS 78, AMA.

63 New Zealand Labour Party, Auckland Women's Branch, Evidence to Committee of Inquiry into Maternity Services, 6 September 1937, MS 78, AMA; see also Mein Smith, *Maternity in Dispute*, p. 85.

64 Richard Barnett, 'Obstetric Anaesthesia and Analgesia in England and Wales 1945–1975', PhD thesis, University College London, 2007, p. 132.

65 NZSPWC minutes, 9 November 1936, MS 1144/7, AMA.

66 Miss Every and Miss Paterson, Obstetrical Branch of the New Zealand Registered Nurses Association, Evidence to Committee of Inquiry into Maternity Services, 22 May 1937, MS 78, AMA.

67 NZSPWC minutes, 19 August 1936, MS 1144/7, AMA. Mitchinson similarly found in Canada in the 1920s that organisations such as the National Council of Women advocated medical assistance during childbirth and that maternity benefits could ensure this for all women: Mitchinson, *Giving Birth in Canada*, p. 170.

68 Elizabeth Hanson, *The Politics of Social Security: The 1938 Act and Some Later Developments*, Auckland University Press, Auckland, and Oxford University Press, Wellington, 1980, p. 32.

69 New Zealand Obstetrical and Gynaecological Society (NZOGS) minutes, 10 March 1938.

70 New Zealand Obstetrical and Gynaecological Society, *A Statement on the Dominion's Need for One Well-equipped Hospital for Obstetrics and Gynaecology to Serve as The One Post Graduate Training School for these Sciences within NZ. Printed at the request of The Women's Associations of New Zealand*, February 1945 (NZOGS Statement, 1945), Dr Doris Clifton Gordon Papers, MS 115 F.1.

71 Mrs Cassey, Women's Auxiliary, Unemployed Workers' Union, Mrs Stewart, Devonport Housewives' Union, Evidence to Committee of Inquiry into Maternity Services, 7 September 1937, MS 78, AMA.

72 Department of Health Annual Report, *AJHR*, H-31, 1940, pp. 6–8.

73 Donley, *Save the Midwife*, pp. 47–48, 118.

74 Doris Gordon, *The Weekly News*, 21 August 1946, p. 15.

75 NZOGS Statement, 1945.

76 Report of NZSPWC interview with Reverend Mr Wood, Chairman Auckland Hospital Board, 9 November 1936, MS 1144/7, AMA.

77 NCW, Auckland Branch minutes, 28 November 1938, MS 879, 4, AMA.
78 Selwyn Kenrick, Evidence to Committee of Inquiry into Maternity Services, 6 September 1937, MS 78, AMA.
79 Joseph Craven, Evidence to Committee of Inquiry into Maternity Services, 7 September 1937, MS 78, AMA.
80 Selwyn Kenrick, Evidence to Committee of Inquiry into Maternity Services, 9 September 1937, MS 78, AMA.
81 NZSPWC minutes, 12 February 1939, MS 1144/7, AMA.
82 Anne Nightingale, interviewed by Deborah Jowitt, 21 February 2003, transcript, p. 6.
83 Mrs Stewart, Devonport Housewives' Union, Evidence to Committee of Inquiry into Maternity Services, 7 September 1937, MS 78, AMA.
84 NZSPWC minutes, 13 November 1939, MS 1144/7, AMA.
85 NCW, Auckland Branch minutes, 28 November 1938, MS 879, 4, AMA.
86 Report of Deputation, 15 December 1936, NZSPWC minutes, 8 February 1937, p. 97, MS 1144/7, AMA.
87 J. O. C. Neill, *Grace Neill. The Story of a Noble Woman, With a Contribution by Miss Flora J. Cameron*, N. M. Peryer, Christchurch, 1961, pp. 55–56.
88 Charlotte Parkes, 'The Impact of the Medicalisation of New Zealand's Maternity Services on Women's Experience of Childbirth, 1904–1937', in Linda Bryder (ed.), *A Healthy Country: Essays on the Social History of Medicine in New Zealand*, Bridget Williams Books, Wellington, 1991, pp. 172–3.
89 Doris Gordon to Douglas Robb, 11 April 1941, cited in *University of Auckland News*, vol. 6, 7, September 1976, p. 8.
90 Charles Hercus, Evidence to Committee of Inquiry into Maternity Services, 21 May 1937, MS 78, AMA.
91 Selwyn Kenrick, Evidence to Committee of Inquiry into Maternity Services, 6 September 1937, MS 78, AMA; NZOGS minutes, 26 February 1937.
92 Agnes Kent-Johnston, Evidence to Committee of Inquiry into Maternity Services, 21 May 1937, MS 78, AMA.
93 Henry Jellett, 'Maternal Welfare, Report of the Consulting Obstetrician, Department of Health Annual Report for 1925', *AJHR*, H-31, 1926, pp. 21–22.
94 Milton J. Lewis, 'Obstetrics: Education and Practice, 1870–1939, Part 2', *Australian and New Zealand Journal of Obstetrics and Gynaecology*, vol. 18, 1978, pp. 165–8.
95 NCW, Auckland Branch minutes, 27 February 1939, MS 879, 4, AMA.
96 Amy May Hutchinson 'Odd Memories at Eighty Odd and Life in 1900: Memories of a Social Worker', p. 4, MS 1340, AMA.

2: NATIONAL WOMEN'S HOSPITAL AND THE POSTGRADUATE SCHOOL OF OBSTETRICS AND GYNAECOLOGY

1 Linda Bryder, 'Gordon, Doris Clifton – Biography', *Dictionary of New Zealand Biography. Te Ara – the Encyclopedia of New Zealand*, updated 1 September 2010, http://www.TeAra.govt.nz/en/biographies/4g14/1. Gordon's letterhead stated: 'Doris Gordon FRCSE, FRCOG, DPH (Women and Children only) / Consultations by appointment only, Stratford': letterhead, 7 March 1946, Plunket Society Archives (PSA) 581, Hocken Library, Dunedin.
2 NZOS Inaugural Meeting minutes, 5 February 1927.
3 Doris Gordon, *Backblocks Baby-doctor: An Autobiography*, Faber & Faber, London, and Whitcombe & Tombs, Auckland, 1955, p. 207.
4 On this campaign, see Mein Smith, *Maternity in Dispute*, pp. 23–40.
5 NZOS minutes, 14 September 1928.
6 Gordon, *Backblocks Baby-doctor*, p. 207 (her emphasis).
7 Doris Gordon to Helen Deem, 30 December 1945, PSA 581, Hocken Library; on Helen Deem, see Linda Bryder, 'Muriel Helen Deem', in Jane Thomson (ed.), *Southern People: A Dictionary of Otago Southland Biography,* Longacre Press in association

8 Henry Jellett, 'Maternal Welfare, Report of the Consulting Obstetrician, Department of Health Annual Report for 1925', *AJHR*, H-31, 1926, p. 21.
9 Lewis, 'Obstetrics: Education and Practice', p. 167.
10 D. W. Carmalt Jones, *Annals of the University of Otago Medical School 1875–1939*, A. H. & A. W. Reed, Wellington, 1945, p. 224.
11 NZOS minutes, 23 February 1929.
12 Page, *The National Council of Women*, p. 73.
13 Carmalt Jones, *Annals*, p. 226.
14 NZOS minutes, 18 February 1930.
15 NZOS minutes, summary of Obstetrical Endowment Appeal, 21 May 1930.
16 Carmalt Jones, *Annals*, p. 228.
17 Ibid., pp. 231–2.
18 Ibid., p. 229; NZOS minutes, 21 May 1930.
19 NZOGS minutes, 1 September 1937 (the one scholar was H. K. Pacey).
20 NZOGS minutes, 7 September 1938.
21 Gordon, *Backblocks Baby-doctor*, p. 215.
22 NZOGS minutes, 16 March 1933.
23 Report by Gordon to NZOGS, NZOGS minutes, 8 March 1940.
24 Keith Sinclair, *A History of the University of Auckland, 1883–1993*, Auckland University Press, Oxford University Press, Auckland, 1983, p. 273.
25 Report by Gordon to NZOGS, NZOGS minutes, 8 March 1940.
26 They included: 1928, R. E. Bridge (resigned); 1929, F. F. Chisholm (resigned); 1930, H. K. Pacey; 1931, D. R. L. Stevenson; 1932, J. A. Stallworthy; 1933, G. R. Stoneham; 1934, R. R. Talbot; 1935, R. W. S. Riley; 1936, W. Hawksworth; 1937, T. A. Macfarlane; 1938, B. W. Grieve; 1939, J. L. Wright; 1939 and 1940, J. Borrie: Dr George Herbert Green Papers (Green Papers), MSS 1433, UOASC.
27 NZOGS minutes, 8 March 1940; *NZH*, 14 January 1947.
28 Gordon, *Backblocks Baby-doctor*, pp. 218–19.

with the Dunedin City Council, Dunedin, 1998, pp. 125–6; on Plunket Society, see Bryder, *A Voice for Mothers*.

29 George Weisz, *Divide and Conquer: A Comparative History of Medical Specialization*, Oxford University Press, Oxford, 2006, p. 207.
30 Ornella Moscucci, *The Science of Woman: Gynaecology and Gender in England, 1800–1929*, Cambridge University Press, Cambridge, 1990, pp. 184, 186.
31 Ibid., p. 180; Jane Lewis, *The Politics of Motherhood: Child and Maternal Welfare in England, 1900–1939*, Croom Helm, London, and McGill-Queen's University Press, Montreal, 1980, p. 126.
32 NZOGS minutes, 23 February 1928, 21 May 1930.
33 AGM, NZOGS minutes, 27 February 1935.
34 Ibid. On double certification, see Weisz, *Divide and Conquer*, p. 207.
35 Charles Hercus, Evidence to Committee of Inquiry into Maternity Services, 21 May 1937, MS 78, AMA.
36 Louis Levy, Report of Conference, NZOGS minute book, 11 December 1940, p. 192; on America, see also Wolf, *Deliver Me From Pain*, p. 83.
37 NZOGS Statement 1945, Dr Doris Clifton Gordon Papers, MS 115 F.1, AMA.
38 Scholars' Conference Report, 8 March 1940, NZOGS minute book, vol. 2, p. 173.
39 NZOGS minutes, 4 September 1940.
40 Ibid.
41 Address by Dr Doris Gordon to the National Council of Women of New Zealand, Auckland Branch, 5 November 1940, Green Papers, MSS 1433, UOASC; reported in *NZH*, 5 November 1940.
42 Gordon to Barrer, 29 November 1944, Doris Clifton Gordon Papers, MS 115, AMA; this was reprinted in the New Zealand Obstetrical and Gynaecological Society Inc., *The Proposed Auckland Hospital for Women to Function as a Post-Graduate School of Obstetrics and Gynaecology and to Assist with the Training of Undergraduates in these Subjects. Printed at the Request of Leaders of Women's Organisations, and to be Read in Conjunction with the Society's Statement Issued in May 1941*,

February 1945, p. 4, Green Papers, MSS 1433, UOASC.
43 Nina Barrer was president of the Masterton branch of the Women's Division of the New Zealand Farmers' Union 1927–30, Dominion vice-president and member of Advisory Board 1925–7. She also became a prominent member of the New Zealand National Party, as a member of the Dominion council 1942–3, and women's vice-president North Island 1944–5: see Christopher van der Krogt, 'Barrer, Nina Agatha Rosamond – Biography', *Dictionary of New Zealand Biography. Te Ara – the Encyclopedia of New Zealand*, updated 1 September 2010, http://www.TeAra.govt.nz/en/biographies/4b6/1.
44 Gordon to Barrer, 29 November 1944, Doris Clifton Gordon Papers, MS 115, AMA; see also Gordon, *Backblocks Baby-doctor*, p. 218.
45 See also Dorothy Page, *Anatomy of a Medical School: A History of Medicine at the University of Otago 1875–2000*, University of Otago Press, Dunedin, 2008, p. 81.
46 Her speeches were printed in the press, *NZH*, 5 November 1940; see also *NZH*, 28 September 1943.
47 *NZH*, 5 November 1940.
48 NZOGS Statement, 1945, Dr Doris Clifton Gordon Papers, MS 115 F.1, AMA.
49 'Abridged Report of a Conference held in the BMA Chambers, 26, The Terrace, Wellington, on 11th Dec. 1940, convened by The New Zealand Obstetrical and Gynaecological Society', Green Papers, MSS 1433, UOASC; Report of Discussion 11 December 1940 in NZOGS minute book, vol. 2, pp. 191–200; Gordon, *Backblocks Baby-doctor*, p. 224.
50 Gordon, *Backblocks Baby-doctor*, p. 243.
51 Ibid., p. 241.
52 Ibid.
53 Derek A. Dow, 'Sir Douglas Robb', in Nicholas Tarling (ed.), *Auckland Minds and Matters*, University of Auckland, Auckland, 2003, pp. 134, 138–9.
54 Gordon, *Backblocks Baby-doctor*, p. 223.
55 Ibid., p. 224.
56 Gordon to Deem, 28 November 1940, AG 7, 586, PSA, Hocken Library.
57 Gordon to Mrs Begg, 28 November 1940, 216, PSA, Hocken Library.
58 Deem to Gordon, 9 December 1940, AG 7, 586, PSA, Hocken Library.
59 NCW, Auckland Branch minutes, 17 April 1941; 28 April 1941; 20 June 1941; 17 November 1941; 24 August 1942, MS 879, AMA.
60 Ibid., 20 September 1943; 27 September 1943, MS 879, AMA.
61 Gordon, *Backblocks Baby-doctor*, pp. 244–5.
62 NCW, Auckland Branch minutes, 3 September 1945, MS 879, AMA.
63 Ibid., 27 September 1948, MS 879, AM; see also Betty Holt, *Women in Council: A History of the National Council of Women of New Zealand*, National Council of Women, Wellington, 1980, p. 84.
64 Shirley Coulter, '25th Birthday of O. and G. Postgraduate School's Beginnings', *University of Auckland News*, vol. 6, 7, September 1976, p. 10.
65 Hunter to Robb, 20 June 1944, Dr Doris Clifton Gordon Papers, MS 115 F.1, AMA.
66 Gordon to Robb, 24 June 1944, Dr Doris Clifton Gordon Papers, MS 115 F.1, AMA.
67 Gordon, *Backblocks Baby-doctor*, p. 246.
68 Gordon to Sir Thomas Hunter, 16 September 1945, NZOGS minute book; see also Gordon, *Backblocks Baby-doctor*, p. 246.
69 Sinclair, *A History of the University of Auckland*, pp. 169, 229.
70 *Otago Daily Times*, 18 February 1946.
71 Harry D. Erlam, *A Notable Result: An Historical Essay on the Beginnings and the First Fifteen Years of the School of Medicine with a Chapter on the History of the Postgraduate School of Obstetrics and Gynaecology by G.H. Green*, University of Auckland, School of Medicine, Auckland, 1983, p. 68.
72 Shaw to Eardley, 20 December 1945,

Notes to Pages 38–42

A4/4/18, RCOG Archives, London.
73 *NZH*, 14 January 1947; Shaw conducted the first examinations in Australia for the Diploma of Membership of the RCOG: Gordon to Sir Thomas Hunter, 3 September 1946, Green Papers, MSS 1433, UOASC.
74 Cecil Lewis, 'A Brief Survey of the History of the Postgraduate School of Obstetrics and Gynaecology and its Prospects in Relation to the Faculty of Medicine', 7 May 1968, Box 257, Archives, Office of the Vice-Chancellor, University of Auckland (UOAA).
75 Sir William Fletcher Shaw, 'Report on the Obstetrical and Gynaecological Services of NZ', Supplement to the *NZMJ*, vol. 47, June 1948, pp. 8, 568–70; Report from Sir William Fletcher Shaw to the President of the Royal College of Obstetricians and Gynaecologists, Adopted by Council 22 March 1947, Green Papers, MSS 1433, UOASC.
76 Erlam, *A Notable Result*, p. 68.
77 Richard Seddon, interviewed by Jenny Carlyon, 2 September 2005, transcript, p. 1; Jack Matthews, interviewed by Penelope Dunkley, 4 February 1991, transcript, p. 10.
78 NZOGS Statement, 1945, Dr Doris Clifton Gordon Papers, MS 115 F.1, AMA.
79 Lilian Knights (Stone), interviewed by Jenny Carlyon, 10 December 2004, transcript, p. 1.
80 Minutes of meeting of Academic Advisory Committee on Chair in Obstetrics and Gynaecology, Auckland University College, 24 May 1946, p. 3, Douglas Robb Papers 7/1, UOASC.
81 Aitken to Douglas Robb, 20 February 1946, Douglas Robb Papers 7/1, UOASC.
82 *NZH*, 6 June 1957.
83 Gordon to Robb, 9 March 1947, Douglas Robb Papers 5/6, UOASC.
84 Ibid., and Gordon to Robb, 2 November 1941, Green Papers, MSS 1433, UOASC.
85 'Obituary: John Arthur Stallworthy', *NZMJ*, vol. 107, 26 January 1994, p. 23; 'Obituary: John Arthur Stallworthy', *The Independent*, 30 November 1993;

'NZ Doctor Led UK Medicine', *NZH*, 1 December 1993.
86 Gordon to Sir Thomas Hunter, 29 December 1943, Green Papers, MSS 1433, UOASC.
87 W. Hawksworth, 'The First Doris Gordon Memorial Oration: Progress of Obstetrics in the Last Twenty-five Years' (delivered New Plymouth, 2 November 1962), *NZMJ*, vol. 62, January 1963, pp. 2–9.
88 Minutes of meeting of Academic Advisory Committee on Obstetrics and Gynaecology, Auckland University College, 18 November 1949, UOAA.
89 Cornwall Hospital and O & G Hospital Green Lane West, Hospital Medical Committee minutes, 19 December 1949, YCBZ 15492 1a, Archives New Zealand, Auckland (ANZA); Minutes of Meeting of Academic Advisory Committee on Obstetrics and Gynaecology, Auckland University College, 5 July 1950, Green Papers, MSS 1433, UOASC.
90 'Obituary: William Hawskworth', *Journal of Obstetrics and Gynaecology of the British Commonwealth*, vol. 73, 1966, pp. 862–3.
91 Minute books, New Zealand Region RCOG, 12 September 1966, B9/4/5, RCOG Archives, London, p. 24. William Hawksworth (1911–1966) was appointed consultant obstetrician and gynaecologist to the United Oxford Hospitals in 1947: see J. Peel (compiler), *The Lives of the Fellows of the Royal College of Obstetricians and Gynaecologists, 1929–1969*, RCOG, London, 1976, pp. 190–2.
92 NCW, Auckland Branch minutes, 28 August 1950, MS 879, AMA.
93 Application for Chair of Obstetrics and Gynaecology, Auckland University College, from Gerald Spence Smyth, Green Papers, MSS 1433, UOASC.
94 Spence Smyth, to Principal, Auckland University College, 27 November 1952, Box 129, UOAA.
95 G. Spence Smyth, Report on the Development of the Department of Post-Graduate Obstetrics and Gynaecology, 1951–1952, Box 129, UOAA.

96 NZH, 16 March 1954. Letter of resignation, 1 March 1954, University of Auckland O&G Academic Advisory Committee, 1954–1962, Box 257, UOAA.
97 Erlam, *A Notable Result*, p. 68.
98 G. Spence Smyth to Green, 12 November 1965; RCOG meeting, London, 14 October 1975, Green Papers, MSS 1433, UOASC.
99 Applications for the Position of Assistant to the Medical Director O & G Hospital Green Lane West, Box 156, UOAA; 'Obituary: Irwin Bruce (Bill) Faris', *NZMJ*, vol. 123, 1319, 30 July 2010, http://journal.nzma.org.nz/journal/123-1319/4241.
100 O & G Hospital Joint Relations Committee, 24 June 1953, Green Papers, MSS 1433, UOASC.
101 Carey to Green, 3 May 1976, Green Papers, MSS 1433, UOASC.
102 University of Auckland O&G Academic Advisory Committee, 1954–1962, 2 December 1954, Box 257, UOAA.
103 Gordon to Barrer, 27 February 1955, Doris Clifton Gordon Papers, MS 116, AMA.
104 For the agreement to appoint and Gordon's dissent, see University of Auckland O&G Academic Advisory Committee, 1954–1962, 2 December 1954, Box 257, UOAA; see also Sinclair, *A History of the University of Auckland*, p. 274.
105 Gordon to Barrer, 27 February 1955, Doris Clifton Gordon Papers, MS 116, AMA.
106 Joan Faulkner-Blake, 'Woman with a Sword', radio broadcast, 21 October 1957, Douglas Robb Papers, 6/2, UOASC.
107 NZOGS AGM, minutes, 16 March 1933; Bryder, 'Gordon, Doris Clifton'.
108 *Auckland Star*, 26 November 1964.
109 For a discussion of 'maternalism', see Bryder, *A Voice for Mothers*, p. xii.
110 Gordon to Mrs Evelyn Lovegrove, 25 November 1955, Joan Donley Papers, UOASC (her underlining).
111 Ibid. Also quoted in *Auckland Star*, 19 September 1979.

3: A TRIPOD: PATIENT CARE, RESEARCH AND TEACHING, THE 1950s TO 1963

1 John Grierson, 'Foreword' and F. L. Clark and G. H. Green, 'Introduction', in F. L. Clark and G. H. Green, *Obstetrical and Gynaecological Unit, Cornwall Hospital, Auckland, NZ, First Clinical Report for the Year Ended 31st March 1949*, Auckland Hospital Board, Auckland, 1950.
2 Geoffrey Chamberlain, *Special Delivery: The Life of the Celebrated Obstetrician William Nixon*, Royal College of Obstetricians and Gynaecologists, London, 2004, p. 93.
3 *Women in Council: Journal of the National Council of Women*, vol. 8, 3, May 1960, p. 4.
4 Grace Pinkerton qualified MRCS LRCP 1952, and registered as a medical practitioner in New Zealand 14 May 1954.
5 O & G Hospital Joint Relations Committee, Applications for the Position of Assistant to the Medical Director O & G Hospital Green Lane West, Box 156, UOAA.
6 Grace Carey (Pinkerton), interviewed by Linda Bryder, 4 July 2004.
7 J. Willocks and A. A. Calder, 'The Glasgow Royal Maternity Hospital 1834–1984: 150 Years of Service in a Changing Obstetric World', *Scottish Medical Journal*, vol. 30, 1985, p. 252.
8 Ian Donald, *Practical Obstetric Problems*, Lloyd-Luke, London, 1st edn, 1955, preface; Lloyd-Luke, London, 3rd edn, 1964, p. vii.
9 Grace Carey (Pinkerton), interviewed by Linda Bryder, 4 July 2004.
10 Elizabeth (Betty) Port, interviewed by Jenny Carlyon, 29 July 2005, transcript, p. 5.
11 *NZH*, 30 August 1946.
12 Ibid.
13 W. H. Cocker to W. Hawksworth, 9 September 1949, Auckland University College, Academic Advisory Committee on O & G, 13 September 1949, Green Papers, MSS 1433, folder 2, UOASC.
14 Ibid.

15. The National government of the 1950s did, however, increase subsidies for private hospitals: see Iain Hay, *The Caring Commodity: The Provision of Health Care in New Zealand*, Oxford University Press, Oxford, 1989, pp. 134–9.
16. Hospital Medical Committe (HMC) minutes, 24 April 1956, 3 December 1957, BAGC A638 38a, ANZA.
17. HMC minutes, 10 December 1962, BAGC A638 22b, ANZA.
18. HMC minutes, 13 December 1955, BAGC A638 37a, ANZA.
19. Letter from L. H. Wright, 8 April 1960, HMC minutes, 2 May 1960, BAGC A638 38b, ANZA.
20. Spence Smyth, Report on the Development of the Department of Post-Graduate Obstetrics and Gynaecology, 1951–1952, Auckland University College, Box 129, UOAA.
21. Carey to Registrar, 25 October 1955, Box 156, UOAA; Carey, Postgraduate School of Obstetrics and Gynaecology, March 1959, p. 2, Box 157, UOAA; one was Dr Rae West: Dr Rae West, interviewed by Scott Morgan, 26 October 2005, transcript, p. 1.
22. Edwin Sayes, email correspondence to Linda Bryder, 27 May 2004.
23. Carey, Postgraduate School of Obstetrics and Gynaecology, March 1959, p. 4, Box 157, UOAA.
24. HMC minutes, 18 June 1962, BAGC A638 39a, ANZA.
25. Ibid.
26. G. H. Green, *Introduction to Obstetrics: A Theory and Practice for Obstetric Nurses*, N. M. Peryer, Christchurch, 1962.
27. For example, G. H. Green, 'Trends in Maternal Mortality', *NZMJ*, vol. 65, February 1966, pp. 80–86; G. H. Green, 'Maori Maternal Mortality in New Zealand', *NZMJ*, vol. 66, May 1967, pp. 295–9.
28. See Bryder, *A History of the 'Unfortunate Experiment'*.
29. Erlam, *A Notable Result*, p. 69.
30. Margaret Liley, unpublished notes, sent to Linda Bryder, 13 September 2005.
31. Sir John Scott, 'Sir Albert William Liley', www.rsnz.org/directory/yearbooks/ybook97/obitLiley.html.
32. Sandoz to Registrar, 3 December 1956, Box 156, UOAA.
33. Foundation Genesis, *Sir William Liley: A Tribute to the Father of Fetology*, Foundation Genesis, Strathfield, New South Wales, 1984, pp. 11–12.
34. Carey to University of Auckland Registrar, 11 October 1956, Box 156, UOAA.
35. Green to University of Auckland Registrar, 8 August 1963, Box 314, UOAA.
36. Mont Liggins, interviewed by Jenny Carlyon, 12 May 2004, transcript, p. 2.
37. Ibid., p. 1.
38. University of Auckland Acting Registrar to Secretary, Auckland Hospital Board, 19 December 1958, Box 157, UOAA.
39. HMC minutes, 16 October 1961, BAGC A638 39a, ANZA.
40. Carey to Green, 3 May 1976, Green Papers, UOASC.
41. 'Obituary: Harvey McKay Carey', *Medical Journal of Australia*, vol. 152, 2 April 1990, p. 379.
42. John Stewart, interviewed by Jenny Carlyon, 9 March 2004, transcript, p. 2.
43. HMC minutes, 30 July 1957, BAGC A638 38a; HMC minutes, 11 June 1960, BAGC A638 38b, ANZA.
44. Cornwall Hospital Medical Committee minutes, 17 June 1948, YCBZ 15492 1a, ANZA.
45. HMC minutes, 13 December 1955, 14 February 1956, BAGC A638 37a, ANZA.
46. Jack Dilworth Matthews, interviewed by Penelope Dunkley, 4 February 1991, transcript, p. 20.
47. HMC minutes, 19 March 1962, BAGC A638 39a, ANZA.
48. HMC minutes, 12 October 1959, BAGC A638 38b, ANZA.
49. HMC minutes, 16 October 1961, BAGC A638 39a, ANZA.
50. HMC minutes, 29 November 1961, BAGC A638 39a, ANZA.
51. HMC minutes, 8 May 1963, BAGC A638 22b, ANZA.
52. HMC minutes, 12 February 1957, BAGC A638 38a, ANZA.

53 Carey to Green, 3 May 1976, Green Papers, UOASC.
54 Jean Donnison, *Midwives and Medical Men: A History of the Struggle for the Control of Childbirth*, Historical Publications, London, 1988, p. 201.
55 Mary Thomas, 'Preface', in Mary Thomas (ed.), *Post-war Mothers: Childbirth Letters to Grantly Dick-Read, 1946–1956*, University of Rochester Press, Rochester, 1997, p. ix.
56 B. V. Kyle and T. J. Buckley, *The Obstetrical and Gynaecological Unit Cornwall Hospital, Green Lane West, Auckland, Third Clinical Report For the Year Ended 31st March 1951*, Auckland Hospital Board, Auckland, 1951, pp. 7, 9, 101, 116.
57 T. R. Plunkett, Postgraduate course in paediatrics, 'Asphyxia Neonatorium', February 1944, AG7 4-275, PSA, Hocken Library (my emphasis).
58 Deputation, Hutt Valley Women's Citizen Guild and the Family Planning Association to Minister of Health, A. H. Nordmeyer, 27 June 1946, H1 13 24626, ANZW.
59 Cited in Caton, *What a Blessing She Had Chloroform*, p. 152.
60 Geoffrey Cumberlege, *Maternity in Great Britain: A Survey of Social and Economic Aspects of Pregnancy and Childbirth Undertaken by a Joint Committee of the Royal College of Obstetricians and Gynaecologists and the Population Investigation Committee*, Oxford University Press, London, 1948, pp. 80, 86.
61 Jenny Kitzinger, 'Strategies of the Early Childbirth Movement: A Case-Study of the National Childbirth Trust', in Garcia et al. (eds), *The Politics of Maternity Care*, pp. 97–98.
62 Deputation, Hutt Valley Women's Citizen Guild and the Family Planning Association to Minister of Health, A. H. Nordmeyer, 27 June 1946, H1 13 24626, ANZ.
63 Cornwall Hospital Medical Committee minutes, 15 March 1948, YCBZ 15492 1a, ANZA.
64 HMC minutes, 20 September 1958, 10 November 1958, BAGC A638 38b, ANZA.
65 Cornwall Hospital Medical Committee minutes, 1 May 1948, YCBZ 15492 1a, ANZA.
66 NZOGS, Report of a Sub-Committee of the Wellington Division on Pain Relief in Obstetrics, *NZMJ*, vol. 50, December 1951, p. 616.
67 T. F. Corkill, 'Chloroform in Obstetrics', *NZMJ*, vol. 49, April 1950, p. 109.
68 HMC minutes, 4 February 1958, BAGC A638 38a, ANZA.
69 Climie to Carey, 2 February 1959, BAGC A638 38b, ANZA.
70 Arnold L. Walker, A. J. Wrigley, A. D. Marston, Katherine M. Hirst and W. J. Martin, *Report on Confidential Enquiries into Maternal Deaths in England and Wales 1952–1954*, Reports on Public Health and Medical Subjects No. 97, HMSO, London, 1957, p. 40; Richard Barnett, 'Obstetric Anaesthesia and Analgesia in England and Wales 1945–1975', PhD thesis, University College London, 2007, pp. 175, 201. See also R. F. J. Hickey and R. B. Dorofaeff, 'A Study of the Effects of Pain Relief in Labour', *NZMJ*, vol. 72, December 1970, pp. 377–82.
71 HMC minutes, 10 November 1958, BAGC A638 38b, ANZA.
72 C. R. Climie, 'Epidural Anaesthesia in Obstetrics', *NZMJ*, vol. 59, March 1960, p. 130.
73 R. B. Parker, 'Maternal Death from Aspiration Asphyxia', *British Medical Journal (BMJ)*, vol. 2, 4983, 7 July 1956, pp. 17–18; on the United States, see also M. Sandelowski, *Pain, Pleasure and American Childbirth: From the Twilight Sleep to the Read Method, 1914–1960*, Greenwood Press, Westport, Connecticut, 1984, p. 93. Wolf found that around 1950 obstetric anaesthesia was implicated in one of every eight deaths in the United States: Wolf, *Deliver Me From Pain*, p. 78.
74 Climie, 'Epidural Anaesthesia in Obstetrics', p. 130; see R. B. Parker, 'Risk from the Aspiration of Vomit during Obstetric Anaesthesia', *BMJ*, vol. 2, 4879, 10 July 1954, pp. 65–69.
75 Hickey and Dorofaeff, 'A Study of

76 T. R. Plunkett, Postgraduate course in paediatrics, 'Asphyxia Neonatorium', February 1944, AG7 4-275, PSA, Hocken Library.

77 Clark and Green, *First Clinical Report*, p. 110.

78 Walker et al., *Report on Confidential Enquiries into Maternal Deaths, 1957*, p. 42.

79 HMC minutes, 2 March 1959, BAGC A638 38b, ANZA; on Mushin, see also 'Obituary: William Woolf Mushin', *Anaesthesia*, vol. 48, 6, June 1993, pp. 461–2.

80 C. R. Climie to Carey, 9 February 1959, HMC minutes, 2 March 1959, BAGC A638 38b, ANZA.

81 Climie, 'Epidural Anaesthesia in Obstetrics', p. 129.

82 Ibid., pp. 127–30.

83 C. R. Climie to Carey, January 1959, HMC minutes, 2 February 1959, BAGC A638 38b, ANZA.

84 C. R. Climie to Carey, 2 February 1959, BAGC A638 38b, ANZA.

85 Richard B. Clark, 'Epidural Anesthesia in Obstetrics: How Did Lumbar Epidural Technique Become the Prime Obstetric Anesthetic in the United States?', *American Society of Anesthesiologists Newsletter*, vol. 62, March 1998, http://www.asahq.org/Newsletters/1998/03_98/Epidural_0398.html.

86 Climie to Carey, 22 April 1960, HMC minutes, 2 May 1960, BAGC A638 38b, ANZA.

87 *NZH*, 1 August 1956; the percentage of deliveries involving instrumental intervention was 3.7 per cent of all hospital deliveries in 1953 in Britain: Barnett, 'Obstetric Anaesthesia and Analgesia', p. 82. Dick-Read's middle and last name were legally hyphenated in 1958: see Thomas (ed.), *Post-war Mothers*, p. 9.

88 H. E. Reiss, 'Francis James Browne, 1879–1963: A Great Obstetrician and a Great Teacher', *Journal of Obstetrics and Gynaecology*, vol. 24, 6, September 2004, pp. 696–9.

89 Francis J. Browne, *Antenatal and Postnatal Care*, J. & A. Churchill, London, 1937; Grantly Dick-Read, *Revelation of Childbirth: The Principles and Practice of Natural Childbirth*, William Heinemann, London, 1943, p. vii.

90 Vera Crowther, 'Correspondence: Maternity and the Working Woman', *Woman To-day*, January 1938, p. 240.

91 T. R. Plunkett, Postgraduate course in paediatrics, 'Asphyxia Neonatorium', February 1944, AG7 4-275, PSA, Hocken Library.

92 Grantly Dick-Read, letter to the editor, 'Obstetric Methods', *Auckland Star*, 13 March 1956.

93 Maurice Bevan-Brown, *The Sources of Love and Fear, with Contributions by Members of the Christchurch Psychological Society*, A. H. & A. W. Reed, Wellington, 1950; Mary Dobbie, *The Trouble with Women: The Story of Parents Centre New Zealand*, Cape Catley, Whatamongo Bay, 1990; Marie Bell, *The Establishment of Parents' Centre: Successful Advocacy for Parents of Children under Three by the Parents' Centre Organisation in its First Decade 1952–1962*, Institute for Early Childhood Studies, Occasional Papers Series 18, Victoria University of Wellington, Wellington, 2006, p. 2.

94 Thomas (ed.), *Post-war Mothers*, p. 73.

95 Dobbie, *The Trouble with Women*, p. 43; Bevan-Brown, *The Sources of Love and Fear*, pp. 53–54.

96 Helen Brew, 'Viewpoints in Antenatal Education. The Parents' Viewpoint', speech at National Women's Hospital 1958, pp. 3, 12, 'Early Wellington Branch', Box 1.0, Federation of New Zealand Parents' Centres (FNZPC) Archives, Wellington; also cited in Karen Guilliland and Sally Pairman, *Women's Business: The Story of the New Zealand College of Midwives 1986–2010*, New Zealand College of Midwives, Christchurch, 2010, p. 187.

97 Dobbie, *The Trouble with Women*, p. 43.

98 *NZH*, 1 August 1956.

99 *Auckland Star*, 24 February 1956.

100 Dobbie, *The Trouble with Women*, p. 43.

101 FNZPC, *First Annual Report 1958*, p. 2, Box 1.1, FNZPC Archives.
102 Dobbie, *The Trouble with Women*, p. 52.
103 *Auckland Star*, 24 February 1956.
104 Letter to the editor, 'Painless Childbirth', *Auckland Star*, 21 February 1956.
105 FNZPC, First Dominion Conference, 29 March 1957, p. 5, Box 1.0, FNZPC Archives, Wellington.
106 Letter to the editor, 'Pangs of Childbirth', *Auckland Star*, 10 February 1956.
107 Climie, 'Epidural Anaesthesia in Obstetrics', p. 129.
108 Wolf, *Deliver Me From Pain*, pp. 84, 110, 119.
109 Donald, *Practical Obstetric Problems*, 1st edn, p. 324.
110 HMC minutes, 10 October 1960, BAGC A638 38b, ANZA.
111 Jellett, *The Causes and Prevention of Maternal Mortality*, p. 223.
112 Kyle and Buckley, *Third Clinical Report*, pp. 7, 9, 101, 116; for Britain, see Barnett, 'Obstetric Anaesthesia and Analgesia', p. 82.
113 G. H. Green, *Obstetrical and Gynaecological Unit, Cornwall Hospital, Auckland, NZ, Second Clinical Report, for the Year Ended 31st March 1950*, Auckland Hospital Board, Auckland, 1951, p. 3.
114 Ibid., 'Review of the Year's Work', p. 11. On this practice, see also Mitchinson, *Giving Birth in Canada*, p. 256. Like his counterparts in Canada (Mitchinson, *Giving Birth in Canada*, p. 258), Green stressed the importance of patient consent in sterilisation: G. H. Green, 'Tubal Ligation', *NZMJ*, vol. 57, February 1958, pp. 470–7.
115 HMC minutes, 10 October 1960, BAGC A638 38b, ANZA.
116 HMC minutes, 21 July 1958, BAGC A638 37a, ANZA; H. P. Dunn, 'Sequelae of Caesarean Section', *NZMJ*, vol. 59, April 1960, pp. 180–3.
117 'Leading Article: Maternal Mortality', *BMJ*, vol. 2, 5039, 3 August 1957, p. 281.
118 HMC minutes, 21 July 1958, BAGC A638 37a, ANZA; Dunn, 'Sequelae of Caesarean Section', pp. 180–3.
119 D. H. Smith and H. M. Carey, 'Continuous Integration of the Foetal Heart Rate', *NZMJ*, vol. 55, February 1956, pp. 309–12; *Auckland Star*, 17 February 1956.
120 Carey to K. Maidment, Principal, Auckland University College, 17 July 1953, Box 129, UOAA.
121 HMC minutes, 12 February 1957, BAGC A638 38a, ANZA. On the development of the fetal heart monitor, see Adrian Grant, 'Monitoring the Fetus During Labour', in Iain Chalmers, Murray Enkin and Marc J. N. C. Keirse (eds), *Effective Care in Pregnancy and Childbirth, vol. 2: Childbirth*, Oxford University Press, Oxford, 1989, p. 848.
122 HMC minutes, 21 July 1958, BAGC A638 37a, ANZA.
123 Dunn, 'Sequelae of Caesarean Section', p. 183; HMC minutes, 2 February 1959, BAGC A638 38b, ANZA.
124 H. A. Brant, 'Childbirth with Preparation and Support in Labour: An Assessment', *NZMJ*, vol. 61, April 1962, pp. 211–19. On the 'Apgar scale', see chapter 5.
125 Dobbie, *The Trouble with Women*, p. 76.
126 Herbert A. Brant and Margaret Brant, *A Dictionary of Pregnancy, Childbirth and Contraception*, Mayflower, London, 1971.
127 Fay Hercock, *Alice: The Making of a Woman Doctor, 1914–1974*, Auckland University Press, Auckland, 1999, p. 139; Helen Smyth, *Rocking the Cradle: Contraception, Sex and Politics in New Zealand*, Steele Roberts, Wellington, 2000, p. 85.
128 Hercock, *Alice*, p. 143.
129 Minutes of Auckland Division of the New Zealand Branch of the British Medical Association, 31 May and 30 August 1961, Box 5, acc. 1224, UOASC.
130 Hercock, *Alice*, p. 147; Minutes of Auckland Division, 7 June 1961, Box 6, UOASC.
131 Dobbie, *The Trouble with Women*, p. 81.
132 Carey to Secretary, Auckland Hospital

Board, 29 January 1960, Box 157, UOAA.
133 Algar Warren, Memorandum to Superintendent-in-chief, 17 November 1960, Extract 1, The Postgraduate School of Obstetrics and Gynaecology and its Relationships with the Auckland Hospital Board and the Auckland School of Medicine, March 1975, Box 157, UOAA.
134 Carey to Registrar, University of Auckland, 7 November 1960, Box 157, UOAA.
135 Warren to Secretary, Auckland Hospital Board, Joint Relations Committee minutes, 18 April 1961, p. 27, Box 157, UOAA.
136 Carey to Green, 3 May 1976, Green Papers, UOASC.
137 Carey to Registrar, University of Auckland, 16 July 1962, Box 257, UOAA.
138 Ibid.; also reported in *NZH*, 22 August 1962.
139 Harvey Carey (ed.), *Modern Trends in Human Reproductive Physiology – 1*, Butterworths, London, 1963.
140 Dobbie, *The Trouble with Women*, p. 81.
141 Sir John Scott, in L. Bryder and D. A. Dow (eds), *The History of Fetal Medicine with a Special Emphasis on Auckland*, Witness Seminar at Old Government House, The University of Auckland, 19 February 2005, The Australian and New Zealand Society of the History of Medicine, Auckland, 2006, p. 44.
142 William Liley to Douglas Robb, 18 May 1965, Douglas Robb Papers, 7/1, UOAA.

4: A WOMAN'S WORLD: MOTHERS, NURSES AND MIDWIVES AT NATIONAL WOMEN'S, THE 1950s TO 1963

1 Janet McCalman, *Sex and Suffering: Women's Health and a Women's Hospital: The Royal Women's Hospital, Melbourne, 1856–1996*, Melbourne University Press, Carlton, Victoria, 1998, p. 280.
2 NMRB existed from 1925 to 1971 when its role was taken over by the Nursing Council of New Zealand.
3 Spence Smyth, Report on the Development of the Department of Post-Graduate Obstetrics and Gynaecology, 1951–1952, Auckland University College, Box 129, UOAA.
4 *NZH*, 26 May 1956.
5 HMC minutes, 12 February 1957, BAGC A638 38a, ANZA.
6 HMC minutes, 8 October 1957, BAGC A638 38a, ANZA; HMC minutes, 3 December 1957, BAGC A638 38a, ANZA.
7 Barry Twydle, interviewed by Jenny Carlyon, 18 September 2004. On Barry Twydle, National Women's first male maternity nurse and later midwife, see also *New Zealand Woman's Weekly (NZWW)*, 7 June 1982, pp. 4–5.
8 NZOGS minutes, 23 September 1936, 26 February 1937, 1 September 1937, 8 April 1942; Dr Craven, Medical Superintendent of Auckland Hospital, also told the 1937 Committee of Inquiry into Maternity that, 'Many of our nurses have told me that they are going to take maternity training because they cannot get a decent job without it': Joseph Craven, Evidence to Committee of Inquiry into Maternity Services, 7 September 1937, MS 78, AMA.
9 See Bryder, *A Voice for Mothers*, p. 59.
10 NZOGS minutes, 25 March 1941, Dr Francis Bennett, 22 October 1941.
11 NZOGS minutes, 22 October 1941.
12 See Melanie Nolan, *Breadwinning: New Zealand Women and the State*, Canterbury University Press, Christchurch, 2000, pp. 225–9. On the 'disastrous shortage of nursing and domestic staff' in maternity hospitals, see also British Medical Association (NZ Branch), *Report of the Committee of Inquiry into Maternity Hospital Staffing, 1946*, British Medical Association (NZ Branch), Wellington, 1947; and 'Editorial: The 1946 Committee of Inquiry into Maternity Hospital Staffing', *NZMJ*, vol. 46, April 1947, pp. 75–77.
13 McCalman, *Sex and Suffering*, p. 257; Madonna May Grehan, 'Professional

Aspirations and Consumer Expectations: Nurses, Midwives and Women's Health', PhD thesis, University of Melbourne, 2009, p. 258, where she states a 1948 inquiry concluded that workforce shortages occurred because midwifery training was undertaken for career advancement, rather than to practise in midwifery, and because many women married immediately after training.

14 Mary Ellen O'Connor, *Freed to Care, Proud to Nurse: 100 Years of the New Zealand Nurses Organisation*, New Zealand Nurses Organisation, Wellington, 2010, p. 103.

15 Cornwall Hospital Medical Committee minutes, 22 November 1948, YCBZ 15492 1a, ANZA.

16 HMC minutes, 8 November 1955, BAGC A638 37a, ANZA.

17 HMC minutes, 12 February 1957, BAGC A638 38a, ANZA.

18 Harvey Carey to Betty Holt, 26 May 1956, NCW, MS 879 21 1956, AMA.

19 Anne Nightingale, interviewed by Deborah Jowitt, 21 February 2003, transcript, p. 5.

20 Noted in HMC minutes, 24 July 1956, BAGC A638 38a, ANZA.

21 Deborah Jowitt, 'The H-Bug Epidemic: The Impact of Antibiotic-resistant Staphylococcal Infection on New Zealand Society and Health 1955–1963', MSc (Midwifery) thesis, Auckland University of Technology, 2004.

22 HMC minutes, 28 August 1956, BAGC A638 38a, ANZA. The controlled trial involved 554 cases in a ward providing showering techniques with a pyrexia incidence of 6.5%, and 518 in the 'control' ward according to the technique laid down by the nursing regulations with a pyrexia incidence of 6.5%: Carey to Douglas Robb, 25 October 1955, Green Papers, MSS 1433, folder 3, UOASC.

23 HMC minutes, 24 July 1956, BAGC A638 38a, ANZA.

24 Carey to Douglas Robb, 25 October 1955, Green Papers, MSS 1433, UOASC.

25 R. Durand, 'Rooming-in – Results of an Inquiry', *NZMJ*, vol. 59, October 1960, pp. 457–8.

26 Louisa Dixon, interviewed by Chanel Clarke, 28 June 2002, National Women's Oral History Project, transcript, p. 5.

27 HMC minutes, 8 November 1955, BAGC A638 38a, ANZA.

28 McCalman, *Sex and Suffering*, p. 257.

29 HMC minutes (Dr Phillips), 24 April 1956, BAGC A638 38a, ANZA.

30 Dobbie, *The Trouble with Women*, p. 51. For debates around 'demand feeding', see Bryder, *A Voice for Mothers*, pp. 118–26.

31 HMC minutes, 12 February 1957, BAGC A638 38a, ANZA.

32 See also Elizabeth Temkin, 'Rooming-in: Redesigning Hospitals and Motherhood in Cold War America', *Bulletin of the History of Medicine*, vol. 76, 2, 2002, pp. 271–98.

33 HMC minutes, 25 October 1955, BAGC A638 37a; HMC minutes, 26 June 1956, BAGC A638 38a, ANZA.

34 HMC minutes, 26 March 1957, BAGC A638 38a; HMC minutes, 15 June 1964, BAGC A638 39b, ANZA.

35 Personal notes from Margaret Liley (née Helen Margaret Irwin Hunt, born 6 January 1928), 16 September 2005, presented following Witness Seminar, Auckland, 2005.

36 HMC minutes, 17 September 1962, BAGC A638 22b, ANZA.

37 Christina A. Jeffery, 'Whanautanga: The Experiences of Maori Women who Gave Birth at National Women's Hospital 1958–2004', MA thesis, University of Auckland, 2005, p. 41.

38 'M.S. Readers Have Their Say', *New Zealand Family Doctor*, November 1958, p. 7.

39 Report on a Maternity Services Survey September 1961, H1 29/21 (27900), ANZW; Elizabeth Orr, 'A Maternity Services Survey', *New Zealand Nursing Journal: Kai Tiaki (NZNJ)*, vol. 55, 9, September 1962, pp. 6–7.

40 Gabrielle Bourke, 'Illuminating the Dark Hour: Auckland's St Helens Hospital, 1906–1990', MA thesis, University of Auckland, 2006, p. 135. Some mothers' misgivings about rooming-in continued in the following years: see Amy Brown, 'The

Maternity Technique, Enjoy Your Stay in Hospital', *Thursday*, 1 October 1970, p. 62.
41 This was spelt out in HMC minutes, 1 December 1958, BAGC A638 38b, ANZA.
42 HMC minutes, 12 February 1957, BAGC A638 38a, ANZA.
43 HMC minutes, 27 March 1956, BAGC A638 38a, ANZA.
44 Mary Dobbie, 'A Wise and Lovable Woman . . . Rissa Scelly 1907–1983', *Parents Centre Bulletin*, vol. 98, 1984, p. 15; HMC minutes, 1 December 1958, BAGC A638 38b, ANZA.
45 HMC minutes, 1 December 1958, BAGC A638 38b, ANZA.
46 Barbara Smith, interviewed by Jenny Carlyon, 17 September 2004, transcript, p. 8; Moira Tretheway, interviewed by Jenny Carlyon, 22 November 2005, transcript, p. 4. See also Val Dickens, interviewed by Jenny Carlyon, 24 November 2005, transcript, pp. 7–8.
47 HMC minutes, 16 May 1962, BAGC A638 22b, ANZA.
48 HMC minutes, 3 December 1957, BAGC A638 38a, ANZA.
49 Else Bryder, personal communication.
50 Margaret Liley, personal communication, 13 September 2005.
51 National Women's Hospital Medical Committee minutes, 11 June 1960, BAGC A638 38b, ANZA.
52 Report on a Maternity Services Survey September 1961, H1 29/21 27900, ANZW; Orr, 'A Maternity Services Survey', pp. 6–7.
53 Dorothy McAleer, interviewed by Jenny Carlyon, 5 September 2004, transcript, p. 10.
54 Else Bryder, personal communication.
55 Jeffery, 'Whanautanga', p. 107.
56 Joyce Hare, interviewed by Chanel Clarke, 31 May 2002, transcript, pp. 9, 12.
57 Dorothy McAleer, interviewed by Jenny Carlyon, 5 September 2004, transcript, p. 3.
58 McCalman, *Sex and Suffering*, p. 293.
59 Chamberlain, *Special Delivery*, pp. 55–56.
60 Jack Dilworth Matthews, interviewed by Penelope Dunkley, 4 February 1991, transcript, p. 14.
61 Isobel Fisher, interviewed by Jenny Carlyon, 7 September 2004, transcript, p. 7.
62 L. Bryder, 'Breastfeeding and Health Professionals in Britain, New Zealand and the United States, 1900–1970', *Medical History*, vol. 49, 2, 2005, pp. 179–96.
63 Report by Medical Director and Matron, 8 October 1952, AG 7 4-114, PSA, Hocken Library.
64 Jack Dilworth Matthews, interviewed by Penelope Dunkley, 12 February 1991, transcript, pp. 17–18.
65 See, for example, Donley, *Save the Midwife*, pp. 1, 11.
66 Report of First Dominion Conference 1957, Box 1.0, FNZPC Archives, Wellington; *Evening Post*, 30 March 1957; *Dominion*, 1 April 1957.
67 Dobbie, *The Trouble with Women*, p. 42.
68 Ibid., p. 48.
69 FNZPC, *First Annual Report 1958*, pp. 2–3, Box 1.1, FNZPC Archives, Wellington.
70 FNZPC Conference, June 1959, p. 57, FNZPC Archives, Wellington.
71 FNZPC News Brief, to all Centres from Hon. Sec. E. J. Campbell, 10 September 1961, Box 123, FNZPC Archives, Wellington.
72 Bryder, *A Voice for Mothers*, pp. 127–9.
73 The Plunket Society had similar concerns mid-century: see Bryder, *A Voice for Mothers*, pp. 126–31.
74 The FNZPC Educational Advisory Council included Dr Enid Cook, psychiatrist, Wellington; Dr Wallace Ironside, head of Department of Psychiatry, Otago Medical School; Professor H. C. D. Somerset, Department of Education, Victoria University of Wellington, and member of the National Council of Adult Education; Dr Maurice Bevan-Brown, psychiatrist, Wellington; Mr Quentin Brew, psychologist, Department of Education, Wellington; Mr A. Grey, lecturer in child development, Auckland Teachers' College; Dr J. Robb, social scientist, Victoria

University of Wellington; Professor Philip Smithells, director, School of Physical Education, University of Otago: FNZPC, *First Annual Report 1958*, p. 1, Box 1.1, FNZPC Archives, Wellington.
75 FNZPC, *First Annual Report 1958*, p. 2, Box 1.1, FNZPC Archives, Wellington.
76 Reported in Minutes of Auckland Division BMA, 28 January 1958, 30 August 1961, NZMA Auckland Division Archives, 1224, Box 5, UOASC; Dobbie, *The Trouble with Women*, p. 78.
77 Barry Twydle, interviewed by Jenny Carlyon, 18 September 2004, transcript, p. 1. From 1977 there were no differences in training between male and female nurses.
78 Dobbie, *The Trouble with Women*, p. 62.
79 HMC minutes, 5 September 1960, BAGC A638 38b, ANZA; Senior Medical Staff, National Women's Hospital (22 names), 'To the Editor: New Nursing Curriculum', *NZMJ*, vol. 59, October 1960, pp. 500–1.
80 Report by Sub-Committee, Wellington Branch Parents' Centre, 5 February 1960, p. 10, Box 1.1, FNZPC Archives, Wellington.
81 Ibid., p.15.
82 Dobbie, *The Trouble with Women*, p. 64; Bonham complained in 1976 that rectal examinations were still being carried out in some hospitals: see Maternity Services Committee, *Maternity Services in New Zealand: A Report by the Maternity Services Committee Board of Health*, Board of Health Report Series No. 26, Government Printer, Wellington, 1976, p. 10.
83 Report by Sub-Committee, Wellington Branch Parents' Centre, 5 February 1960, p. 10, Views of the Director of Nursing, p. 15, Box 1.1, FNZPC Archives, Wellington.
84 Kathleen A. Latch, Hon. Sec., National Council of Women, Auckland Branch, to Secretary, Nurses' and Midwives' Board, 27 June 1956, copy forwarded by Carey to University Registrar, Box 156, UOAA.
85 NCW, Auckland Branch minutes, 24 August 1959, MS 879, 39, AMA.
86 Dobbie, *The Trouble with Women*, p. 70.
87 *NZH*, 6 December 1959.
88 'Maternity Services in New Zealand: Report by a Sub-Committee of the Wellington Branch of the National Council of Women', 5 February 1960, p. 22, Box 1.1: Early Federation Files, Executive minutes 1957–64–75, FNZPC Archives, Wellington.
89 Ibid., pp. 24, 26; see also Dobbie, *The Trouble with Women*, pp. 65–66; and O'Connor, *Freed to Care, Proud to Nurse*, pp. 124, 148.
90 'Are New Zealand's Maternity Services Perfect? Report by a Committee', *Women's Viewpoint*, vol. 1, 1 June 1960, p. 35 (Organ of the NCW Auckland Branch); NCW, Auckland Branch minutes, 22 February 1960, MS 879, 40, AMA.
91 Dobbie, *The Trouble with Women*, p. 67.
92 *Auckland Star*, 21 March 1960.
93 W. R. Aitchison to Director-General of Health, 26 August 1960, H1 29/21 27900, ANZW.
94 Dobbie, *The Trouble with Women*, pp. 65, 71 (her emphasis). Bidets were eventually included in each ward of the new National Women's Hospital: Med sup memo (Bidet Pans) to Secretary, Auckland Hospital Board, 12 March 1964, HMC minutes, 20 May 1964, BAGC A638 39b, ANZA.
95 Dobbie, *The Trouble with Women*, p. 65.
96 Green to Mrs Helen Brew, 16 June 1960, Box 2.1, FNZPC Archives, Wellington.
97 H. B. Turbott, memo, 30 June 1960, H 13 27353, 'Maternal 1953–61', ANZW.
98 H. G. R. Mason, memo to Secretary, Board of Health, 6 July 1960, H1 29/21 27900, ANZW.
99 Dobbie, *The Trouble with Women*, p. 70.
100 Beverley Ross, Oamaru Mothers' Group, 1960, H1 27900, ANZW.
101 *Dominion*, 19 September 1960.
102 Ibid.

103 Sec. Board of Health to NCW Dominion Secretary, 2 March 1962, H1 1936 29/21 30145, ANZW.
104 Beverley Ross, Oamaru Mothers' Group to Don McKay, Minister of Health, 24 May 1962, and reply, 6 June 1962, H1 1936 29/21 30145, ANZW.
105 She was still on the committee during the Maternity Services survey, 1969–72: Maternity Services Committee, *Maternity Services in New Zealand*, p. 2.
106 New Zealand Federation of University Women, Report on a Maternity Services Survey, September 1961, p. 1, H1 29/21 27900, ANZW; Orr, 'A Maternity Services Survey', p. 6.
107 Orr, 'A Maternity Services Survey', pp. 6–7.
108 Leavitt, *Brought to Bed*, p. 192.
109 Bryder, *A Voice for Mothers*, p. 132; Dobbie, *The Trouble with Women*, p. 21.
110 HMC minutes, 14 September 1954, BAGC A638 37a, ANZA.
111 *NZH*, 27 January 1960.
112 HMC minutes, 10 October 1960, BAGC A638 38b, ANZA.
113 *Auckland Star*, 5 January 1960.
114 Bourke, 'Illuminating the Dark Hour', p. 131.
115 Joan Dodd, interviewed by Jenny Carlyon, 17 September 2004, transcript, pp. 1–2.

5: FROM PREMATURE NURSERY TO PAEDIATRIC DEPARTMENT, 1950s TO 1963

1 Gordon to Deem, 28 November 1940, Doris Gordon papers, MS 115, AM.
2 See Bryder, *A Voice for Mothers*, pp. 86–91.
3 Plunket Society, Auckland Branch, *Annual Report for 1926*, p. 34, cited in Linda Bryder, *Not Just Weighing Babies: Plunket in Auckland, 1908–1998*, Pyramid Press, Auckland, 1998, p. 38.
4 Ibid., p. 35.
5 *New Zealand Observer*, 1931, cited in Bryder, *Not Just Weighing Babies*, p. 40; and Bryder, *A Voice for Mothers*, p. 87.
6 *Weekly News*, 5 June 1946.
7 Plunket Society, *Proceedings of 1922 Annual Conference*, Dunedin, p. 24.
8 Jeffrey P. Baker, *The Machine in the Nursery: Incubator Technology and the Origins of Newborn Intensive Care*, Johns Hopkins University Press, Baltimore, 1996, p. 2.
9 See Peter M. Dunn, 'The Development of Newborn Care in the UK since 1930, American Academy of Pediatrics Thomas E. Cone, Jr. Lecture on Perinatal History', *Journal of Perinatology*, vol. 18, 6, 1, 1998, p. 472; Baker, *The Machine in the Nursery*, p. 2; Alan Browne (ed.), *Masters, Midwives and Ladies-in-Waiting: The Rotunda Hospital 1745–1995*, A. & A. Farmar, Dublin, 1995, p. 119.
10 Bryder, *Not Just Weighing Babies*, p. 38; Plunket Society, Auckland Branch, *Annual Report for 1926*, p. 11.
11 See Bryder, *Not Just Weighing Babies*, p. 40.
12 Ludbrook to Deem, 19 July 1948, AG 7, 581, PSA, Hocken Library.
13 Ibid.
14 Cornwall Hospital Medical Committee minutes, 14 July 1948, 23 August 1948, YCBZ 15492 1a, ANZA.
15 Jack Matthews, interviewed by Penelope Dunkley, 4 May 1991, transcript, p. 9, OHInt-0131/07, Neonatal Nursing Oral History Project, Alexander Turnbull Library, Wellington.
16 Green, *Second Clinical Report*, p. 13; Kyle and Buckley, *Third Clinical Report*, p. 11.
17 Kyle and Buckley, *Third Clinical Report*, pp. 11, 143. The definition of prematurity had been given by Moncrieff in 1936: see John O. Forfar, *Child Health in a Changing Society*, Oxford University Press, Oxford, 1988.
18 Green, *Second Clinical Report*, p. 13.
19 Cornwall Hospital Medical Committee minutes, 22 May 1950, YCBZ 15492 1a, ANZA.
20 Jack Matthews, interviewed by Penelope Dunkley, 12 May 1991, transcript, p. 1.
21 HMC minutes, 16 July 1962, BAGC A638 22b, ANZA.
22 Jack Matthews, interviewed by Penelope

23 Dunkley, 4 May 1991, transcript, p. 24.
Ibid., p. 12.
24 Clark and Green, *First Clinical Report*, p. 126.
25 Jack Matthews, interviewed by Penelope Dunkley, 4 May 1991, transcript, pp. 24–25.
26 *Auckland Star*, 27 July 1955.
27 Ross N. Howie, '"Historical Events at National Women's Hospital": Comments on the Booklet (Aug. 2004 version) Circulated at the Hospital's Farewell Function 24 Sep. 2004', 1 October 2004 (in author's possession).
28 Jack Matthews, interviewed by Penelope Dunkley, 4 May 1991, transcript, pp. 23, 25.
29 See also McCalman, *Sex and Suffering*, pp. 245, 409, note 88; Reuben Hertzberg, 'Michael Hugh Mulvihille Ryan', *Australian Journal of Ophthalmology*, vol. 10, 1982, pp. 3–4.
30 Study cited in W. J. Hope-Robertson, 'Retrolental Fibroplasia', *NZMJ*, vol. 54, October 1955, p. 537.
31 Ibid., pp. 538–9; Neil C. Begg and Rowland P. Wilson, 'Retrolental Fibroplasia: Report of a Case', *NZMJ*, vol. 52, February 1953, pp. 30–34.
32 Browne, *Masters, Midwives and Ladies-in-Waiting*, p. 140.
33 Dunn, 'The Development of Newborn Care', p. 472.
34 Jack Matthews, interviewed by Penelope Dunkley, 12 May 1991, transcript, p. 2.
35 'Obituary: V. Mary Crosse OBE, MD, MMSA, DObstRCOG, DPH', *BMJ*, vol. 2, 5859, 21 April 1973, p. 183.
36 University of Auckland O & G Academic Advisory Committee minutes, 14 August 1962, Minutes 1954–1962, Box 257, UOAA.
37 HMC minutes, 14 February 1956, BAGC A638 37a, ANZA.
38 HMC minutes, 12 February 1957, BAGC A638 38a, ANZA.
39 Dunn, 'The Development of Newborn Care', p. 473. See also D. A. Christie and E. M. Tansey (eds), *Origins of Neonatal Intensive Care in the UK: A Witness Seminar held at the Wellcome Institute for the History of Medicine, London, 27 April 1999*, vol. 9, Wellcome Trust, London, 2001, p. 36.
40 Professor Tom Oppé, in Christie and Tansey (eds), *Origins of Neonatal Intensive Care*, p. 36.
41 'Obituary: Louis K. Diamond', *Transfusion*, vol. 42, October 2002, pp. 1381–2.
42 Clark and Green, *First Clinical Report*, p. 96.
43 Dunn, 'The Development of Newborn Care', p. 473; 'Obituary: Louis K. Diamond'.
44 Green, *Second Clinical Report*, p. 13.
45 B. W. Grieve, 'Haemolytic Disease of the Newborn: Obstetric Aspects', *NZMJ*, vol. 52, June 1953, pp. 164, 167.
46 HMC minutes, 27 March 1956, BAGC A638 38a, ANZA.
47 HMC minutes, 2 July 1957, BAGC A638 38a, ANZA.
48 Ross Howie, 'Prenatal Glucocorticoids in Preterm Birth: A Paediatric View of the History of the Original Studies by Ross Howie, 2 June 2004', in L. A. Reynolds and E. M. Tansey (eds), *Prenatal Corticosteroids for Reducing Morbidity and Mortality after Preterm Birth: The Transcript of a Witness Seminar held by the Wellcome Trust Centre for the History of Medicine at UCL, London, on 15 June 2004*, vol. 25, Wellcome Trust, London, 2005, appendix 2, p. 89.
49 D. C. A. Bevis, 'Blood Pigments in Haemolytic Disease of the Newborn', *Journal of Obstetrics and Gynaecology of the British Empire*, vol. 63, 1956, pp. 68–75; A. H. C. Walker, 'Liquor Amnii Studies in the Prediction of Haemolytic Disease of the Newborn', *BMJ*, vol. 2, 5041, 17 August 1957, pp. 376–8.
50 HMC minutes, 3 August 1959, BAGC A638 38b, ANZA.
51 HMC minutes, 14 March 1961, BAGC A638 39a, ANZA.
52 A. W. Liley, 'Intrauterine Transfusion of Foetus in Haemolytic Disease', *BMJ*, vol. 2, 5365, 2 November 1963, pp. 1107–9; G. H. Green, A. W. Liley and G. C. Liggins, 'The Place of Foetal Transfusion in Haemolytic Disease:

A Report of 22 Transfusions in 16 Patients', *Australian and New Zealand Journal of Obstetrics and Gynaecology*, vol. 5, 1965, pp. 53–59; A. W. Liley, 'The Development of the Idea of Fetal Transfusion', *American Journal of Obstetrics and Gynecology*, vol. 3, 1971, pp. 302–4.

53 'National Women's Hospital Research Projects', December 1962 (report given to author by Professor John France).

54 HMC minutes, 16 June 1962, BAGC A638 22b, ANZA.

55 Green to University of Auckland Registrar, 8 August 1963, Box 314, UOAA.

56 Barbara J. Hawgood, 'Physiologists: Professor Sir William Liley (1929–83): New Zealand Perinatal Physiologist', *Journal of Medical Biography*, vol. 13, 2, May 2005, p. 85.

57 *NZH*, 19 September 1973.

58 Liley, 'Intrauterine Transfusion of Foetus in Haemolytic Disease' (acknowledgements), p. 1109; see also Bryder and Dow (eds), *The History of Fetal Medicine with a Special Emphasis on Auckland*, pp. 22, 23.

59 *NZH*, 19 September 1973.

60 Moira Tretheway, interviewed by Jenny Carlyon, 22 November 2005, transcript, p. 6.

61 Reported in *The Times*, 24 September 1963.

62 *NZH*, 19 September 1973; see also 'The Miraculous Blood Transfusion', *Weekly News*, 30 December 1964.

63 Monica J. Casper, *The Making of the Unborn Patient: A Social Anatomy of Fetal Surgery*, Rutgers University Press, New Brunswick, 1998, p. 34. 'Whenua' is Maori for both land and placenta, revealing a spiritual connection between the land and the womb.

64 John Stallworthy, *43rd RCOG Annual Report*, 1971, pp. 70–71, A4/17/7, RCOG Archives, London. (New Zealand might look small on the map but in fact it is c. 268,000 square kilometres compared to the UK's c. 244,000 sq. km.)

65 Casper, *The Making of the Unborn Patient*, pp. 30, 56.

66 University of Auckland, Department of Obstetrics and Gynaecology, *Annual Report of the Superintendent-in-chief, Auckland Hospital Board, for Year Ending 31 March 1966*, p. 43.

67 D. T. Zallen, D. A. Christie and E. M. Tansey (eds), *The Rhesus Factor and Disease Prevention: The Transcript of a Witness Seminar held by the Wellcome Trust Centre for the History of Medicine at UCL, London, on 3 June 2003*, vol. 22, Wellcome Trust, London, 2004, p. 57.

68 Dubow, *Ourselves Unborn*, p. 5.

69 University meeting with Medical Research Council, 25 July 1968, Box 208, UOAA.

70 Bonham to Kirkness, 23 May 1968, Box 208, UOAA.

71 Browne, *Masters, Midwives and Ladies-in-Waiting*, pp. 118, 133.

72 Dunn, 'The Development of Newborn Care', p. 473.

73 HMC minutes, 8 February 1960, BAGC A638 38b, ANZA.

74 HMC minutes, 26 June 1956, BAGC A638 38a, ANZA.

75 V. Apgar, 'A Proposal for a New Method of Evaluation of the Newborn Infant', *Anesthesia and Analgesia Current Research*, vol. 32, 1953, p. 260.

76 HMC minutes, 10 October 1960, BAGC A638 38b, ANZA.

77 HMC minutes, 16 October 1961, BAGC A638 39a, ANZA.

78 Ibid. That anaesthetists were still involved in resuscitation in 1969 is evidenced by an article in the *NZMJ* written by National Women's senior anaesthetist Ian Hutchison: I. L. G. Hutchison, 'Neonatal Resuscitation Table', *NZMJ*, vol. 70, September 1969, pp. 175–8.

79 HMC minutes, 19 March 1962, BAGC A638 39a, ANZA.

80 HMC minutes, 27 August 1962, BAGC A638 39a, ANZA.

81 Medical Superintendent memo to Secretary, HMC, 6 August 1962, HMC minutes, 27 August 1962, BAGC A638 39a, ANZA.

82 R. R. A. Coombs, A. E. Mourant and R. R. Race, 'A New Test for the

Detection of Weak and "Incomplete" Rh Agglutinins', *British Journal of Experimental Pathology*, vol. 26, 1945, pp. 255–66; Grieve, 'Haemolytic Disease of the Newborn', p. 166; HMC minutes, 17 September 1962, BAGC A638 22b, ANZA.

83   HMC minutes, 17 September 1962, BAGC A638 22b, ANZA.

6: A BRIGHT NEW AGE: ADVANCES IN REPRODUCTIVE MEDICINE, 1964–1980s

1   Carroll Wall, 'The Glamorous Gynaecologists: An Anarchy of the Heart', *Metro*, June 1984, pp. 32–50.
2   'The New National Women's Hospital, Auckland', *NZMJ*, vol. 63, April 1964, pp. 241–2; 'Official Opening of National Women's Hospital Souvenir Issue', *Health and Service*, vol. 18, 4, 1964, p. 21; reprinted in Robb's memoirs, *Medical Odyssey*, p. 81.
3   'National Women's Hospital, Auckland', *NZNJ*, vol. 75, April 1964, p. 10.
4   'The New National Women's Hospital, Auckland', *NZMJ*, vol. 63, April 1964, pp. 241–2.
5   Summary of a one-hour TV documentary on National Women's, 'A Far Cry', by Shirley Maddock, *New Zealand Listener*, 11 December 1964, p. 3; National Women's Hospital, *Annual Report for Year Ending March 1965*, p. 3.
6   Dorothy McAleer, interviewed by Jenny Carlyon, 5 September 2004, transcript, p. 2.
7   John Stallworthy later wrote that he and Peel had supported Bonham's appointment as the best candidate: Sir John Stallworthy to Green, 14 April 1976, Green Papers, MSS 1433, folder 1, UOASC; on visit, see 'News from Divisions: Auckland', *NZMJ*, vol. 69, May 1969, p. 314.
8   Chamberlain, *Special Delivery*, p. 105.
9   University of Auckland O & G Academic Advisory Committee minutes, 3 July 1963, Minutes 1954–1962, Box 257, UOAA.
10 Dennis G. Bonham, 'The Evolution of Obstetrics and Gynaecology', *NZMJ*, vol. 63, November 1964, p. 711.
11 Sir John Scott, *University News*, vol. 35, 5, 2005, pp. 20–21.
12 Delivery staff meeting, 6 July 1979, in 'Changing Trends, Attitudes, Structure and Design in Delivery Suite National Women's Hospital', 1962–88 (supplied to author by Glenda Stimpson).
13 Jeffery, 'Whanautanga', p. 89.
14 University of Auckland Postgraduate School of Obstetrics and Gynaecology at National Women's Hospital New Zealand, *Annual Report for Year Ended December 1967*, pp. 5–11.
15 Nancie Bonham, personal communication.
16 D. G. Bonham, 'Report on Study Leave Oct–Dec 1969', p. 21, Senate Papers, UOAA.
17 'News: New Perinatal Society', *NZMJ*, vol. 93, 25 March 1981, p. 199.
18 D. G. Bonham, 'Post-graduate School of Obstetrics & Gynaecology and its Relationship to the Auckland Hospital Board', March 1975 (file given to author by Professor John France).
19 HMC minutes, 20 May 1964, BAGC A638 39b, ANZA. On perinatal meetings as a great learning occasion, see also Pat Clarkson, interviewed by Jenny Carlyon, 7 December 2005, transcript, p. 26; on visitors' impressions, see also Paul Lancaster, in Bryder and Dow, *The History of Fetal Medicine*, pp. 12–13.
20 Sinclair, *A History of the University of Auckland*, p. 275.
21 Bonham, 'The Evolution of Obstetrics and Gynaecology', pp. 709–15, 710.
22 Memo to Secretary, Auckland Hospital Board, on Definitive Office and Research Accommodation for the Professorial Unit of Obstetrics & Gynaecology, NWH, 25 May 1964.
23 University of Auckland, Department of Obstetrics and Gynaecology, *Annual Report of the Superintendent-in-chief, Auckland Hospital Board, for Year Ending 31 March 1966*, p. 43; University of Auckland, Department of Obstetrics and Gynaecology, *Report for the Year*

23. *Ending December 1964*; *Report for the Year Ending December 1965* (NB: after this, the annual reports used the title 'School' and not 'Department').
24. G. C. Liggins, 'A Brief Autobiography of Professor Sir Graham Liggins FRS', unpublished manuscript, p. 23 (in author's possession).
25. Cornwall Hospital, Medical Committee minutes, 20 July 1950, YCBZ 15492 1a; 2 October 1950, YCBZ 15492 1a, ANZA; McCalman, *Sex and Suffering*, p. 357.
26. Margaret Marsh and Wanda Ronner, *The Empty Cradle: Infertility in America from Colonial Times to the Present*, Johns Hopkins University Press, Baltimore, 1996, pp. 152, 173; Margaret Marsh and Wanda Ronner, *The Fertility Doctor: John Rock and the Reproductive Revolution*, Johns Hopkins University Press, Baltimore, 2008.
27. McCalman, *Sex and Suffering*, p. 357.
28. Marsh and Ronner, *The Empty Cradle*, pp. 170, 172, 183.
29. J. E. Giesen, 'Practical Aspects in the Treatment of Sterility', *NZMJ*, vol. 50, August 1951, pp. 331, 334–6; on Giesen, see 'Obituary: James Edmett Giesen', *NZMJ*, vol. 91, 14 May 1980, p. 357.
30. Cornwall Hospital Medical Committee minutes, 20 July 1950, YCBZ 15492 1a; 2 October 1950, YCBZ 15492 1a, ANZA.
31. Marsh and Ronner, *The Empty Cradle*, pp. 139, 147.
32. Gemzell visited Auckland in 1967: see *Auckland Star*, 21 October 1967.
33. HMC minutes, 19 March 1962, BAGC A638 39a, ANZA.
34. McCalman, *Sex and Suffering*, p. 356.
35. *Auckland Star*, 21 December 1967.
36. *The Times*, 28 July 1965.
37. Algar Warren, Medical Superintendent, National Women's Hospital, *Annual Report of the Superintendent-in-chief, Auckland Hospital Board, for Year Ending 31 March 1966*, p. 40.
38. University of Auckland Registrar, 17 December 1964, Box 188, UOAA; HMC minutes, 15 December 1964, BAGC A638 39b, ANZA. In 1970 Ibbertson was appointed foundation professor of endocrinology at the University of Auckland and set up an endocrinology laboratory at Auckland Hospital.
39. University of Auckland Postgraduate School of Obstetrics and Gynaecology at National Women's Hospital New Zealand, *Annual Report for Year Ended Dec. 1966*, p. 8.
40. *Auckland Star*, 28 September 1967.
41. University of Auckland Postgraduate School of Obstetrics and Gynaecology at National Women's Hospital New Zealand, *Annual Report for Year Ended Dec. 1966*, p. 8; Bernadette Noble, 'Infertility and a New Miracle in Search for Motherhood', *Thursday*, 20 February 1969, p. 17.
42. 'News: Medical Research Council: National Hormone Committee', *NZMJ*, vol. 76, 9 March 1977, p. 201. A 1980 study placed the multiple pregnancy risk in using clomiphene at 8 per cent, while that for HPG was 20 per cent: see D. G. Bonham, D. J. Court, F. M. Graham, J. D. Hutton, G. C. Liggins, A. W. Liley, C. D. Mantell and E. B. Nye, 'Obstetric and Gynaecological Disorders: Advances in Treatment', *New Ethicals*, September 1980, p. 79.
43. Noble, 'Infertility and a New Miracle in Search for Motherhood', p. 17.
44. Report, February 1975, HMC minutes, 20 March 1975, BAGC A638 41a, ANZA.
45. R. McKenzie, 'Laparoscopy', *NZMJ*, vol. 74, August 1971, p. 91.
46. G. T. Thomas, 'Laparoscopy in Southland', *NZMJ*, vol. 91, 9 January 1980, pp. 10–12.
47. Report, February 1975, HMC minutes, 20 March 1975, BAGC A638 41a, ANZA.
48. Marsh and Ronner, *The Empty Cradle*, pp. 190, 200, 217, 223.
49. Bonham to Honeyman, AHB, 1 June 1983, UOAA.
50. David Cole to C. J. Maiden, 23 June 1983, UOAA.
51. Bonham to Aitken, 18 October 1982; Bonham to Honeyman, 1 June 1983, UOAA.
52. Marsh and Ronner, *The Empty Cradle*, p. 231.
53. Bonham to Aitken, 18 October 1982, UOAA.

54 Dennis Bonham, 'Leading Article: Advances in the Management of Infertility', *NZMJ*, vol. 97, 14 March 1984, pp. 146–7.
55 C. R. Stewart, K. R. Daniels and D. H. Boulnois, 'The Development of a Psychosocial Approach to Artificial Insemination by Donor Sperm', *NZMJ*, vol. 95, 8 December 1982, p. 855; see also K. R. Daniels, 'The Practice of Artificial Insemination of Donor Sperm in New Zealand,' *NZMJ*, vol. 98, 10 April 1985, pp. 235–9.
56 Robyn Scott-Vincent, 'Infertility: New Hope . . . For Some', *NZWW*, 17 March 1986, pp. 53–55; see also Department of Justice, Law Reform Division, *New Birth Technologies: An Issues Paper on AID, IVF and Surrogate Motherhood, March 1985*, Department of Justice, Wellington, p. 15.
57 Daniels, 'The Practice of Artificial Insemination', p. 237; A. B. MacLean, D. R. Aickin and J. J. Evans, 'Artificial Insemination by Donor', *NZMJ*, vol. 97, 25 July 1984, p. 485.
58 Personal correspondence from Rebecca Hamilton, 21 November 2006; also referred to in *New York Times*, 20 January 2006 and *Toronto Globe and Mail*, 30 September 2006: 'Rebecca Hamilton, a law student at Harvard who created a documentary about searching for her donor father in New Zealand. The documentary helped rally support for a law there prohibiting anonymous donation.'
59 Richard Fisher, interviewed by Jenny Carlyon, 26 October 2006, transcript, p. 10.
60 Bonham, 'Leading Article: Advances in the Management of Infertility', pp. 146–7.
61 H. P. Dunn, 'Correspondence: Artificial Insemination by Donor', *NZMJ*, vol. 97, 26 September 1984, p. 658.
62 Richard Fisher, interviewed by Jenny Carlyon, 26 October 2006, transcript, p. 11.
63 *Daily Mail*, 27 July 1978.
64 McCalman, *Sex and Suffering*, p. 360.
65 Pauline Ray, 'When Babies are Inconceivable', *New Zealand Listener*, 25 June 1983, pp. 20–21; *NZH*, 14 April 1983.
66 *Auckland Star*, 27 July 1983.
67 Wall, 'The Glamorous Gynaecologists', p. 36.
68 Bonham, 'Leading Article: Advances in the Management of Infertility', pp. 146–7.
69 Department of Justice, Law Reform Division, *New Birth Technologies: An Issues Paper on AID, IVF and Surrogate Motherhood, March 1985*, p. 32.
70 F. M. Graham, J. T. France and J. Clark, 'The Development of a Programme for in Vitro Fertilisation in New Zealand', *NZMJ*, vol. 98, 27 March 1985, pp. 177–81.
71 *NZH*, 23 December 1983.
72 Wall, 'The Glamorous Gynaecologists', p. 36.
73 Ibid.
74 *Auckland Star*, 14 July 1984.
75 *NZH*, 14 April 1983; Wall, 'The Glamorous Gynaecologists', p. 36.
76 K. R. Daniels, 'Demand for and Attitudes towards in Vitro Fertilisation: A Survey of Obstetricians and Gynaecologists', *NZMJ*, vol. 100, 11 March 1987, p. 148; Anne Clark, John C. Peek, Peter Forbes-Smith, Rodney C. Bycroft, Moya Shaw and Frederick M. Graham, 'Social and Reproductive Characteristics of the First 100 Couples Treated by in Vitro Fertilisation Programme at National Women's Hospital, Auckland', *NZMJ*, vol. 100, 24 June 1987, pp. 380–2.
77 Scott-Vincent, 'Infertility: New Hope . . . For Some', p. 55.
78 'Politics and Health: In-vitro Programme', *NZMJ*, vol. 99, 28 May 1986, p. 377.
79 *Weekend Herald*, 20 August 2005, p. 20.
80 Richard Fisher, interviewed by Jenny Carlyon, 26 October 2006, transcript, p. 10.
81 H. P. Dunn, 'Correspondence: In Vitro Fertilisation and Artificial Insemination by Donor', *NZMJ*, vol. 97, 25 April 1984, p. 273.
82 Norman E. MacLean, 'Correspondence: In Vitro Fertilisation and Ethics', *NZMJ*, vol. 97, 27 June 1984, p. 417.

83 F. M. Graham, 'Correspondence: In Vitro Fertilisation', *NZMJ*, vol. 97, 8 August 1984, p. 540.
84 Mary Warnock (chair), *Report of the Committee of Inquiry into Human Fertilisation and Embryology*, HMSO, London, 1984; 'News: Human Fertilisation Report', *NZMJ*, vol. 97, 22 August 1984, p. 571.
85 *The Times*, 27 June 1984.
86 D. Brahams, 'Medicine and the Law: In Vitro Fertilisation and Related Research: Why Parliament Must Legislate', *The Lancet*, vol. 2, 24 September 1983, pp. 726–7.
87 'Position Paper: Issues Arising from in Vitro Fertilisation, Artificial Insemination by Donor and Related Problems in Biotechnology', *NZMJ*, vol. 98, 22 May 1985, pp. 396–8.
88 Bonham, 'Leading Article: Advances in the Management of Infertility', p. 147.
89 Roger Cooter, 'The Ethical Body', in Roger Cooter and John Pickstone (eds), *Companion to Medicine in the Twentieth Century*, Routledge, London, 2002, pp. 451–69.

7: THE NEW PATIENT AND PERINATAL MEDICINE

1 Wall, 'The Glamorous Gynaecologists', p. 37.
2 Sir George Douglas Robb, 'Strong Medicine', *The Times*, 18 May 1966.
3 *Auckland Star*, 20 November 1980.
4 Jane Harding, in Bryder and Dow (eds), *The History of Fetal Medicine*, p. 5.
5 Maternity Services Committee, *Special Care Services for the Newborn in New Zealand: A Report of the Maternity Services Committee*, Board of Health Report Series No. 29, Wellington, 1982, p. 64; 'Prenatal Glucocorticoids in Preterm Birth: A Paediatric View of the History of the Original Studies by Ross Howie, 2 June 2004', in L. A. Reynolds and E. M. Tansey (eds), *Prenatal Corticosteroids for Reducing Morbidity and Mortality after Preterm Birth: The Transcript of a Witness Seminar held by the Wellcome Trust Centre for the History of Medicine at UCL, London, on 15 June 2004*, vol. 25, Wellcome Trust, London, 2005, Appendix 2, p. 94.
6 Ross Howie, 'Tangaroa and Beyond: The Newborn Service', Talk given to Auckland Medical History Society, 4 July 2002, and revised draft, 27 March 2004 (in author's possession); Ross Howie to Secretaries of the Maternity Services and Child Health Committees, 10 March 1981, ABQU 632 Acc W4550 5 29-21 (1978–81), ANZW.
7 'Application to the Medical Research Council of New Zealand [MRCNZ] by the Postgraduate School of Obstetrics and Gynaecology in the University of Auckland for the Triennium 1970–2 for Group Projects in Fetal and Neonatal Health, Biochemistry and Medical Data Processing and Analysis, February 1969', p. 14 (in author's possession).
8 J. C. Maclaurin, 'Some Aspects of Neonatal Paediatrics', *Scottish Medical Journal*, vol. 14, 1969, p. 323.
9 Dunn, 'The Development of Newborn Care', p. 473.
10 Matthews, memo to Medical Superintendent, 5 May 1967, HMC minutes, 15 May 1967, BAGC A638 40a, ANZA.
11 Howie, '"Historical Events at National Women's Hospital"'.
12 Postgraduate School of Obstetrics and Gynaecology at National Women's Hospital, *Annual Report for Year Ending December 1967*, p. 7; 'University Report, Appendix A: Fetal and Neonatal Health Projects', Report to the Medical Research Council of New Zealand, for year ending December 1967, p. 8.
13 Ross Howie, interviewed by Jenny Carlyon, 9 December 2004, transcript, p. 1.
14 HMC minutes, 27 March 1969, BAGC A638 40b, ANZA; Postgraduate School of Obstetrics and Gynaecology at National Women's Hospital, *Annual Report for Year Ending December 1968*, p. 15.
15 Ross Howie to Lois Reynolds, 26 August 2005, in Reynolds and Tansey (eds), *Prenatal Corticosteroids*, p. 15, footnote

30; G. A. Gregory, J. A. Kitterman, R. H. Phibbs, W. H. Tooley and W. K. Hamilton, 'Treatment of the Idiopathic Respiratory-distress Syndrome with Continuous Positive Airway Pressure', *New England Journal of Medicine*, vol. 284, 1971, pp. 1333–40.

16 Dunn, 'The Development of Newborn Care', p. 474.

17 Howie, notes provided to author, 18 April 2009.

18 HMC minutes, 4 December 1974, BAGC A638 41a, ANZA.

19 Howie, notes provided to author, 18 April 2009.

20 Ministry of Health, *Inquiry under S.47 of the Health and Disabilities Services Act 1993 into the Provision of Chest Physiotherapy Treatment Provided to Pre-term Babies at National Women's Hospital between April 1993 and December 1994*, Ministry of Health, Wellington, 1999 (chair Helen Cull, Cull Report), pp. 11, 23, 29; http://www.moh.govt.nz/notebook/nbbooks.nsf/0/ AFD2CAA0D6BDBC0B4C2567 C300827D77/$file/chesphys1.pdf. See chapter 11 below.

21 On Liggins, see also Sir Peter Gluckman and Tatjana Buklijas, 'Sir Graham Collingwood (Mont) Liggins 24 June 1926–24 August 2010', *Biographical Memoirs of Fellows of the Royal Society*, 2013, http://dx.doi.org/10.1098/rsbm.2012.0039.

22 Letter from Professor Sir Graham (Mont) Liggins to Sir Iain Chalmers (6 April 2004), in Reynolds and Tansey (eds), *Prenatal Corticosteroids*, Appendix 1, p. 85; Liggins' submission read by Ross Howie, in Bryder and Dow (eds), *The History of Fetal Medicine*, p. 33.

23 Gluckman and Burklijas, 'Sir Graham Collingwood (Mont) Liggins', p. 10.

24 Ibid., p. 8.

25 Postgraduate School of Obstetrics and Gynaecology at National Women's Hospital, *Annual Report for Year Ending December 1964*; Liggins, 'A Brief Autobiography of Professor Sir Graham Liggins FRS', p. 22.

26 Liggins to Chalmers, in Reynolds and Tansey (eds), *Prenatal Corticosteroids*, Appendix 1, p. 86.

27 Postgraduate School of Obstetrics and Gynaecology at National Women's Hospital, *Annual Report for 1966*.

28 Liggins to Chalmers, in Reynolds and Tansey (eds), *Prenatal Corticosteroids*, Appendix 1, p. 86; Tilli Tansey, 'Premature Sheep and Dark Horses: Wellcome Trust Support for Mont Liggins' Work, 1968–76', in Reynolds and Tansey (eds), *Prenatal Corticosteroids*, Appendix 3, p. 97; Gluckman and Buklijas, 'Sir Graham Collingwood (Mont) Liggins', p. 10.

29 Postgraduate School of Obstetrics and Gynaecology at National Women's Hospital, *Annual Report for 1968*.

30 See F. Peter Woodford, *The Ciba Foundation: An Analytical History 1949–1974*, Associated Scientific Publishers, Amsterdam, 1974.

31 C. W. G. Redman, 'Geoffrey Sharman Dawes', in Royal College of Physicians, *Lives of the Fellows*, http://munksroll.rclondon.ac.uk/Biography/Details/1197; Sir Graham Liggins, 'Geoffrey Sharman Dawes, CBE, 21 January 1918–6 May 1996', *Biographical Memoirs of Fellows of the Royal Society*, 44, November 1998, pp. 110–25.

32 G. E. W. Wolstenholme and Maeve O'Connor (eds), *Foetal Autonomy: A Ciba Foundation Symposium*, J. & A. Churchill, London, 1969, preface, p. x.

33 Ibid., p. 142.

34 Ibid., pp. 142–3.

35 Mont Liggins (from tape recording), in Reynolds and Tansey (eds), *Prenatal Corticosteroids*, p. 9.

36 Ibid., p. 9. See also Liggins, 'A Brief Autobiography of Professor Sir Graham Liggins FRS', p. 30. Mary Ellen Avery was later (from 1974) professor of paediatrics at Harvard Medical School.

37 R. A. de Lemos, D. W. Shermeta, J. H. Knelson, R. Kotas and M. E. Avery, 'Acceleration of Appearance of Pulmonary Surfactant in the Fetal Lamb by Administration of Corticosteroids', *American Review of Respiratory Disease*, vol. 102, 1970, pp. 459–61.

38 HMC minutes, 20 February 1969, BAGC

A638 40 b, ANZA; Liggins to Chalmers, in Reynolds and Tansey (eds), *Prenatal Corticosteroids*, Appendix 1, p. 87.
39 Howie, in Bryder and Dow (eds), *The History of Fetal Medicine*, p. 33; Howie, in Reynolds and Tansey (eds), *Prenatal Corticosteroids*, Appendix 2, p. 90.
40 MRCNZ, *Research Review 1973*, p. 131; Gluckman and Buklijas, 'Sir Graham Collingwood (Mont) Liggins', p. 13.
41 G. C. Liggins and R. N. Howie, 'A Controlled Trial of Antepartum Glucocorticoid Treatment for Prevention of the Respiratory Distress Syndrome in Premature Infants', *Pediatrics*, vol. 50, 4, 1972, pp. 515–25; MRCNZ, *Research Review 1973*, p. 131.
42 G. C. Liggins and R. N. Howie, 'Prevention of Respiratory Distress Syndrome by Antepartum Corticosteroid Therapy', in Physiological Society, Barcroft Sub-committee, R. S. Comline et al. (eds), *Foetal and Neonatal Physiology, Proceedings of the Sir Joseph Barcroft Centenary Symposium, 1972*, Cambridge University Press, Cambridge, 1973, pp. 613–17.
43 MRCNZ, *Research Review 1979*, p. 137.
44 Liggins to Chalmers, in Reynolds and Tansey (eds), *Prenatal Corticosteroids*, Appendix 1, p. 87; Liggins and Howie, 'A Controlled Trial of Antepartum Glucocorticoid Treatment', pp. 515–25.
45 Liggins to Chalmers, in Reynolds and Tansey (eds), *Prenatal Corticosteroids*, Appendix 1, p. 87; R. N. Howie and G. C. Liggins, 'Clinical Trial of Antepartum Betamethasone Therapy for Prevention of Respiratory Distress in Pre-term Infants', in A. Anderson, R. W. Beard, J. M. Brudenell and P. M. Dunn (eds), *Preterm Labour: Proceedings of the Fifth Study Group of the Royal College of Obstetricians and Gynaecologists*, The College, London, 1978, pp. 281–9.
46 MRCNZ, *Research Review 1973*, p. 131.
47 MRCNZ, *Research Review 1977*, p. 111; MRCNZ, *Research Review 1978*, p. 72; MRCNZ, *Research Review 1979*, p. 137.
48 Stuart R. Dalziel, Natalie Walker, Varsha Parag and Colin Mantell et al., 'Cardiovascular Risk Factors after Antenatal Exposure to Betamethasone: 30-year Follow-up of a Randomised Controlled Trial', *The Lancet*, vol. 365, 9474, 28 May–3 June 2005, pp. 1856–62; reported in Liggins Institute, *Dialogue*, vol. 10, 6, 2005, pp. 1, 7; Stuart R. Dalziel, Varsha Parag, Anthony Rodgers and Jane E. Harding, 'Cardiovascular Risk Factors at Age 30 Following Pre-term Birth', *International Journal of Epidemiology*, vol. 36, 2007, pp. 907–15.
49 Collaborative Group on Antenatal Steroid Therapy, 'Effects of Antenatal Dexamethasone Administration in the Infant: Long-term Follow-up', *Journal of Pediatrics*, vol. 104, 1984, pp. 259–67.
50 N. R. C. Roberton, 'Advances in Respiratory Distress Syndrome', *BMJ*, vol. 284, 27 March 1982, pp. 917–18.
51 Iain Chalmers, in Reynolds and Tansey (eds), *Prenatal Corticosteroids*, p. 56.
52 National Institutes of Health, 'Consensus Statement: Effect of Corticosteroids for Fetal Maturation on Perinatal Outcomes, 28 February–2 March 1994', *Consensus*, vol. 12, 1994, pp. 1–24, cited by Stephen Hanney, in Reynolds and Tansey (eds), *Prenatal Corticosteroids*, p. 72.
53 Patricia Crowley, in Reynolds and Tansey (eds), *Prenatal Corticosteroids*, p. 27.
54 Liggins, 'A Brief Autobiography', p. 31.
55 'Witness' seminars bring together major players in an important medical development of the twentieth century to reflect upon the influences that brought about that development. See, for example, Christie and Tansey (eds), *Origins of Neonatal Intensive Care*; Reynolds and Tansey (eds), *Prenatal Corticosteroids*.
56 Patricia Crowley and Jane Harding, in Reynolds and Tansey (eds), *Prenatal Corticosteroids*, pp. 23, 33.
57 See, for example, Ross N. Howie, 'Of Perinates and Other People', *Newsletter of the Perinatal Society of Zealand*, August 2004.
58 Maclaurin, 'Some Aspects of Neonatal Paediatrics', p. 321.

59 Richard Cooke, in Christie and Tansey (eds), *Origins of Neonatal Intensive Care*, p. 56.
60 Iain Chalmers citing Liggins, in Reynolds and Tansey (eds), *Prenatal Corticosteroids*, p. 39, footnote 85.
61 Iain Chalmers and Mary Ellen Avery, in Reynolds and Tansey (eds), *Prenatal Corticosteroids*, pp. 39–40.
62 *NZH*, 2 July 1980; *NZH*, 3 July 1980; *Auckland Star*, 3 July 1980; *NZH*, 19 September 1980 (where it was announced they were leaving the hospital).
63 Liggins Institute, *Dialogue*, vol. 2, 3, 2002, p. 1.
64 See, for example, 'Obituary: Sir Graham Liggins 1926–2010', *New Zealand Listener*, 4 September 2010, p. 10; *University of Auckland News*, vol. 40, 16, 3 September 2010, p. 6.
65 MRCNZ, *Research Review 1973*, p. 118.
66 'Discovering the Greatest Secret of Birth', *NZH*, 12 April 1980.
67 Trish Gribben, 'Towards Better Birth', *New Zealand Listener*, 30 October 1976, p. 14.
68 *NZH*, 15 June 1991.
69 'Obituary: Sir Graham Liggins', *The Economist*, 2 September 2010, http://www.economist.com/node/16941245.
70 G. S. Dawes, 'Chairman's Closing Remarks', in Wolstenholme and O'Connor (eds), *Foetal Autonomy*, p. 316.
71 *The West Australian*, 23 November 1967.
72 Clare Hanson, *A Cultural History of Pregnancy: Pregnancy, Medicine and Culture, 1750–2000*, Palgrave Macmillan, New York, 2004, pp. 154, 156.
73 Malcolm Nicolson and John E. E. Fleming, *Imaging and Imagining the Fetus: The Development of Obstetric Ultrasound*, Johns Hopkins University Press, Baltimore, 2013, p. 80.
74 I. Donald, J. MacVicar and T. G. Brown, 'Investigation of Abdominal Masses by Pulsed Ultrasound', *The Lancet*, vol. 1, issue 7032, 1958, p. 1188–95.
75 I. Donald, 'On Launching a New Diagnostic Science', *American Journal of Obstetrics and Gynecology*, vol. 1, 1969, pp. 609–28, 618, cited in Oakley, *The Captured Womb*, p. 157; and Casper, *The Making of the Unborn Patient*, p. 84.
76 E. M. Tansey and D. A. Christie, *Looking at the Unborn: Historical Aspects of Obstetric Ultrasound, Wellcome Witnesses to Twentieth Century Medicine, March 1998*, vol. 5, The Wellcome Trust, London, 2000, p. 40; 'Real-time image allows the acquisition and display of images to occur so rapidly that their formation and display appear to be simultaneous', ibid., p. 72; see also Hanson, *A Cultural History of Pregnancy*, p. 136.
77 Browne, *Masters, Midwives, and Ladies-in-waiting*, p. 26.
78 HMC minutes, 15 June 1964, BAGC A638 39b, ANZA.
79 Postgraduate School of Obstetrics and Gynaecology at National Women's Hospital, *Annual Report for Year Ending December 1968*, p. 9.
80 F. Fraser to Ian Donald, 25 March 1970, British Medical Ultrasound Society Archives, cited in Nicolson and Fleming, *Imaging and Imagining the Fetus*, p. 210.
81 HMC minutes, 19 October 1972, BAGC A638 21a, ANZA.
82 *NZH*, 22 February 1973.
83 HMC minutes, 16 September 1976, BAGC A638 41a, ANZA.
84 Maternity Services Committee, *Maternity Services in New Zealand*, p. 67.
85 HMC minutes, 25 October 1979, BAGC A638 21b, ANZA.
86 *Auckland Star*, 14 June 1980.
87 HMC minutes, 25 November 1982, BAGC A638 22a, ANZA.
88 Ibid.
89 HMC minutes, 19 May 1983, BAGC A638 22a, ANZA.
90 HMC minutes, 10 May 1983, BAGC A638 22a, ANZA.
91 Ann Oakley, 'The History of Ultrasonography in Obstetrics', *BIRTH*, vol. 13, Special Supplement, December 1986, pp. 8–13.
92 Leigh Parker, 'Scans... How Safe for Babies?', *NZWW*, 9 October 1989, pp. 18–19.

93 'Ultrasound Panel Discussion', Auckland, 7 June 1990, and submission by West Auckland Women's HealthWatch, p. 2, Joan Donley Papers, MSS & Archives 1007/15, item 2/5/B/1 pt. 2, UOASC.
94 J. P. Neilson and C. R. Whitfield, 'Ultrasound in Obstetrics', *The Lancet*, 11 July 1981, p. 94; J. P. Neilson and Valerie D. Hood, 'Ultrasound in Obstetrics and Gynaecology: Recent Developments', *British Medical Bulletin*, vol. 36, 1980, pp. 249–55.
95 Louis M. Hellman, Gillian M. Duffus, Ian Donald and Bertil Sunden, 'Safety of Diagnostic Ultrasound in Obstetrics', *The Lancet*, vol. 1, 7657, 1970, pp. 1133–5.
96 Nicolson and Fleming, *Imaging and Imagining the Fetus*, pp. 222–5.
97 HMC minutes, 25 November 1982, BAGC A638 22a, ANZA.
98 Jim Neilson and Adrian Grant, 'Ultrasound in Pregnancy', in Iain Chalmers, Murray Enkin and Marc J. N. C. Keirse (eds), *Effective Care in Pregnancy and Childbirth, vol. 1: Pregnancy*, Oxford University Press, Oxford, 1989, p. 420.
99 Lesley McCowan, interviewed by Jenny Carlyon, 19 December 2005, transcript, p. 11; 'Special Scan Saved My Son', *NZWW*, 5 September 1988, p. 10; H. S. Bada, W. Hajiar, C. Chua and D. S. Sumner, 'Non-invasive Diagnosis of Neonatal Asphyxia and Intraventricular Haemorrhage by Doppler Ultrasound', *Joural of Pediatrics*, vol. 95, 1979, pp. 775–9.
100 'Special Scan Saved My Son', *NZWW*, 5 September 1988, p. 10; J. P. Neilson, 'Doppler Ultrasound', *British Journal of Obstetrics and Gynaecology*, vol. 94, 1987, pp. 929–34.
101 Judith Lumley, 'Foetal Monitoring: A Look at the Evidence', *New Doctor (Journal of the Doctors' Reform Society of Australia)*, vol. 15, 1980, pp. 45–48. See also Judith Lumley and Jill Astbury, *Birth Rites, Birth Rights: Childbirth Alternatives for Australian Parents*, Nelson, Melbourne, 1980; and Kerreen M. Reiger, *Our Bodies,*
Our Babies: The Forgotten Women's Movement, Melbourne University Press, Melbourne, 2001, p. 280.
102 Fiona Bolwell and Patricia Jones, 'Letter to the Editor: Amniocentesis', *New Zealand Listener*, 8 October 1988, pp. 16–17. (Pathologist David Becroft responded that this was not a rigid policy, and that women under the age of 37 were tested if there were special circumstances, although he also commented on the current shortage of resources for more tests.)
103 Letter to Secretary Auckland Hospital Board, 12 September 1969, HMC minutes, 18 September 1969, BAGC A638 40b, ANZA.
104 Browne, *Masters, Midwives, and Ladies-in-waiting*, p. 133.
105 J. R. Martin, 'A Double Catheter Technique for Exchange Transfusion in the Newborn Infant', *NZMJ*, vol. 77, March 1973, pp. 167–9.
106 Matthews, memo to Medical Superintendent, 5 May 1967, HMC minutes, 15 May 1967, BAGC A638 40a, ANZA.
107 'The Miraculous Blood Transfusion', *Weekly News*, 30 December 1964, p. 2. The first sixteen patients (with an addendum including the first 30) were reported by Green, Liley and Liggins, 'The Place of Foetal Transfusion in Haemolytic Disease'.
108 'Editorial: Intrauterine Transfusion', *BMJ*, 11 March 1967, pp. 583–4.
109 'Leading Article: Intrauterine Transfusion', *Scottish Medical Journal*, vol. 12, 1967, pp. 293–4.
110 *NZH*, 19 September 1973.
111 MRCNZ, *Research Review 1976*, p. 115.
112 University Report, Appendix A: Fetal and Neonatal Health Projects: Report to the MRCNZ for year ended December 1967, p. 12; Martin, 'A Double Catheter Technique', pp. 167–9; Ross Howie, notes on Witness Seminar, 14 February 2005, p. 4.
113 'The Rh Factor; No Longer a Nightmare for the Pregnant', *Thursday*, 17 April 1970, pp. 53, 62.
114 HMC minutes, 18 October 1973, BAGC A638 21a, ANZA, reported

in the *NZMJ*: Sandra Kinnock and A. W. Liley, 'The Performance of an anti D Immunoprophylaxis Scheme', *NZMJ*, vol. 80, 23 October 1974, pp. 337–43.
115 'Fetal Health Project', MRCNZ, *Research Review 1973*, 1974, p. 102.
116 Howie, notes on Witness Seminar, 14 February 2005, p. 2.
117 J. R. Martin, 'Phototherapy, Phenobarbitone and Physiological Jaundice in the Newborn Infant', *NZMJ*, vol. 79, 12 June 1974, pp. 1022–4; Howie, notes on Witness Seminar, 14 February 2005.
118 Neil Pattison, interviewed by Jenny Carlyon, 30 March 2006, transcript, p. 4.
119 Matthews, memo to Medical Superintendent, 5 May 1967, HMC minutes, 15 May 1967, BAGC A638 40a, ANZA.
120 Howie, Appendix 2, in Reynolds and Tansey, *Prenatal Corticosteroids*, p. 94; Howie, in Bryder and Dow, *The History of Fetal Medicine*, pp. 31–32.
121 MRCNZ, *Research Review 1976*, pp. 111–12.
122 HMC minutes, 12 May 1977, BAGC A638 41b, ANZA.
123 Ibid.
124 Howie, 'Of Perinates and Other People', p. 3; P. A. Dunkley, 'Premature and Plural – Be Prepared', *NZNJ*, August 1967, pp. 8–12.
125 Dunkley, in Bryder and Dow, *The History of Fetal Medicine*, p. 38.
126 *NZH*, 11 December 1973; *Auckland Star*, 4 September 1980; *NZH*, 5 September 1980; *NZH*, 8 September 1980; *Auckland Star*, 16 September 1980.
127 HMC minutes, 28 April 1977, BAGC A638 41b, ANZA.
128 *Auckland Star*, 13 August 1980.
129 *NZH*, 2 December 1979.
130 Anne Recordon, interviewed by Jenny Carlyon, 30 November 2005, transcript, p. 5.
131 HMC minutes, 8 May 1980, BAGC A638 21b, ANZA; Report by I. L. G. Hutchison, 1980, Box 401, UOAA.
132 John Armstrong, *Under One Roof: A History of Waikato Hospital*, Waikato Health Memorabilia Trust, Hamilton, 2009, pp. 303–4.
133 *Auckland Star*, 9 September 1980; *NZH*, 10 September 1980; *NZH*, 19 September 1980.
134 Ross N. Howie, 'Newborn Services in Crisis, New Zealand 1980', 13 September 2010, unpublished paper in author's possession.
135 Maternity Services Committee, *Special Care Services for the Newborn in New Zealand*.
136 Howie, personal notes in author's possession, 18 April 2009.
137 'News from Divisions: Auckland', *NZMJ*, vol. 99, 23 July 1986, p. 558; in the 1980s National Women's Hospital had ten ventilator cots, about half the number the neonatal paediatricians thought they should have: see Auckland Health Board, 1991 Report on Development of Maternity Services, Appendix 7.
138 Barbara Anderson, letter to the editor, 'Don't Rubbish State Hospitals', *Auckland Star*, 28 March 1979.
139 Baker, *The Machine in the Nursery*.
140 MRCNZ, *Research Review 1976*, p. 113.
141 MRCNZ, *Research Review 1973*, p. 133.
142 Maternity Services Committee, *Special Care Services for the Newborn in New Zealand*, pp. 8, 9, 11.
143 J. E. Clarkson, 'Leading Article: Is Neonatal Intensive Care Effective?', *NZMJ*, vol. 96, 13 April 1983, pp. 242–3.
144 'Position Paper: Retinopathy of Prematurity: A Statement by the Committee on the Fetus and Newborn of the Paediatric Society of New Zealand', *NZMJ*, vol. 98, 12 June 1985, pp. 446–7.
145 B. A. Darlow, 'Viewpoint: How Small is Too Small – A Reappraisal', *NZMJ*, vol. 98, 24 July 1985, pp. 596–8. (In 2001 Darlow was appointed Cure Kids Chair of Paediatric Research, University of Otago, Christchurch.)
146 Ibid.
147 Stephen R. Munn, 'Correspondence: Very Premature Infants', *NZMJ*, vol. 98, 28 August 1985, p. 710.
148 David Rothman, *Strangers at the*

Bedside: A History of How Law and Bioethics Transformed Medical Decision Making, Basic Books, New York, 1991, pp. 190–221.
149 Simon Rowley, interviewed by Jenny Carlyon, 2 November 2005, transcript, pp. 6–7.
150 Knight was at the Barcroft Symposium in 1972 at which Liggins presented the data: Bryder and Dow, *The History of Fetal Medicine*, p. 43; David Knight, interviewed by Jenny Carlyon, transcript, 2 October 2004, p. 8.

8: CONTRACEPTION, STERILISATION AND ABORTION

1 *NZH*, 16 November 1964; *Auckland Star*, 16 November 1964.
2 See Claire Gooder, 'A History of Sex Education in New Zealand, 1939–1985', PhD thesis, University of Auckland, 2010.
3 *NZH*, 16 November 1964; *Auckland Star*, 16 November 1964.
4 Chamberlain, *Special Delivery*, p. 55.
5 HMC minutes, 18 July 1966, BAGC A638 40a, ANZA.
6 HMC minutes, 29 April 1971, 18 November 1971, BAGC A638 40b, ANZA.
7 Smyth, *Rocking the Cradle*, p. 85.
8 Ibid., p. 127.
9 Hercock, *Alice*, pp. 179–80.
10 Smyth, *Rocking the Cradle*, pp. 126–7.
11 Ibid., pp. 106, 109.
12 Board of Health Maternity Services Committee minutes, 10 March 1971, AAFB 632 Acc W2788 25 29/21, ANZW.
13 *Zealandia*, 29 October 1970, p. 1.
14 J. T. France, 'Improving the Rhythm Method: An Outline of the Research into Ovulation at National Women's Hospital, Auckland', *Choice*, vol. 9, 2, May 1971, pp. 5–7.
15 *NZH*, 25 November 1972.
16 Smyth, *Rocking the Cradle*, p. 103.
17 H. P. Dunn, 'Natural Family Planning', *NZMJ*, vol. 82, 24 December 1975, pp. 407–8.
18 H. P. Dunn, 'Letter to the Editor: Few Restrictions in Natural Family Planning', *NZMJ*, vol. 97, 25 July 1984, p. 498.
19 Smyth, *Rocking the Cradle*, pp. 94–99.
20 D. G. Bonham, 'The Control of Population', Talk to the Medical Association of New Zealand, Palmerston North, February 1971, 'Board of Health Maternity', AAFB 632 Acc W2788 25 29/21, ANZW.
21 MRCNZ Application for Project of Programme Grant, Dennis Geoffrey Bonham (Form MRC/1), 1973, p. 3 (in author's possession).
22 Lara V. Marks, *Sexual Chemistry: A History of the Contraceptive Pill*, Yale University Press, New Haven, 2001, p. 164; 'Editorial: Mortality Rates With Oral Contraception', *NZMJ*, vol. 86, 14 December 1977, p. 525.
23 'Contraceptive Controversy', *New Zealand Listener*, 8 March 1980, pp. 32–33.
24 New Zealand Contraception and Health Study Group, 'New Zealand Contraception and Health Study: Design and Preliminary Report', *NZMJ*, vol. 99, 23 April 1986, pp. 283–6; also reported in Phillida Bunkle, 'Calling the Shots? The International Politics of Depo-Provera', in Rita Arditti, Renate Duelli Klein and Shelley Minden (eds), *Test-Tube Women: What Future for Motherhood?*, Pandora Press, London, 1984, p. 172.
25 Jill Rakusen, 'Depo-Provera – Third World Women Not Told This Contraceptive is on Trial', and Janet Hadley, 'The Case against Depo-Provera', in Sue O'Sullivan (ed.), *Women's Health: A Spare Rib Reader*, Pandora, London, 1987, pp. 164–6, 170.
26 *Auckland Star*, 12 March 1980; *Auckland Star*, 15 March 1980. On the British Campaign Against Depo-Provera (set up in the late 1970s), see Jill Rakusen, 'Depo-Provera: The Extent of the Problem', in Helen Roberts (ed.), *Women, Health and Reproduction*, Routledge & Kegan Paul, London, 1981, pp. 75–108.
27 Ruth Bonita, 'Contraceptive Research: For Whose Protection?', *Broadsheet*, vol. 76, January/February 1980, pp. 6–8;

also cited in Phillida Bunkle, *Second Opinion: The Politics of Women's Health in New Zealand*, Oxford University Press, Auckland, p. 66.

28 P. J. Scott, 'Memorandum to the Director, Medical Research Council of New Zealand from the Standing Committee on Therapeutic Trials, re. The New Zealand Contraception and Health Study Protocol', 1984.

29 'Contraceptive Controversy', *New Zealand Listener*, 8 March 1980, p. 33.

30 Sandra Coney, 'Fertility Action 1984–', in Anne Else (ed.), *Women Together: A History of Women's Organisations in New Zealand: Nga Ropu Wahine o te Motu*, Historical Branch, Department of Internal Affairs, Daphne Brasell Associates Press, Wellington, 1993, pp. 284–6.

31 Submission from Fertility Action to the Committee of Inquiry into the Treatment of Cervical Cancer at National Women's Hospital, including a section on 'Drug Company Funded Research – Upjohn's New Zealand Contraception and Health Study', UOAA, pp. 31–32.

32 Peggy Foster, *Women and the Health Care Industry: An Unhealthy Relationship?*, Open University Press, Buckingham, 1995, p. 21.

33 'Editorial: Intrauterine Devices', *NZMJ*, vol. 86, 26 October 1977, pp. 387–8.

34 Ian Dowbiggin, *The Sterilization Movement and Global Fertility in the Twentieth Century*, Oxford University Press, Oxford, 2008, p. 139; see also A. Tone, *Devises and Desires: A History of Contraceptives in America*, Hill & Wang, New York, 2001, pp. 279–83.

35 Phillida Bunkle, 'Dalkon Shield Disaster', *Broadsheet*, vol. 122, September 1984, p. 22; Bunkle, *Second Opinion*, pp. 116–18. The articles were: R. W. Jones, 'Correspondence: Septic Abortion and IUD', *NZMJ*, vol. 80, 28 August 1974, p. 186; R. W. Jones, 'Performance of the Dalkon Shield Intrauterine Device', *NZMJ*, vol. 82, 13 August 1975, pp. 85–87.

36 'Politics and Health: Dalkon Shield Campaign', *NZMJ*, vol. 98, 26 June 1985, p. 505.

37 E. L. Jones (Fertility Action), 'Correspondence: Dalkon Shield', *NZMJ*, vol. 98, 24 July 1985, p. 609.

38 Coney, 'Fertility Action', p. 284.

39 Ibid., pp. 284–6.

40 Helen Roberts, Lesley McCowan, Christine Roke, Hilary Liddell, Lynda Batcheler and Jennifer Wilson, 'Correspondence: Contraceptive Choice', *NZMJ*, vol. 100, 11 February 1987, p. 80; see also *NZH*, 26 November 1988.

41 *NZH*, 8 December 1987; Smyth, *Rocking the Cradle*, pp. 196–7.

42 John D. Baeyertz, 'Correspondence: Contraceptive Choice', *NZMJ*, vol. 100, 25 March 1987, p. 188; Sandra Coney, 'Correspondence: Contraceptive Choice', *NZMJ*, vol. 100, 13 May 1987, p. 296; Sandra Coney, 'Correspondence: Contraceptive Choice', *NZMJ*, vol. 100, 27 May 1987, p. 325; G. W. Smith and G. A. Hoogland, 'Correspondence: Contraceptive Choice', *NZMJ*, vol. 100, 8 July 1987, p. 428; Helen Roberts et al., 'Correspondence: Risks of Oral Contraceptives', *NZMJ*, vol. 100, 8 July 1987, pp. 430–1; Lesley McCowan, 'Correspondence: Contraceptive Choice', *NZMJ*, vol. 100, 12 August 1987, p. 503; Lesley McCowan, 'Correspondence: Safety of IUDs', *NZMJ*, vol. 100, 12 August 1987, p. 503.

43 Sterilisation or 'tubal ligation' by the 1970s was performed either by laparoscopy, which involved a small quantity of gas being introduced into the abdomen to help in observation and then the fallopian tubes being sealed off by electrocoagulation, or laparotomy where the fallopian tubes were tied off and cut or cauterised. See Sue McCauley, 'Everything You Wanted to Know about Sterilisation that Your Doctor Didn't Tell You', *Thursday*, 12 April 1973, p. 20.

44 'Editorial: Sterilisation as a Medical-Legal Problem', *NZMJ*, vol. 52, June 1953, pp. 153–6.

45 NZOS minutes, 14 September 1932.

46 Mrs Elsie Marion Barnes, Evidence to

the Committee of Inquiry into Cervical Treatment at National Women's Hospital, Day 45, 9 November 1987, pp. 3846–52, ANZA.
47 *Auckland Star*, 19 February 1974.
48 'Curing the Hysterectomy Hangups', October 1981, pamphlet reprinted from *Thursday* magazine; Bryder, *A History of the 'Unfortunate Experiment'*, p. 10; on the USA, see also Dowbiggin, *The Sterilization Movement*, p. 174.
49 Dowbiggin, *The Sterilization Movement*, p. 171.
50 P. J. Dempsey and R. M. Davie, 'Correspondence: Sterilisation of Women', *NZMJ*, vol. 84, 22 September 1976, pp. 251–2.
51 'Leading Article: Legality of Sterilization', *BMJ*, vol. 1, 5698, 21 March 1970, pp. 704–5; Pauline Jackson, Betson Phillips, Elizabeth Prosser, H. O. Jones, V. R. Tindall, D. L. Crosby, I. D. Cooke, J. M. McGarry and R. W. Rees, 'A Male Sterilization Clinic', *BMJ*, vol. 4, 31 October 1970, pp. 295–7.
52 'From the London Mail: Vasectomy', *NZMJ*, vol. 76, December 1972, p. 442.
53 Dowbiggin, *The Sterilization Movement*, pp. 152, 156, 168; presumably the fact they were married made it respectable.
54 A. Duke, 'Correspondence: Voluntary Sterilisation in the Male', *NZMJ*, vol. 71, June 1970, pp. 392–3.
55 Smyth, *Rocking the Cradle*, p. 145.
56 D. Urquhart-Hay, 'Voluntary Sterilisation in the Male', *NZMJ*, vol. 71, April 1970, pp. 230–2; D. Urquhart-Hay, 'Correspondence: Ethics and Vasectomy', *NZMJ*, vol. 81, 25 June 1975, pp. 568–9.
57 Memo to Medical Superintendent Auckland Hospital, 21 August 1970, HMC minutes, 17 September 1970, BAGC A638 40b, ANZA.
58 'Vasectomy and Hysterectomy: The Psychology of Sex Organ Surgery', *Thursday*, 9 December 1971, p. 54.
59 D. G. Bonham, 'The Control of Population', Talk to the Medical Association of New Zealand, Palmerston North, February 1971, AAFB 632 Acc W2788 25 29/21, 'Board of Health Maternity', ANZW.
60 Terry Bell and John Evans, 'Vasectomy, the "Snip and Tie" Operation is Booming', *Thursday*, 6 December 1973, p. 21.
61 Smyth, *Rocking the Cradle*, p. 148.
62 Board of Health Maternity Services Committee minutes, 10 March 1971, AAFB 632 Acc W2788 25 29/21, ANZW.
63 'Contraceptive Controversy', *New Zealand Listener*, 8 March 1980, pp. 32–33.
64 'The Abortion Doctors: A Nationwide Survey of Certifying Consultants under the CS & A Act', *Broadsheet*, vol. 68, April 1979, p. 21.
65 J. H. Taylor, memo to Acting Medical Superintendent, 5 July 1979, HMC minutes, 24 May 1979, BAGC A638 21b, ANZA.
66 HMC minutes, 25 October 1979, BAGC A638 21b, ANZA.
67 Peter Jackson and J. Lew Lander, 'Female Sterilisation: A Five-year Follow-up in Auckland', *NZMJ*, vol. 91, 27 February 1980, pp. 140–3; also reported in *NZH*, 10 March 1980.
68 Cornwall Hospital Medical Committee minutes, 25 November 1946, YCBZ 15492 1a, ANZA.
69 HMC minutes, 14 September 1954, BAGC A638 37a, ANZA.
70 Leslie Reagan, *When Abortion was a Crime: Women, Medicine, and Law in the United States, 1867–1973*, University of California Press, Berkeley, 1997, p. 190.
71 John Taylor, interviewed by Jenny Carlyon, 18 May 2004, transcript, p. 8; see also 'Obituary: John Heywood Taylor', *NZMJ*, vol. 122, 1296, 5 June 2009, http://www.nzma.org.nz/journal/122-1296/xxxx/.
72 H. P. Dunn, 'Therapeutic Abortion in New Zealand', *NZMJ*, vol. 68, October 1968, pp. 253–8; also reported in *NZH*, 31 October 1968.
73 HMC minutes, 10 May 1968, BAGC A638 37a, ANZA.
74 Alison McCulloch, *Fighting to Choose: The Abortion Rights Struggle in New Zealand*, Victoria University Press, Wellington, 2013, p. 105.

75 HMC minutes, 18 July 1966, 17 May 1967, BAGC A638 40a, ANZA.
76 HMC minutes, 17 July 1967, BAGC A638 40a: Gluckman's report, 5 December 1967, J. S. B. Lindsay memo to Medical Superintendent, 18 January 1968, HMC minutes, 20 March 1968, BAGC A638 40a, ANZA.
77 'Case 28', Gluckman's report, 5 December 1967, BAGC A638 40a, ANZA. On his work in the clinic, see also L. K. Gluckman, 'Some Unanticipated Complications of Therapeutic Abortion', *NZMJ*, vol. 74, August 1971, pp. 72–78. On abortion stories prior to 1978, see also Margaret Sparrow, *Abortion Then and Now: New Zealand Abortion Stories from 1940 to 1980*, Victoria University Press, Wellington, 2010.
78 Reagan, *When Abortion was a Crime*, p. 218.
79 Professor Werry memo, 20 July 1972, HMC minutes, 19 October 1972, BAGC A638 21a, ANZA.
80 HMC minutes, 19 October 1972, BAGC A638 21a, ANZA.
81 HMC minutes, 16 November 1972, BAGC A638 21a, ANZA.
82 Reported in *NZH*, 26 July 1972.
83 *NZH*, 26 February 1974.
84 Reagan, *When Abortion was a Crime*, p. 244.
85 *NZH*, 20 February 1974.
86 Memo, 'Family Planning Advisory Officer', 6 April 1974, HMC minutes, 23 May 1974, BAGC A638 21a, ANZA.
87 Royal Commission of Inquiry into Contraception, Sterilisation, and Abortion in New Zealand, *Report of the Royal Commission of Inquiry into Contraception, Sterilisation, and Abortion in New Zealand*, Government Printer, Wellington, 1977 (McMullin Report), p. 149.
88 Pauline Ray, 'Abortion: A Shift of Opinion', *Thursday*, August 1973, p. 33; *NZH*, 14 August 1973.
89 HMC minutes, 21 March 1974, BAGC A638 21a, ANZA.
90 Ray, 'Abortion: A Shift of Opinion'.
91 R. W. Jones, 'Antenatal Diagnosis of Certain Genetic and Biochemical Disorders', report presented to HMC; HMC minutes, 18 October 1973, BAGC A638 21a, ANZA.
92 HMC minutes, 22 November 1973, BAGC A638 21a, ANZA.
93 David Becroft, Pathologist-in-charge, Princess Mary Laboratory, Auckland Hospital, memo to Bonham, 30 August 1973; A. M. O. Veale, Professor of Human Genetics and Community Health, to Bonham, 18 September 1973, HMC minutes, 18 October 1973, BAGC A638 21a; *Auckland Star*, 7 February 1973.
94 Sir William Liley, 'Development of Life', reprinted in Foundation Genesis, *Sir William Liley*, pp. 27–41. See also Albert W. Liley, 'The Foetus in Control of his Environment', in Thomas W. Hilgers and Denis J. Horan (eds), *Abortion and Social Justice*, Sheed & Ward, New York, 1972, p. 27; A. W. Liley, 'The Foetus as Personality', *Australian and New Zealand Journal of Psychiatry*, vol. 6, 1972, pp. 99–105; A. W. Liley, 'A Case against Abortion', *Liberal Studies*, Whitcombe & Tombs, Auckland, 1971; Marilyn Pryor and Des Dalgety, 'From New Zealand', in Foundation Genesis, *Sir William Liley*, (Dalgety and Pryor were successive presidents of SPUC), p. 6.
95 N. C. Begg, review of H. M. I. Liley and Beth Day, *Modern Motherhood*, 1968, in *NZMJ*, vol. 69, April 1969, p. 251.
96 'Obituary: Albert William Liley', *NZMJ*, vol. 96, 10 August 1983, pp. 631–2.
97 'The Unborn Child', *Health*, 1971, pp. 12–13, cited in Casper, *The Making of the Unborn Patient*, p. 60.
98 Linda Gordon, *The Moral Property of Women: A History of Birth Control Politics in America*, University of Illinois Press, Urbana, 2002, p. 306.
99 'Obituary: Albert William Liley', p. 631; Sir John Scott wrote in his obituary of Liley, 'Although brought up in a Methodist/Anglican tradition, he held no specific religious beliefs': 'Obituary: Sir Albert William Liley', http://www.rsnz.org/directory/yearbooks/ybook97/obitLiley.html.

100 Casper, *The Making of the Unborn Patient*, p. 62.
101 Donald used this form of words more than once: see Nicolson and Fleming, *Imaging and Imagining the Fetus*, p. 244.
102 *NZH*, 8 July 1972.
103 Dowbiggin, *The Sterilization Movement*, pp. 185–6.
104 *NZH*, 17 April 1973.
105 *NZH*, 15 May 1974.
106 McMullin Report, p. 360.
107 Gordon, *The Moral Property of Women*, pp. 310–13.
108 'Proceedings: Society for the Protection of the Unborn Child, Annual General Meeting, 10 July 1972', *NZMJ*, vol. 76, November 1972, pp. 355–7.
109 On 8 July 1972. For a critique of Liley's involvement in SPUC, see Jocelyn Brooks, *Ill Conceived: Law and Abortion Practice in New Zealand*, Caveman Press, Dunedin, 1981, pp. 36–40.
110 *NZH*, 16 June 1983.
111 Casper, *The Making of the Unborn Patient*, pp. 66, 67.
112 See tributes in Foundation Genesis, *Sir William Liley*.
113 *NZH*, 27 September 1973.
114 Sandra Coney and Phillida Bunkle, 'An Unfortunate Experiment at National Women's', *Metro*, June 1987, p. 49; Bryder, *A History of the 'Unfortunate Experiment'*, p. 53.
115 G. H. Green, 'The Foetus Began to Cry . . . Abortion' (Part 1), *NZNJ*, vol. 63, 7, 1970, pp. 11–12; (Part 2), *NZNJ*, vol. 63, 9, 1970, pp. 6–7; (Part 3), *NZNJ*, vol. 63, 9, 1970, pp. 11–12.
116 Paul Patten, interviewed by Jenny Carlyon, 28 October 2004, transcript, p. 1.
117 Opening reported in *Auckland Star*, 22 May 1974; *NZH*, 23 May 1974 (Werry was one of the operating physicians).
118 'Editorial: The Pattern of Abortion', *NZMJ*, vol. 93, 24 September 1980, p. 237.
119 *Auckland Star*, 11 October 1974; also discussed in McCulloch, *Fighting to Choose*, pp. 85–86.
120 M. A. F. Baird, 'Morbidity of Therapeutic Abortion in Auckland', *NZMJ*, vol. 83, 9 June 1976, pp. 395–9.
121 McCulloch, *Fighting to Choose*, p. 106.
122 Smyth, *Rocking the Cradle*, p. 243.
123 Medical Council Central Ethical Committee, 6 May 1977, Box 245, UOAA.
124 Maternity Services Committee minutes, 8 May 1969, p. 8, H1 Acc W26 76 Box 20, 29/21 35171, 'Maternity Services Committee, 1968–69', ANZW.
125 N. W. Williamson, 'Viewpoint: Abortion: A Legal View', *NZMJ*, vol. 72, October 1970, pp. 257–9.
126 B. Corkill, 'Correspondence: Abortion Questionnaire and the Royal College of Obstetricans and Gynaecologists', *NZMJ*, vol. 74, December 1971, pp. 410–11.
127 R. A. M. Gregson and Janet R. M. Irwin, 'Opinions on Abortion from Medical Practitioners', *NZMJ*, vol. 73, May 1971, pp. 267–73.
128 Reagan, *When Abortion was a Crime*, p. 217.
129 See also Hayley Marina Brown, '"A Woman's Right to Choose": Second Wave Feminist Advocacy of Abortion Law Reform in New Zealand and New South Wales from the 1970s', MA thesis, University of Canterbury, Christchurch, 2004.
130 *NZH*, 26 May 1972.
131 *NZH*, 26 February 1974; see also Brown, '"A Woman's Right to Choose"', pp. 115–41; A. F. C. Rogers and Judith F. Lenthall, 'Characteristics of New Zealand Women Seeking Abortion in Melbourne, Australia', *NZMJ*, vol. 81, 26 March 1975, pp. 282–6.
132 Brown, '"A Woman's Right to Choose"', p. 144.
133 McMullin Report, p. 180; 'Report: Contraception, Sterilisation, and Abortion in New Zealand', *NZMJ*, vol. 85, 25 May 1977, pp. 441–5.
134 Maureen Molloy, 'Rights, Fact, Humans and Women: An Archaeology of the Royal Commission on Contraception, Sterilisation and Abortion in New Zealand', *Women's Studies Journal*, vol. 12, 1, August 1996, p. 76.
135 Smyth, *Rocking the Cradle*, p. 154.
136 'Editorial: Abortion Again', *NZMJ*,

137 *Auckland Star*, 5 September 1978.
138 *Auckland Star*, 12 September 1978; *Auckland Star*, 23 August 1978.
139 'Editorial: The Pattern of Abortion', *NZMJ*, vol. 93, 24 September 1980, pp. 237-8.
140 Liam Wright, 'Correspondence: Abortion', *NZMJ*, vol. 93, 14 January 1981, p. 23.
141 *Auckland Star*, 10 January 1979.
142 *Auckland Star*, 19 September 1979.
143 'News: Abortion Supervisory Council', *NZMJ*, vol. 90, 26 September 1979, p. 29.
144 *NZH*, 11 December 1980.
145 Smyth, *Rocking the Cradle*, p. 156.
146 'News: Abortions in 1981', *NZMJ*, vol. 95, 8 September 1982, p. 633; 'News: Abortion 1982', *NZMJ*, vol. 96, 9 November 1983, p. 944; 'News: Abortion in 1983', *NZMJ*, vol. 97, 26 September 1984, p. 652.
147 Heather J. White, S. C. Hawes and D. Heginbotham, *Report of the Abortion Supervisory Committee for the Year Ended 31 March 1986*, Wellington, Abortion Supervisory Committee, 1986, pp. 5-6.
148 Sarah E. Clarkson, 'Viewpoint: On Being a Certifying Abortion Consultant: An Ethical Dilemma', *NZMJ*, vol. 91, 14 May 1980, pp. 346-7.
149 E. G. McQueen, 'Correspondence: Medical Ethics', *NZMJ*, vol. 96, 12 October 1983, p. 774; Norman. E. MacLean, 'Correspondence: Doctors for Life', *NZMJ*, vol. 96, 26 October 1983, p. 812; Norman E. MacLean, 'Correspondence: Euthanasia', *NZMJ*, vol. 99, 23 April 1986, p. 291; Norman E. MacLean, 'Correspondence: Abortion and Certifying Consultants', *NZMJ*, vol. 100, 24 June 1987, p. 390; Norman E. MacLean, 'Correspondence: Abortion', *NZMJ*, vol. 100, 22 July 1987, p. 464.
150 Norman E. MacLean, 'Correspondence: Abortion for Fetal Abnormality', *NZMJ*, vol. 90, 25 July 1979, p. 75.
151 Liam Wright, 'Correspondence: Abortion and the Holocaust', *NZMJ*, vol. 88, 23 August 1978, p. 150; Smyth, *Rocking the Cradle*, pp. 155, 244.

vol. 90, 24 October 1979, p. 353.
152 White et al., *Report of the Abortion Supervisory Committee for the Year Ended 31 March 1986*, p. 7; Jennie Nicol, 'Abortion Services in New Zealand: A Report prepared for the Women, Children and Family Health Programme to Aid in Planning and Policy Formulation', Department of Health, Wellington, September 1987, pp. 47, 48.
153 Nicol, 'Abortion Services in New Zealand', pp. 2, 3.
154 E. J. Moss, Deputy Head Orderly, National Women's Hospital, Report on Epsom Day Hospital, p. 3 (in author's possession).
155 *Broadsheet*, vol. 68, April 1979, p. 20.
156 *Auckland Star*, 12 July 1979.
157 Wichtel, 'Delivering with Style', p. 14.
158 *NZH*, 14 November 1979.
159 John Taylor, interviewed by Jenny Carlyon, 18 May 2004, transcript, p. 7.
160 Brian Stevens Assessors Ltd to Chief Executive, Auckland Hospital Board, 26 May 1987; Brown, 'A Woman's Right to Choose', p. 157; Jenny Rankine, 'More Anti-abortion Arson', *Broadsheet*, vol. 150, 1987, p. 9; McCulloch, *Fighting to Choose*, p. 248.
161 *Central Leader*, 12 December 1990.
162 *Auckland Star*, 19 September 1979.

9: OBSTETRICS AND THE WINDS OF CHANGE, 1964–1980s

1 Maternity Services Committee, *Obstetrics and the Winds of Change*, Board of Health, Wellington, 1979; copy found in 'Maternity Services', ABQU 632 Acc W4550 5 29-21 (1978–79), ANZW; also cited in Joan Donley, *Herstory of N.Z. Homebirth Association*, New Zealand Homebirth Association, Auckland, 1992, p. 10.
2 Board of Health, Maternity Services Committee minutes, 8 May 1969, H1 Acc W26 76 Box 20, 29/21 35171, ANZW.
3 Sir Arnold L. Walker, A. J. Wrigley, G. S. Organe, Marjorie Kuck and M. A. Heasman, *Confidential Maternal*

Mortality Report for 1961–63, No. 115, HMSO, London, 1966, Preface, p. iii.
4 Ibid., p. 1.
5 I. W. Barrowclough, 26 July 1973, 'Maternal and Child Welfare', ABQU 632 Acc W4415/21 13/6/18, ANZW. Ironically, in 1982 he was at the receiving end of an inquiry into a maternal death: see Bryder, *A History of the 'Unfortunate Experiment'*, p. 133.
6 'Birth and Death: Secret Figures Doctored?', *New Zealand Truth*, 28 August 1973.
7 'Why Did Your Mum Die?', *Sunday News*, 9 December 1973.
8 *Dominion*, 5 April 1974.
9 *The Week*, 1 October 1976.
10 Bonham to R. Dickie, Department of Health, 13 February 1978, 'Maternal and Child Welfare', ABQU 632 Acc W4415/21 13/6/18, ANZW.
11 Maternity Services Committee, *Maternity Services in New Zealand*.
12 *The Times*, 6 December 1963; Neville R. Butler and Dennis G. Bonham, *Perinatal Mortality: The First Report of the 1958 British Perinatal Mortality Survey under the Auspices of the National Birthday Trust Fund*, E. & S. Livingstone, Edinburgh, 1963. Bonham also contributed a chapter on caesarean sections to the second report. See Neville R. Butler and Eva D. Alberman (eds), *Perinatal Problems. The Second Report of the 1958 British Perinatal Mortality Survey under the Auspices of the National Birthday Trust Fund*, E. & S. Livingstone, Edinburgh, 1969. See also Williams, *Women and Childbirth in the Twentieth Century*, pp. 196–217.
13 Chamberlain, *Special Delivery*, p. 66.
14 Oakley, *The Captured Womb*, pp. 205–6.
15 Donley, *Save the Midwife*, p. 76; Oakley, *The Captured Womb*, p. 216.
16 Maternity Services Committee, *Maternity Services in New Zealand*; also reported as 'Maternity Services', *NZMJ*, vol. 83, 25 August 1976, pp. 158–9.
17 Maternity Services Committee, *Maternity Services in New Zealand*, p. 55.
18 Ibid., p. 5.
19 D. R. Aickin, 'The Making of an Obstetrician', *NZMJ*, vol. 81, 12 February 1975, pp. 92–95.
20 Joan Donley, 'Having the Baby at Home', *Broadsheet*, September 1985, p. 17; Donley, *Save the Midwife*, p. 63.
21 *NZH*, 2 November 1976.
22 *Auckland Star*, 9 April 1979: 'Muldoon told members of the Save the Mater Committee at the weekend that the age of the private maternity home is dead.'
23 *NZH*, 5 October 1976.
24 Ibid.
25 Ibid.
26 Faris, memo to Medical Superintendent, 10 February 1977, HMC minutes, 21 April 1977, BAGC A638 41b, ANZA. The discussions were also cited in *NZH*, 19 October 1976; in Jenny Wheeler, 'Home or Hospital Birth? The Case for Both ...', *NZWW*, 30 October 1978, p. 28; and in Donley, 'Having the Baby at Home', p. 17.
27 *NZH*, 22 October 1976; see also A. J. Henderson, 'Childbirth – A Natural Function? A Report on One Hundred and Fifty Consecutive Cases of Relaxed Childbirth', *NZMJ*, vol. 53, February 1954, pp. 511–14; A. J. Henderson, 'Correspondence: Perinatal Mortality', *NZMJ*, vol. 98, 11 December 1985, p. 1059.
28 'Obituary: Sir Frank Rutter', *NZH*, 2 November 2002.
29 *NZH*, 16 November 1976.
30 Maternity Services Committee, *Special Care Services for the Newborn in New Zealand*, pp. 22–25. A decade later, Middlemore was upgraded to equal National Women's facilities when it opened a new neonatal unit: see *Health Watch: Auckland Area Health Board News Update*, 2, February 1992, p. 4.
31 John Parboosingh, Marc J. N. C. Keirse and Murray Enkin, 'The Role of the Obstetric Specialist', in Chalmers, Enkin and Keirse (eds), *Effective Care in Pregnancy and Childbirth*, vol. 1, p. 193.
32 Donley, *Save the Midwife*, p. 110.
33 Sue Kedgley, *Mum's the Word: The Untold Story of Motherhood in New Zealand*, Random House, Auckland, 1996, p. 244; also cited in

David McLoughlin, 'The Politics of Childbirth: Midwives versus Doctors', *North & South*, August 1993, p. 57.
34 Bonham, 'The Evolution of Obstetrics and Gynaecology', p. 711.
35 N. Morris, 'Human Relations in Obstetric Practice', *The Lancet*, vol. 1, 23 April 1960, pp. 913–15; Central Health Services Council, Standing Maternity and Midwifery Advisory Committee, *Human Relations in Obstetrics*, HMSO, London, 1961.
36 Bonham, 'The Evolution of Obstetrics and Gynaecology', p. 711.
37 Dobbie, *The Trouble with Women*, p. 104.
38 Ibid., pp. 83, 84, 109.
39 Chamberlain, *Special Delivery*, p. 61.
40 David Knight, interviewed by Jenny Carlyon, 2 October 2004, transcript, p. 27.
41 Dobbie, *The Trouble with Women*, p. 104.
42 'Editorial: The Future of Obstetrics', *NZMJ*, vol. 73, March 1971, pp. 157–8; see also Aickin, 'The Making of an Obstetrician', p. 94.
43 Maternity Services Committee, *Maternity Services in New Zealand*, pp. 79–80.
44 Helen Jenkins and Jocelyn Tracey, 'Comparison of Te Puke Maternity Hospital and National Women's Hospital, Community Health Project 1977/28', Medical School, University of Auckland, 1977, p. 22.
45 Ibid., p. 26.
46 Faris, memo to Medical Superintendent, 10 February 1977, HMC minutes, 21 April 1977, BAGC A638 41b, ANZA.
47 HMC minutes, 12 May 1977, BAGC A638 41b, ANZA.
48 *NZH*, 21 March 1980; Anne Cartwright, *The Dignity of Labour? A Study of Childbearing and Induction*, Tavistock, London, 1979.
49 *Auckland Star*, 14 November 1974.
50 C. M. Purdue to Judge Cartwright, 25 June 1987, BAGC A638 35a, ANZA. Daphne de Jong, National President of Feminists for Life, outlined the motivations for the Bill in an article in the *New Zealand Listener*, and Green was probably the 'senior consultant' who was quoted in the article supporting patients' rights to have a say in how services were administered: Daphne de Jong, 'Birth Rights', *New Zealand Listener*, 18 June 1977, pp. 20–21.
51 In a 1958 article Green had stressed the importance of patient consent for sterilisation: 'He [the doctor] should make sure that the patient is mentally able to give consent and that such consent is fully and fairly given without influence of others': Green, 'Tubal Ligation', p. 477.
52 de Jong, 'Birth Rights'; C. M. Purdue to Judge Cartwright, 25 June 1987, BAGC A638 35a, ANZA; Chief Executive AHB, memo to Medical Superintendent, 27 September 1977, copy of letter 9 September 1977 from National President, Feminists for Life (NZ) Inc. with 'Maternity Patient's Bill of Rights' prepared by that organisation: HMC minutes, 13 October 1977, BAGC A638 41b, ANZA. Approved in principle by the National Council of Women in 1978: see Holt, *Women in Council*, p. 84.
53 HMC minutes, 13 October 1977, BAGC A638 41b, ANZA.
54 Maternity Services Committee, *Obstetrics and the Winds of Change*.
55 Tabled and discussed at HMC meeting: HMC minutes, 19 June 1980, BAGC A638 21B, ANZA.
56 HMC minutes, 26 April 1979, BAGC A638 21b, ANZA.
57 *Auckland Star*, 28 February 1979.
58 'A Very Grateful Patient', *Auckland Star*, 27 February 1979.
59 HMC minutes, 24 May 1979, BAGC A638 21b, ANZA.
60 Ibid.
61 HMC minutes, 16 March 1964, BAGC A638 22b, ANZA.
62 Bonham, 'The Evolution of Obstetrics and Gynaecology', p. 712.
63 HMC minutes, 20 May 1964, BAGC A638 39b, ANZA.
64 Bonham, memo to Medical Advisory Committee, 14 July 1964; HMC minutes, 20 July 1964, BAGC A638 39b, ANZA.

65 Ibid.
66 HMC minutes, 17 August 1964, BAGC A638 39b, ANZA.
67 Grantly Dick-Read, *Childbirth Without Fear: The Principles and Practice of Natural Childbirth*, Revised and Enlarged, Harper & Bros, New York, 1953, p. 224.
68 Ibid.
69 Algar Warren, Medical Superintendent, National Women's Hospital, *Annual Report of the Superintendent-in-chief, Auckland Hospital Board, for Year Ending 31 March 1966*, p. 41.
70 Jenkins and Tracey, 'Comparison of Te Puke Maternity Hospital and National Women's Hospital', Appendix: 'Programme for Preparation for Parenthood'.
71 *Auckland Star*, 4 July 1983.
72 *Plunket News*, vol. 6, 1, February 1968, p. 7.
73 A. M. (tutor specialist), Delivery Staff meeting, 14 August 1979 (files given to author by Glenda Stimpson).
74 *NZH*, 30 November 1973.
75 Bernie Kyle, interviewed by Jenny Carlyon and Linda Bryder, 27 May 2004, transcript, p. 16.
76 *NZH*, 30 November 1973.
77 Margaret Macdonald, 'Dr Pat Dunn and the Male Mastery of Birth', *Metro*, February 1991, p. 132.
78 Ibid., p. 130.
79 H. P. Dunn, 'Come Back, Left-Lateral!', *NZMJ*, vol. 89, 14 March 1979, p. 180.
80 Macdonald, 'Dr Pat Dunn and the Male Mastery of Birth', p. 130. At the beginning of 1979 he himself estimated 10,000: Dunn, 'Come Back, Left-Lateral!', p. 180.
81 D. G. Bonham, 'Leading Article: Caesarean Birth', *NZMJ*, vol. 96, 23 March 1983, p. 206.
82 Judith Walzer Leavitt, *Make Room for Daddy: The Journey from Waiting Room to Birthing Room*, University of North Carolina Press, Chapel Hill, 2009, p. 270.
83 HMC minutes, 12 February 1981, BAGC A638 21c, ANZA; HMC minutes, 23 April 1981, BAGC A638 21c, ANZA.
84 Ibid.
85 Letter from hospital solicitor (Mr Walker), 11 May 1981, HMC minutes, 21 May 1981, BAGC A638 21c, ANZA.
86 This was the thesis put forward in a anthropological study of fathers and childbirth, influenced by Foucauldian theories: see Richard K. Reed, *Birthing Fathers: The Transformation of Men in American Rites of Birth*, Rutgers University Press, New Brunswick, 2005, pp. 30, 77, 101.
87 R. F. (tutor specialist), 'Gowns for Husbands', Delivery suite staff meeting, 12 October 1981, in 'Changing Trends, Attitudes, Structure and Design in Delivery Suite National Women's Hospital', 1962–88 (supplied to author by Glenda Stimpson).
88 Sheila Kitzinger, 'Childbirth and Society', in Chalmers, Enkin and Keirse (eds), *Effective Care in Pregnancy and Childbirth*, vol. 1, p. 104.
89 Marc J. N. C. Keirse, Murray Enkin and Judith Lumley, 'Social and Professional Support during Childbirth', in Chalmers, Enkin and Keirse (eds), *Effective Care in Pregnancy and Childbirth*, vol. 2, p. 809.
90 Leavitt, *Make Room for Daddy*, p. 289.
91 Elizabeth Wood (later a charge nurse), interviewed by Jenny Carlyon, 18 November 2005, transcript, p. 10.
92 Simon Rowley, interviewed by Jenny Carlyon, 2 November 2005, transcript, p. 19.
93 A. W. Liley, memo to Acting Medical Superintendent, 26 May 1977: HMC minutes, 14 July 1977, BAGC A638 41b, ANZA.
94 Supervisor, Delivery Suite 2, memo, June 1977; Principal Nurse, memo to Acting Medical Superintendent, 2 June 1977; Acting Medical Superintendent, memo to Liley, 8 June 1977. On Stimpson's long career at National Women's, see *Midwifery News*, September 2002, pp. 16–17.
95 Ibid.
96 Val Dickens, interviewed by Jenny Carlyon, 24 November 2005, transcript, p. 11.
97 HMC minutes, 25 October 1979, BAGC A638 21b, ANZA; HMC minutes,

13 December 1979, BAGC A638 21b, ANZA.
98 HMC minutes, 18 September 1980, BAGC A638 21c, ANZA.
99 HMC minutes, 8 May 1980, BAGC A638 21b, ANZA; S. E. Reid to I. L. G. Hutchison, 15 April 1980, ABQU 632 Acc W4550 5 29-21 (1978–81), ANZW.
100 *Auckland Star*, 19 March 1980.
101 HMC minutes, 8 May 1980, 19 June 1980, BAGC A638 21b, ANZA; *Auckland Star*, 9 July 1980.
102 Madeleine H. Shearer, 'Maternity Patients' Movements in the United States 1820–1985', in Chalmers, Enkin and Keirse (eds), *Effective Care in Pregnancy and Childbirth*, vol. 1, p. 121.
103 Leavitt, *Make Room for Daddy*, pp. 275–80.
104 Delivery Suite meeting minutes, 3 April 1984 (files supplied to author by Glenda Stimpson).
105 Wichtel, 'Delivering with Style', p. 34.
106 M. A. Sinclair, Manager, Delivery Suite, to Joan Donley (then convener, Child Birth Committee, Auckland Women's Health Council), 8 February 1989, Joan Donley Papers, MSS & Archives 2007/15, item 5/2/B/4 pt. 4, UOASC.
107 Delivery Suite meeting minutes, 9 May 1984, in 'Changing Trends, Attitudes, Structure and Design in Delivery Suite National Women's Hospital', 1962–88.
108 Department of Health, Annual Report, *AJHR*, H-31, 1960, p. 9; *NZH*, 16 May 1968.
109 D. I. Pool, *Te Iwi Maori: A New Zealand Population, Present and Projected*, Auckland University Press, Auckland, 1991, p. 153.
110 Jeffery, 'Whanautanga', p. 29.
111 Ibid., pp. 46, 74.
112 Ibid., p. 81.
113 Ibid., pp. 87, 90–91.
114 Ibid.
115 Ibid., p. 108.
116 Gabrielle Collison, National Women's Hospital, Auckland, New Zealand, A Position Paper, July 1988 (document supplied to author by David Knight), pp. 37–38.
117 Aroha Harris and Mary Jane Logan McCallum, '"Assaulting the Ears of Government": The Indian Homemakers' Clubs and the Maori Women's Welfare League in their Formative Years', in Carol Williams (ed.), *Indigenous Women and Work: From Labor to Activism*, University of Illinois Press, Urbana, 2012, pp. 226–39.
118 Royal New Zealand Plunket Society, Auckland Branch, *Annual Report for 1988*, p. 4.
119 Wichtel, 'Delivering with Style', pp. 14–16; *Auckland Star*, 15 September 1989; Gabrielle Collison, interviewed by Jenny Carlyon, 16 May 2006, transcript, p. 2.
120 Rosy Fenwicke, *In Practice: The Lives of New Zealand Women Doctors in the 21st Century*, Random House, Auckland, 2004, p. 32.
121 Liddell in Fenwicke, *In Practice*, p. 69.
122 Ibid., pp. 70–71.
123 Hilary Liddell, interviewed by Jenny Carlyon, 1 April 2005, transcript, p. 13. See also 'Unsung Successes at National Women's', *NZH*, 26 November 1988.
124 Lesley McCowan, interviewed by Jenny Carlyon, 19 December 2005, transcript, pp. 1–2, 15; Lesley McCowan, Hilary Liddell, Cindy Farquhar, Lynda Batchelor [*sic*], 'Correspondence: Dennis Bonham', *NZMJ*, vol. 103, 14 November 1990, p. 543. See also interview with John France, who also believed that Bonham was at the forefront of women's health issues: John France, interviewed by Jenny Carlyon, 9 December 2004, transcript, p. 20; John Werry, transcript of his speech at Bonham's funeral, 6 May 2005, p. 3 (in author's possession).
125 Rosemary McLeod, 'The Importance of Being Sandra Coney', *North & South*, July 1988, p. 60; Jenny Carlyon, notes from Jenny Carlyon's interview with Nancie Bonham, 6 April 2004.
126 Werry, transcript of his speech at Bonham's funeral, 6 May 2005, p. 3.
127 As a fifth-year medical student in 1956, Jennifer Wilson chose to do her public health dissertation at National Women's: see Jennifer C. Wilson, 'Hypertension of Pregnancy: A Study of Foetal Mortality and Maternal

Prognosis in Pre-eclampsia and Essential Hypertension of Pregnancy carried out at National Women's Hospital, Auckland', Preventive Medicine dissertation, University of Otago, 1956.
128 Lynda Batcheler, interviewed by Jenny Carlyon, 31 March 2006, transcript, p. 3.
129 *NZH*, 4 August 1956.
130 *Dialogue: The Liggins Institute*, vol. 13, December 2006, p. 4.
131 HMC minutes, 21 May 1981, BAGC A638 21c, ANZA.
132 HMC minutes, 7 July 1981, BAGC A638 21c, ANZA. On Cecelia Liggins, see also *Dialogue: The Liggins Institute*, vol. 6, July 2003, p. 3.
133 Barry Twydle, interviewed by Jenny Carlyon, 18 September 2004, transcript, p. 6.
134 Val Dickens, interviewed by Jenny Carlyon, 24 November 2005, transcript, p. 22; 'Obituary: Lady Celia Margaret Liggins, 1925–2003', *O & G: Royal Australian and New Zealand Society of Obstetricians and Gynaecologists*, vol. 5, 3, September 2003, p. 229.
135 *Maternal Mortality Newsletter*, vol. 6, May 1979.

10: FEMINISTS, MIDWIVES AND NATIONAL WOMEN'S HOSPITAL

1 See, for example, Judi Strid, 'Midwifery in Revolt', *Broadsheet*, November 1987, pp. 14–17.
2 Sally Abel, 'Midwifery and Maternity Services in Transition: An Examination of Change following the Nurses Amendment Act 1990', PhD thesis, University of Auckland, 1997, p. 73.
3 Cited by Sandra Coney, 'From Here to Maternity', *Broadsheet*, October 1984, p. 5.
4 *Auckland Star*, 9 July 1980.
5 Professor Dennis Bonham, interviewed by Sandra Coney, 9 December 1986, transcript, Cartwright Inquiry Exhibit, UOAA; Dennis Bonham, Submission to Cartwright Inquiry, p. 27, UOAA.
6 Sandra Coney, *The Unfortunate Experiment: The Full Story behind the Inquiry into Cervical Cancer Treatment*, Penguin, Auckland, 1988, pp. 20–21.
7 Coney, evidence to Cartwright Inquiry, cited in *NZH*, 11 December 1987; *Dominion*, 11 December 1987.
8 Coney, Fertility Action Submission to Cartwright Inquiry, Day 64, 10 December 1987, pp. 5571–2, ANZA.
9 'A New Feature: Healthy Women: This Month: Childbirth', *Broadsheet*, December 1974, p. 30.
10 Sandra Coney, 'Alienated Labour – Foetal Monitoring', *Broadsheet*, May 1979, pp. 16–17, 38–39. See also Adrienne Rich, *Of Woman Born: Motherhood as Experience and Institution*, Norton, New York, 1976. Coney's October 1984 article in *Broadsheet*, 'From Here to Maternity', shows the intellectual influence of Ann Oakley who wrote a book entitled *From Here to Maternity* in 1974.
11 Bunkle, *Second Opinion*, pp. viii–ix (her emphasis).
12 Strid, 'Midwifery in Revolt', p. 15.
13 Joan Donley, 'Healthy Women', *Broadsheet*, October 1981, p. 40.
14 Maternity Services Committee, *Maternity Services in New Zealand*, pp. 38, 44; 'Maternity Services', *NZMJ*, vol. 83, 25 August 1976, pp. 158–9.
15 Sandra Coney, 'Taking Childbirth Back', *Broadsheet*, May 1977, pp. 22–23, 25.
16 Maternity Services Committee, *Mother and Baby at Home: The Early Days*, Board of Health, Wellington, 1982, p. 10.
17 Ibid.
18 Camille Guy, '"I've Enjoyed My Life . . . Hard as it's Been at Times": Vera Jane Ellis Crowther', *Broadsheet*, September 1976, pp. 16–17, 25. Ellis Crowther died in 1983: 'Vera Ellis Crowther 1897–1983: Farewell to a Friend', *Parents Centre Bulletin*, Summer 1983, p. 14.
19 *NZH*, 30 December 1989; NZCOM National Newsletter, November/December 1997, p. 9.
20 Pauline Ray, 'Midwives' Tales', *New Zealand Listener*, 5 November 1983, p. 17.
21 Pauline Ray, 'Whose Body is it? Whose

22. Baby is it?', *New Zealand Listener*, 15 March 1980, p. 22.
22. 'Obituary: Joan Donley', *NZH*, 17 December 2005.
23. Dr Diana Nash, 'Foreword', in Donley, *Save the Midwife*, p. 8, reprinted in Donley, *Birthrites*, p. 8.
24. Patricia A. Sargison, *Notable Women in New Zealand Health: Te Hauora ki Aotearoa: O na Wahine Rongonui*, Longman Paul, Auckland, 1993, p. 71; Wheeler, 'Home or Hospital Birth?'
25. Donley, 'Having the Baby at Home', p. 17.
26. Glynette Gainforte, in Guilliland and Pairman, *Women's Business*, p. 203.
27. Rachel Clarke, 'National Homebirth Conference Report', *New Zealand College of Midwives Journal*, vol. 18, April 1998, p. 25.
28. Donley, *Herstory of N.Z. Homebirth Association*, p. 3.
29. Rea Daellenbach, 'The Paradox of Success and the Challenge of Change: Home Birth Associations of Aotearoa / New Zealand', PhD thesis, University of Canterbury, 1999, p. 106.
30. Ibid., p. 127.
31. Ibid., p. 108.
32. 'Helen Brew: Closer to those Born at Home, a Star Talks', *Thursday*, 19 January 1976, pp. 30–31.
33. *Auckland Star*, 15 February 1979; on the film, see also Frances Parkin, 'Giving Birth Back to Mothers', *New Zealand Listener*, 16 April 1977, p. 18.
34. Mrs Diony Young, 'Parents' Right to Choose Family Centered Maternity Care? Or Change and Choices in Child Rearing?', Address to Christchurch Parents' Centre, 15 January 1979, p. 3, Board of Health – 'Maternity Services', ABQU 632 Acc W4550 5 29-21 (1978–79), ANZW.
35. Adrian Charles Laing, *R. D. Laing: A Biography*, Chester Springs, Pennsylvania, and Peter Owen, London, 1994, p. 190.
36. John Clay, *R. D. Laing: A Divided Self*, Hodder & Stoughton, London, 1996, p. 162.
37. Laing, *R.D. Laing*, p. 192.
38. 'Where to be born?' (meeting notes), debate chaired by Colin Mantell, 10 November 1976, Joan Donley Papers, MSS & Archives 2007/15, item 5/6/A/1, UOASC.
39. Sandra Coney, 'Radicalising Childbirth', *Broadsheet*, March 1974, p. 13.
40. Vanya Hogg, 'I put babies first, says doctor', *Auckland Star*, 4 October 1978.
41. Wheeler, 'Home or Hospital Birth?'
42. Charles M. Jockel, 'Correspondence: Home Confinements', *NZMJ*, vol. 90, 8 August 1979, p. 119.
43. *Auckland Star*, 4 July 1983.
44. *North Shore Times Advertiser*, 10 April 1979; *Auckland Star*, 19 September 1979.
45. Wheeler, 'Home or Hospital Birth?'
46. Guilliland and Pairman, *Women's Business*, p. 176; Daellenbach, 'The Paradox of Success', p. 111.
47. Linda Daly-Peoples, 'The Politics of Childbirth', *Broadsheet*, April 1977, pp. 14–21, 24.
48. Ibid., p. 24.
49. Donley, *Herstory*, pp. 11–12.
50. *Auckland Star*, 12 February 1982; Donley, *Herstory*, p. 14.
51. Ibid. (reprinted from NZHBA, *National Newsletter*, vol. 5, March 1982).
52. Dobbie, *The Trouble with Women*, pp. 126–7.
53. Sian Burgess, interviewed by Jenny Carlyon, 17 November 2005, transcript, p. 8.
54. Ibid., p. 9.
55. Guilliland and Pairman, *Women's Business*, p. 483.
56. Ray, 'Midwives' Tales', p. 16.
57. Abel, 'Midwifery and Maternity Services in Transition', p. 73; Guilliland and Pairman, *Women's Business*, p. 490; Donley, *Herstory*, p. 25.
58. *Auckland Star*, 16 February 1983.
59. Donley, *Herstory*, p. 40.
60. 'Preface', Donley, *Save the Midwife*, p. 12. Her description of obstetricians as 'generals' was later repeated by L. Haines, 'Another Unfortunate Experiment', *New Zealand Listener*, 31 January 2009, p. 15, and Mark Henaghan, *Health Professionals and Trust: A Cure for Healthcare Law and Policy*, Routledge, London, 2012, p. 89.

61 Peggy Anne Field, 'Impressions of Women's Health in New Zealand', *Midwifery*, vol. 6, 1990, p. 185.
62 Joan Mackay to Nancie Bonham, 11 October 2003, enclosing letter from D. G. Bonham to B. J. Mackay, 20 October 1983 (held by Nancie Bonham).
63 Helen Clark to Joan Donley, 26 March 1985, Joan Donley Papers, MSS & Archives 2007/15, item 5/6/A/1, UOASC.
64 Joan Donley, 'The New Women's Board of Health', *NZ Women's Health Network Newsletter*, April 1985, n.p.; *NZ Women's Health Network Newsletter*, no. 50, August 1985, n.p.; see also Bryder, *A History of the 'Unfortunate Experiment'*, pp. 116–17.
65 Health Benefits Review, *Choices for Health Care: Report of the Health Benefits Review*, Health Benefits Review, Wellington, 1986, pp. 5–56.
66 Hay, *The Caring Commodity*, p. 161.
67 *Journal of General Practice*, 4, August 1987, p. 1. For a full account of this episode in the history of National Women's Hospital, see Bryder, *A History of the 'Unfortunate Experiment'*.
68 Coney and Bunkle, 'An Unfortunate Experiment at National Women's'; Jan Corbett, 'Second Thoughts on the Unfortunate Experiment at National Women's', *Metro*, July 1990, p. 55; Committee of Inquiry into Allegations Concerning the Treatment of Cervical Cancer at National Women's Hospital and into Other Related Matters, *Report of the Committee of Inquiry into Allegations Concerning the Treatment of Cervical Cancer at National Women's Hospital and into Other Related Matters*, Government Printing Office, Auckland, 1988 (Cartwright Report).
69 W. A. McIndoe, M. R. McLean, R. W. Jones and P. R. Mullins, 'The Invasive Potential of Carcinoma in Situ of the Cervix', *Obstetrics and Gynecology: Journal of the American College of Obstetricians and Gynecologists*, vol. 64, 1984, pp. 451–8.
70 See Bryder, *A History of the 'Unfortunate Experiment'*, pp. 32–35.
71 See Graeme Overton, 'The 1987 National Women's Hospital (NWH) "Unfortunate Experiment": Accusations of Unethical Experiments and Under-treatment, Resulting in Excess Deaths from Cervical Cancer: Facts and Fables', *NZMJ*, vol. 123, 1319, 30 July 2010, pp. 101–5, http://journal.nzma.org.nz/journal/123-1319/4244/.
72 Thomas McKeown, *The Role of Medicine: Dream, Mirage or Nemesis?*, Basil Blackwell, Oxford, 1979; Thomas McKeown and E. G. Knox, 'The Framework Required for Validation of Prescriptive Screening', in Thomas McKeown (ed.), *Screening in Medical Care: Reviewing the Evidence: A Collection of Essays with a Preface by Lord Cohen of Birkenhead*, Nuffield Provincial Hospitals Trust, Oxford University Press, London, 1968, pp. 159–73; Bryder, *A History of the 'Unfortunate Experiment'*, pp. 13–14.
73 A. L. Cochrane, *Effectiveness and Efficiency: Random Reflections on Health Services*, Nuffield Hospitals Trust, London, 1972, pp. 26–27, 36. See also L. Bryder, 'Debates about Cervical Screening: An Historical Overview', *Journal of Epidemiology and Community Health*, vol. 62, 2008, pp. 284–7.
74 Cartwright Report, pp. 33–34.
75 Malcolm Coppleson, 'Colposcopy', in John Stallworthy and Gordon Bourne (eds), *Recent Advances in Obstetrics and Gynaecology*, Churchill Livingstone, Edinburgh, 12th edn, 1977, p. 178. See also Goran Larrson, *Conization for Preinvasive and Early Invasive Carcinoma of the Uterine Cervix*, Acta Obstetricia et Gynecologica Scandanavica, Supplement 114, Lund, 1983; and L. W. Coppleson and B. W. Brown, 'Control of Carcinoma of Cervix: Role of the Mathematical Model', in Malcolm Coppleson (ed.), *Gynecologic Oncology: Fundamental Principles and Clinical Practice*, vol. 1, Churchill Livingstone, New York, 1981, p. 390; Bryder, *A History of the 'Unfortunate Experiment'*, pp. 28–29, 35, 85; Linda

Bryder, 'A Response to Criticisms of the History of the "Unfortunate Experiment" at National Women's Hospital', *NZMJ*, vol. 123, 1319, 30 July 2010, http:/journal.nzma.org.nz/journal/123-1319/4240/.

76 Leopold G. Koss, 'Dysplasia: A Real Concept or a Misnomer?', *Obstetrics and Gynecology: Journal of the American College of Obstetricians and Gynecologists*, vol. 51, 198, p. 374; Bryder, *A History of the 'Unfortunate Experiment'*, p. 79.

77 World Health Organization International Agency for Research on Cancer, *IARC Handbooks on Cancer Prevention, vol. 10, Cervix Cancer Screening*, IARC Press, Lyon, 2005, p. 214; Angela Raffle and Muir Gray, *Screening: Evidence and Practice*, Oxford University Press, Oxford, 2007, pp. 20, 25; 'Editorial: Adverse Pregnancy Outcomes after Treatment for Cervical Intraepithelial Neoplasia', *BMJ*, vol. 337, 2008, pp. 769–70; M. Arbyn, M. Kyrgiou, C. Simeons, A. O. Raifu, G. Koliopoulos, P. Martin-Hirsch, W. Prendiville and E. Paraskevaidis, 'Perinatal Mortality and Other Severe Adverse Pregnancy Outcomes Associated with Treatment of Cervical Intraepithelial Neoplasia: Meta-analysis', *BMJ*, vol. 337, 2008, pp. 798–802; S. Albrechtsen, S. Rasmussen, S. Thoreson, L. M. Irgens and O. E. Iversen, 'Pregnancy Outcome in Women Before and After Cervical Conisation: Population Based Cohort Study', *BMJ*, vol. 337, 2008, pp. 803–5; 'Editorial: Managing Low Grade and Borderline Cervical Abnormalities', *BMJ*, vol. 339, 28 July 2009, p. 3014, doi: http://dx.doi.org/10.1136/bmj.b3014; see also Bryder, *A History of the 'Unfortunate Experiment'*, pp. 43, 100–1.

78 Lisa Saffron, 'Cervical Cancer – The Politics of Prevention', *Spare Rib*, vol. 129, April 1983, reprinted in Sue O'Sullivan (ed.), *Women's Health: A Spare Rib Reader*, Pandora, London, 1987, pp. 42–49; Jean Robinson, 'Cervical Cancer: Doctors Hide the Truth', *Spare Rib*, vol. 154, 1985, reprinted in O'Sullivan (ed.), *Women's Health*, pp. 49–51.

79 Tina Posner, 'What's in a Smear? Cervical Screening, Medical Signs and Metaphors', *Science as Culture*, vol. 2, 2, 11, 1991, p. 173.

80 These claims relating to recruitment appeared in Margaret R. E. McCredie, Katrina J. Sharples, Charlotte Paul, Judith Baranyai, Gabriele Medley, Ronald W. Jones and David C. G. Skegg, 'Natural History of Cervical Neoplasia and Risk of Invasive Cancer in Women with Cervical Intraepithelial Neoplasia 3: A Retrospective Cohort Study', *The Lancet Oncology*, vol. 9, 5, 2008, pp. 425–34; see Bryder, *A History of the 'Unfortunate Experiment'*, p. 35; Bryder, 'A Response to Criticisms', pp. 14–21.

81 Dennis Bonham, Submission to Cartwright Inquiry, p. 1809, UOAA.

82 Stanley C. Simmons to Katherine O'Regan, 26 March 1991, A426/37, RCOG Archives, London.

83 G. C. Liggins, 'The George Addlington Syme Oration: Winds of Change', *Australia and New Zealand Journal of Surgery*, vol. 61, March 1991, p. 169.

84 Cartwright Report, pp. 167, 171.

85 Ministry of Women's Affairs, *Newsletter*, 7, December 1987–January 1988.

86 Sandra Coney, 'Cartwright Ten Years On: Access to Health Care the Over-Riding Issue', 1997, http://www.womens-health.org.nz/cartwright-ten-years-on.html.

87 Pat Rosier, 'Broadcast: A Feminist Victory', *Broadsheet*, vol. 161, September 1988, pp. 6–7.

88 Theresa Gattung, 'When the Music Stops', *North & South*, April 2013, p. 69.

89 *Sunday Star*, 6 August 1989.

90 *NZH*, 6 August 1988.

91 Corbett, 'Second Thoughts on the Unfortunate Experiment', p. 59.

92 Coney, *The Unfortunate Experiment*, p. 266.

93 *Auckland Star*, 7 October 1988.

94 *Auckland Star*, 14 March 1989.

95 *NZH*, 6 August 1988; *Central Leader*, 16 August 1988.

96 Secretary Auckland Women's Health Council to the Chancellor, University of Auckland, 8 February 1989, Joan Donley Papers, MSS & Archives 2007/15, item 9/1/A/1 pt. 4, UOASC.
97 Donley to Mantell, 11 November 1989, Joan Donley Papers, MSS & Archives 2007/15, item 10/5/B/4, UOASC.
98 D. A. Lewis, for Maternity Action Alliance, Auckland, to Mantell, 17 November 1989, Joan Donley Papers, MSS & Archives 2007/15, item 10/5/B/4, UOASC.
99 Karen Guilliland, Chair, National Midwives Section NZNA, 21 November 1989, Joan Donley Papers, MSS & Archives 2007/15, item 9/1/A/1 pt. 4, UOASC.
100 Wendy Savage, *A Savage Enquiry: Who Controls Childbirth?*, Virago, London, 1986; 'News: Dr Wendy Savage Vindicated', *NZMJ*, vol. 99, 10 September 1986, p. 685.
101 Wendy Savage, 'Family Planning in a Hospital Clinic', *NZMJ*, vol. 83, 28 April 1976, pp. 261–5.
102 *Sunday Star*, 23 October 1988.
103 *Sunday Star*, 9 February 1992.
104 'Medicolegal: Medical Council Charges Professor Bonham', *Sunday Star*, 1 July 1990; *Sunday Star*, 15 July 1990; *NZH*, 15 October 1990.
105 *Sunday Star*, 9 December 1990.
106 Lesley McCowan, Hilary Liddell, Cindy Farquhar and Lynda Batchelor [sic], 'Correspondence: Dennis Bonham', *NZMJ*, vol. 103, 14 November 1990, p. 543.
107 'An Unfortunate Experiment', *NZH*, 14 May 2005.
108 Guilliland and Pairman, *Women's Business*, p. 576.
109 Bonham to R. Dickie, Department of Health, 13 February 1978, 'Maternal and Child Welfare', ABQU 632 Acc W4415/21 13/6/18, ANZW.
110 'New Zealand: Scandal Puts Hospitals under Pressure', *Time (International)*, Special Issue on 'Women: The Road Ahead', Summer 1990, pp. 22–23; see also Donley's article on the Inquiry in *Advance [To an Independent NZ: To Socialism: Communism*, NZ Periodical], vol. 52, March 1989, pp. 6–7.
111 Abel, 'Midwifery and Maternity Services in Transition', pp. 97–98.
112 Ibid., p. 81; Daellenbach, 'The Paradox of Success', p. 157.
113 New Zealand College of Midwives, 'Letters: Midwives' New Baby: An Open Letter to NZNA members', *NZNJ*, April 1989, p. 3.
114 Grehan, 'Professional Aspirations and Consumer Expectations', p. 277; Kerreen Reiger, 'The Politics of Midwifery in Australia: Tensions, Debates and Opportunities', *Annual Review of Health Social Sciences*, vol. 10, 2000, pp. 53–64.
115 Helen Clark, speech notes to open the NZCOM National Conference, Dunedin, 18 August 1990, p. 1, Joan Donley Papers, MSS & Archives 1007/15, item 5/6/A/1, UOASC. Speech also cited in Guilliland and Pairman, *Women's Business*, p. 557, footnote 71, and Daellenbach, 'The Paradox of Success', p. 168.
116 Clark, speech notes, p. 2.
117 Philippa Mein Smith, 'Midwifery Re-innovation in New Zealand', in Jennifer Stanton (ed.), *Innovations in Health and Medicine: Diffusion and Resistance in the Twentieth Century*, Routledge, New York, 2002, pp. 178–9.
118 Clark, speech notes, p. 3; see also Department of Health, Report to Social Services Committee on Nurses Amendment Bill, 10 April 1990, p. 4, ABGX, 16127, W4731, 130, Session 2, 3, ANZW.
119 Clark, speech notes, p. 6.
120 McLoughlin, 'The Politics of Childbirth', p. 65.
121 Clark, speech notes, p. 9.
122 Guilliland and Pairman, *Women's Business*, p. 189.
123 Abel, 'Midwifery and Maternity Services in Transition', pp. 101, 110.
124 Pamela Stirling, 'Hard Labour', *New Zealand Listener*, 12 March 1990, p. 15; see also Diana Nash, 'Foreword', in Donley, *Save the Midwife*, p. 8.
125 Kedgley, *Mum's the Word*, pp. 284–5.
126 Medical School, University of Auckland,

      14 October 1988, Box 432, UOAA.
127 Derek North, Response of the School of Medicine to the University Council Sub-committee (Ryburn Committee) on the Cartwright Report, p. 8, Box 432, UOAA.
128 McLoughlin, 'The Politics of Childbirth', p. 57.
129 Ibid., p. 59; see also Strid, 'Midwifery in Revolt', p. 15.

11: A HOSPITAL IN TROUBLE, 1990–2004

1 *A+ Newsletter*, August 1993, pp. 9, 11.
2 Auckland Healthcare Services Ltd, *National Women's Hospital Clinical Review*, April 1995, Review (chair: Professor Jeffrey Robinson, 'Robinson Review'), pp. 3, 14. This was also reported in *NZH*, 31 March 1995, when a draft review was published for consultation. Review committee members included Tony Baird, Joan Pierson, Jane Harding, Derek North, Teresa Bradfield, Malcolm Leuchars and Jane Hanley.
3 See, for example, R. Klein, *The New Politics of the NHS: From Creation to Reinvention*, Radcliffe Publishing, Oxford, 2010.
4 *Auckland Star*, 15 September 1989.
5 Mary Birdsall and Neil Pattison, 'Introduction', National Women's Hospital, *Annual Report 1991*, p. 2.
6 *NZH*, 19 January 1988.
7 Anne Nightingale, interviewed by Jenny Carlyon, 27 September 2004, transcript, p. 13.
8 *People's Voice*, 25 June 1990, p. 3.
9 'Baby Boom: Who Can't Count? Why Can't the Maternity Services Cope?', *NZNJ*, November 1990, p. 17.
10 Stirling, 'Hard Labour', p. 14.
11 'Baby Boom', p. 19.
12 *Auckland Star*, 25 September 1990.
13 *Central Leader*, 3 October 1990.
14 *NZH*, 15 February 1993.
15 'Baby Boom', p. 19.
16 See, for example, 'Disgust over National Women's Dirt', *NZH*, 25 April 1996.
17 Jeffery, 'Whanautanga', p. 122.
18 *NZH*, 19 January 1988.
19 *NZH*, 6 July 1995.
20 *Project 95*, vol. 1, 3, October 1995, p. 5; *NZH*, 15 September 1995.
21 *NZH*, 7 September 1996.
22 Brett Reid, 'From Here to Maternity – National Women's Takes a "Leap Forward"', *New Zealand General Practice*, 28 August 1990, p. 8.
23 'Baby's Birth Ruined by Lazy Fathers', *East City News*, 28 February 1991.
24 Ibid.
25 *East City News*, 7 March 1991.
26 *Eastern Courier*, 27 March 1991.
27 *Central Leader*, 10 July 1991.
28 Jeffery, 'Whanautanga', p. 131.
29 Cartwright Report, pp. 171–3, 213. See also Bryder, *A History of the 'Unfortunate Experiment'*, p. 178.
30 Williams, in Guilliland and Pairman, *Women's Business*, p. 179.
31 Coney, 'Fertility Action 1984–', p. 286.
32 *NZH*, 11 August 1989; see also Donley, *Herstory*, pp. 38–39.
33 Lynda Williams, 'Dreaming the Impossible Dream: The Fate of Patient Advocacy', in Sandra Coney (ed.), *Unfinished Business: What Happened to the Cartwright Inquiry*, Women's Health Action, Auckland, 1993, pp. 90, 95; see also *Sunday Star*, 1 August 1993.
34 *East & Bays Courier*, 6 December 1995, p. 7.
35 Cited in Kathy Glasgow, 'Maternity "shambles"', *New Zealand Health Review*, vol. 1, 1, Autumn 1998, pp. 9–10.
36 'Pioneering Work Continues', *University of Auckland News*, vol. 24, 1, February 1994, p. 2; Bryder, *A History of the 'Unfortunate Experiment'*, pp. 130–5, 181.
37 Robinson Review, p. 39.
38 National Women's Hospital, *Annual Report 1996*, p. 5; National Women's Hospital, *Annual Report 1997*, p. 6.
39 Auckland Maternity Services Consumer Council, Newsletter no. 1, August 1990.
40 Maternity Benefits Tribunal, *Report and Recommendations of the Maternity Benefits Tribunal*, Ministry of Health, Wellington, 1993, submissions, pp. 1–7.
41 Guilliland and Pairman, *Women's Business*, p. 245.

42 Karen Guilliland and Sally Pairman, 'The Midwifery Partnership – A Model for Practice', paper to NZCOM Conference, Rotorua, 12–14 August 1994, p. 2, published as Karen Guilliland and Sally Pairman, *The Midwifery Partnership: A Model for Practice*, Department of Nursing and Midwifery, Victoria University of Wellington, Wellington, 1995; Sally Pairman, 'Developing & Crafting a Vision: A Strategic Plan for Midwifery', *New Zealand College of Midwives Journal*, 18, April 1998, pp. 6–7.
43 'Dedication to Joan Donley', Guilliland and Pairman, *Women's Business*, p. 2.
44 Guilliland, cited in McLoughlin, 'The Politics of Childbirth', p. 66.
45 Stirling, 'Hard Labour', p. 12.
46 'Mother Care', *Consumer*, no. 356, January/February 1997, p. 5.
47 Robinson Review, p. 19.
48 Abel, 'Midwifery and Maternity Services in Transition', p. 3; Sarah Stewart, 'Midwifery in New Zealand: A Cause for Celebration', *MIDIRS Midwifery Digest*, vol. 11, 3, September 2001, pp. 319–20.
49 McLoughlin 'The Politics of Childbirth', p. 59.
50 M. A. H. Baird to Sian Burgess, 20 October 1997, Joan Donley Papers, MSS & Archives 2007/15, item 1/2/B/1, UOASC.
51 Gillian Turner, personal communication to author, 21 June 2006.
52 Guilliland and Pairman, *Women's Business*, p. 116.
53 Karen Guilliland, 'Learning from Midwives', *NZNJ*, October 1996, p. 23; also cited in Mein Smith, 'Midwifery Re-innovation in New Zealand', p. 181.
54 H. J. W. S. to Sheryl Smail, 1 September 1994 (files provided to author by Glenda Stimpson).
55 Glenda Stimpson, submission, 3 November 1992 (files provided to author by Glenda Stimpson). The hourly rates were $139.60 versus $15–17: Maternity Benefits Tribunal, *Report and Recommendations of the Maternity Benefits Tribunal*, pp. 26–27.
56 Robinson Review, p. 29.
57 Stewart, 'Midwifery in New Zealand: A Cause for Celebration', pp. 319–20.
58 James King, comments on National Women's Hospital, *Annual Report for 1993*, p. 4.
59 Ibid., p. 6.
60 Peter Stone, interviewed by Jenny Carlyon, 22 November 2005, transcript, p. 11.
61 National Women's Hospital, *Annual Clinical Report 2000*, p. 61.
62 'Your Choices in Childbirth', *Consumer*, no. 324, March 1994, p. 7. In 2005 a new independent group, the Perinatal and Maternal Mortality Review Committee, was set up.
63 Anne Nightingale, interviewed by Jenny Carlyon, 27 September 2004, transcript, pp. 10, 16.
64 *NZH*, 3 January 1995. On Sutherland's concerns, see also McLoughlin, 'The Politics of Childbirth', p. 66.
65 The Royal New Zealand College of Obstetricians and Gynaecologists gained the 'Royal' prefix in 1984 after the formation of the New Zealand College in 1982, which replaced the New Zealand Council of the RCOG. It became part of the Royal Australian and New Zealand College of Obstetricians and Gynaecologists in 1998.
66 *NZH*, 3 January 1995.
67 *NZH*, 26 January 1995.
68 Ibid.
69 *Sunday News*, 9 February 1997.
70 *Evening Post*, 18 October 1997; *NZH*, 25 October 1997.
71 *Sunday Star-Times*, 12 April 1998.
72 *New Zealand College of Midwives National Newsletter*, vol. 7, December 1997.
73 *NZH*, 20 December 1997.
74 *Sunday Star-Times*, 28 October 1997.
75 *Evening Post*, 20 April 1998.
76 McLoughlin, 'The Politics of Childbirth', p. 56; see also 'Mother Care', p. 5.
77 Glenn Blanchette, 'The Changing Landscape of Maternity Services', in Robin Gauld (ed.), *Continuity and Chaos: Health Care Management and Delivery in New Zealand*, Otago University Press, Dunedin, 2003, p. 138.

78 McLoughlin, 'The Politics of Childbirth', p. 56; 'Mother Care', p. 5; Bruce Ansley, 'Babies at Risk', *New Zealand Listener*, 5 April 1997, p. 22; Guilliland and Pairman, *Women's Business*, p. 249.
79 'Your Choices in Childbirth', p. 8.
80 This became section 88 of the 2000 Public Health and Disability Act.
81 Blanchette, 'The Changing Landscape of Maternity Services', pp. 140–1; see also Anton Wiles, 'Maternity – A Drastic Cut in Options for Women', *New Zealand Medical Association Newsletter*, 14 November 1997, pp. 3–4; 'Fleeing in Droves from Maternity', *New Zealand Doctor*, 10 December 1997, p. 3.
82 Ansley, 'Babies at Risk', p. 22.
83 Glasgow, 'Maternity "shambles"', p. 9.
84 Karen Guilliland, 'National Director's Forum', *New Zealand College of Midwives National Newsletter*, vol. 7, December 1997, p. 8.
85 Bruce Ansley, 'Another Unfortunate Experiment?', *New Zealand Listener*, 14 August 1999, p. 21.
86 Liane Topham-Kindley, 'Never Say Die: GPOs Meet for CME Talks', *New Zealand Doctor*, 6 October 2004, p. 9; *NZH*, 19 November 2005; *Sunday Star-Times*, 5 February 2006.
87 Gillian Turner, 'Introduction', National Women's Hospital, *Annual Report 1996*, p. 5; Peter Stone and David Knight, 'Introduction', National Women's Hospital, *Annual Clinical Report 2000*, p. 3.
88 Robinson Review, p. 12.
89 *NZH*, 31 March 1995.
90 *NZH*, 17 June 1995.
91 *A+ Newsletter*, July 1995, p. 3.
92 McCalman, *Sex and Suffering*, pp. 343–5.
93 *Project 95*, vol. 1, 3, October 1995, p. 5.
94 Review of Maternity Services at National Women's Hospital, June–August 1996, Report and Summary of Recommendations (files provided to author by Glenda Stimpson).
95 Marjet Pot, interviewed by Jenny Carlyon, 26 July 2006, transcript, p. 1.
96 Review of Obstetric and Gynaecological Staffing at National Women's, September 1997 (review supplied to author by Professor Jeffrey Robinson).
97 Gillian Turner, 'Introduction', National Women's Hospital, *Annual Report 1997*, p. 6.
98 Aroha Harris, *Measuring the Effectiveness of Health Services for Maori Consumers*, Ministry of Health, Wellington, 1994.
99 *The Newz, What's the Buzz*, issue 6, 1 October 1997, p. 1; issue 20, 20 April 1999, p. 1.
100 On 'Birthcare', see Kim Paterson, 'Birth . . . the Way You Want It', *NZWW*, 13 July 1987, pp. 56–57.
101 Peter Stone and David Knight, 'Introduction', National Women's Hospital, *Annual Clinical Report 1999*, p. 4; Mark Revington, 'Born Free', *New Zealand Listener*, 14 August 1999, pp. 18–21.
102 *The Newz, What's the Buzz*, issue 45, March/April 2003.
103 Robinson Review, pp. 36–37.
104 Cecil Lewis, 'A Brief Survey of the History of the Postgraduate School of Obstetrics and Gynaecology and its Prospects in Relation to the Faculty of Medicine', 7 May 1968, Box 257, UOAA.
105 Notes by G.H.G. on the present situation of the Postgraduate School of Obstetrics and Gynaecology, 15 April 1968, Green Papers, MSS 1433, folder 4, UOASC.
106 David S. Cole to Vice-Chancellor Dr Maiden, Re. Conditions of Appointment Professor D. G. Bonham, 21 October 1977, Box 245, UOAA.
107 Bonham, Mantell, Green, Liggins, Liley and France to Vice-Chancellor, 31 January 1979, Green Papers, MSS 1433, folder 4, UOASC.
108 Bonham to Registrar, Warwick Nicoll, 10 April 1987, Box 415, UOAA.
109 Cole to Registrar, Warwick Nicoll, 13 September 1988, Box 415, UOAA.
110 'Department of Obstetrics and Gynaecology University Academic Unit', National Women's Hospital, *Annual Clinical Report 1998*, p. 136.
111 'Research Centre in Reproductive

112 'Department of Obstetrics and Gynaecology University Academic Unit', National Women's Hospital, Annual Report 1995, p. 90; 'University Department of Obstetrics and Gynaecology', National Women's Hospital, Annual Report 1996, p. 97.
113 On international trends in these areas, see also Barbara Bridgman Perkins, *The Medical Delivery Business: Health Reform, Childbirth, and the Economic Order*, Rutgers University Press, New Brunswick, 2004, p. 131.
114 Sheryl Smail, 'Foreword', National Women's Hospital, Annual Report 1993, p. 4.
115 Auckland Healthcare Services Ltd, Provision of Women's Health Services in the Acute Services Building on the Grafton site, November 1999, Appendix 1, Lesley McCowan, Peter Stone, Janet Rowan, to Carolynn Whiteman, 15 November 1999 (document provided to author by Peter Stone).
116 Gillian Turner, 'Introduction', National Women's Hospital, Annual Report 1997, p. 7; 'Focus on the Foetus', *Ingenio, Magazine of the University of Auckland*, Autumn 2003, pp. 14–16.
117 Quoted in the centre's magazine, *Dialogue*, vol. 2, 3, 2002, p. 1.
118 Ibid.
119 'Focus on the Foetus', pp. 14–16.
120 *The Newz: What's the Buzz*, issue 35, July/August 2001.
121 Turner, 'Introduction', National Women's Hospital, Annual Report 1996, p. 6.
122 *Sunday Star-Times*, 27 July 1997; 'Prem Babies – Should They be Saved?', *NZWW*, 10 March 1997, pp. 32–33.
123 Cull Report, p. 21.
124 'Prem Babies – Should They be Saved?', p. 32; Cull Report, p. 21.
125 'Prem Babies – Should They be Saved', p. 32.
126 Cull Report, p. 22.
127 *Sunday Star-Times*, 4 July 1999.
128 See, for example, N. Finer and J. Boyd, 'Chest Physiotherapy in the Neonate: A Control Study', *Pediatrics*, vol. 61, 1978, pp. 282–5; D. I. Tudehope and C. Bagley, 'Techniques of Physiotherapy in Intubated Babies with Respiratory Distress Syndrome', *Australian Paediatric Journal*, vol. 16, 1980, pp. 226–8.
129 Cull Report, p. 11.
130 This article appeared in *Archives of Disease in Childhood*, vol. 67, 1992, pp. 307–11.
131 Cull Report, p. 11.
132 Sandra Coney, 'Physiotherapy Technique Banned in Auckland', *The Lancet*, vol. 345, 25 February 1995, p. 510.
133 'ACC' is shorthand for compensation from the Accident Compensation Corporation which administered it. On the legislation which introduced this see pp. 132–3.
134 Cull Report, p. 18.
135 National Women's Hospital, Annual Clinical Report 2000, p. 5.
136 Sandra Coney, 'New Zealand Inquires Further into Baby Deaths', *The Lancet*, vol. 354, 31 July 1999, p. 406.
137 *NZH*, 13 November 2000; *NZH*, 27 November 2002.
138 *NZH*, 27 November 2002.
139 A. N. Williams and R. Sunderland, 'Neonatal Shaken Baby Syndrome: An Aetiological View from Down Under', *Archives of Disease in Childhood: Fetal Neonatal Edition*, vol. 87, 2002, F29–30; L. Rosenbloom and S. Ryan, 'Correspondence: Commentary', *Archives of Disease in Childhood: Fetal Neonatal Edition*, vol. 87, 2002. The authors cited J. E. Harding, F. K. I. Miles, D. M. O. Becroft, B. C. Allen and D. B. Knight, 'Chest Physiotherapy May be Associated with Brain Damage in Extremely Premature Infants', *Journal of Pediatrics*, vol. 132, 1998, pp. 440–4; D. B. Knight, D. J. Bevan, J. E. Harding, R. L. Teele, C. A. Kuschel, M. R. Battin and R. S. H. Rowley, 'Chest Physiotherapy and Porencephalic Lesions in Very Preterm Infants', *Journal of Paediatrics and Child Health*, vol. 37, 2001, pp. 554–8; V. J. Flenady and P. H. Gray, 'Chest Physiotherapy for Preventing Morbidity in Babies

being Extubated from Mechanical Ventilation', *The Cochrane Library*, Oxford, Update Software, 2000: issue 4. See also Jean Robinson, 'Shaken Baby Syndrome: Caused by Hospital Care', *AIMS Journal*, Spring 2003, vol. 15, 1, http://www.aims.org.uk/Journal/Vol15No1/ShakenBabySyndrome.htm; D. B. Knight, 'Letter: Shaken Baby Syndrome – Lessons to be Learnt', *Archives of Disease in Childhood: Fetal Neonatal Edition*, vol. 88, 2003, F161–F162, doi:10.1136/fn.88.2.F161-a.

140 Edmund Hey and Iain Chalmers, 'Mis-investigating Alleged Research Misconduct can Cause Widespread, Unpredictable Damage', *Journal of the Royal Society of Medicine*, vol. 103, 2010, pp. 132–7, doi: 10.1258/jrsm.2010.09k045; Jonathan Gornall, 'The Role of the Media in the Stoke CNEP Saga', *Journal of the Royal Society of Medicine*, vol. 103, 5, 2010, pp. 173–177, doi: 10.1258/jrsm.2010.10k011; Teresa Wright, 'The Stoke CNEP Saga – How it Damaged All Involved', *Journal of the Royal Society of Medicine*, vol. 103, 7, 2010, pp. 277-82, doi: 10.1258/jrsm.2010.10k012.

141 *NZH*, 12 March 2002.

142 A. J. Gunn, P. D. Gluckman and T. R. Gunn, 'Selective Head Cooling in Newborn Infants Following Perinatal Asphyxia: A Safety Study', *Pediatrics*, vol. 102, 4, 1998, pp. 885–992, doi:10.1542/peds.102.4.885.

143 *NZH*, 12 March 2002; on Tania Gunn's legacy, see 'Obituary: Tania Gunn', *University of Auckland News*, April 1999, p. 15.

144 *NZH*, 7 May 2004; A. Gunn, P. D. Gluckman, J. S. Wyatt, M. Thoresen and A. D. Edwards, 'Selective Head Cooling after Neonatal Encephalopathy', *The Lancet*, vol. 365, 2005, pp. 1619–20, doi:10.1016/S0140-6736(05)66505-1.

145 Robinson Review, p. 40.

146 Grehan, 'Professional Aspirations and Consumer Expectations', p. 279.

147 *Weekend Herald*, 19–20 February 2000; *NZH*, 8 May 2001; *Auckland City Harbour News*, 21 February 2003.

148 *NZH*, 7 December 2003.

149 *NZH*, 14 January 1995.

150 Anne Manchester, 'Four Auckland Hospitals Become One: The New Auckland City Hospital the Largest Public Building in the Country, is Certainly Impressive, but Adapting to New Systems and a New Hospital Culture Continues to be Challenging for Nurses', *NZNJ*, October 2004, pp. 24–26.

151 Kay Hyman, 'Foreword', *National Women's Annual Clinical Report 2005*, p. 3.

152 Hilary Liddell, interviewed by Jenny Carlyon, 1 April 2005, transcript, pp. 15–16.

153 Cynthia Farquhar, interviewed by Jenny Carlyon, April 2005, transcript, p. 9.

CONCLUSION

1 Abel, 'Midwifery and Maternity Services in Transition', pp. 85–86.

2 FNZPC, *First Annual Report 1958*, pp. 2–3, Box 1.1, FNZPC Archives, Wellington.

3 Pamela Wood, 'Guest Editorial', *New Zealand College of Midwives (Inc.) Journal*, vol. 31, October 2004, pp. 4–6.

4 J. Stojanovic, '"Leaving your dignity at the door": Maternity in Wellington 1950–1970', *New Zealand College of Midwives (Inc.) Journal*, vol. 31, October 2004, pp. 12–18; Jane Stojanovic, 'Midwifery in New Zealand, 1904–1971', *Birthspirit Midwifery Journal*, vol. 5, February 2010, p. 59.

5 Papps and Olssen, *Doctoring Childbirth and Regulating Midwifery in New Zealand*.

6 Donley, *Save the Midwife*, pp. 1, 11.

7 See also Grehan, 'Professional Aspirations and Consumer Expectations', pp. 254, 298, 312, 319.

8 *NZH*, 9 July 1970.

9 Douglas Robb, 'Strong Medicine', *The Times*, 18 May 1966.

10 Gluckman and Buklijas, 'Sir Graham Collingwood (Mont) Liggins', p. 14.

11 Ibid.

12. M. E. J. Lean, J. I. Mann, J. A. Hoek, R. M. Elliott and G. Schofield, 'Translational Research: From Evidence Based Medicine to Sustainable Solutions for Public Health Problems', *BMJ*, vol. 337, 27 September 2008, pp. 705–6.
13. Wall, 'The Glamorous Gynaecologists'.
14. 'Introduction', Jo Garcia, Robert Kilpatrick and Martin Richards (eds), *The Politics of Maternity Care: Services for Childbearing Women in Twentieth-century Britain*, Oxford University Press, Oxford, 1990, p. 2. (The actual title was *Human Relations in Obstetrics*.)
15. Strid, 'Midwifery in Revolt', p. 16.
16. Pauline Bart, 'Seizing the Means of Reproduction: An Illegal Feminist Abortion Collective – How and Why it Worked', in Helen Roberts (ed.), *Women, Health and Reproduction*, Routledge & Kegan Paul, London, 1981, p. 113.
17. Gail Young, 'A Woman in Medicine: Reflections from the Inside', in Roberts (ed.), *Women, Health and Reproduction*, p. 159.
18. Sheila Kitzinger, 'Foreword', in Reiger, *Our Bodies, Our Babies*, p. v.
19. National Women's Hospital, *Annual Report 1996*, p. 6.

BIBLIOGRAPHY

ARCHIVES

Archives New Zealand, Auckland Regional Office (ANZA)
Auckland Hospital Board, Green Lane and Cornwall Park Hospital Committee minutes, 1946–1952; Hospital Medical Committee minutes, 1954–87.

Archives New Zealand, Wellington (ANZW)
Board of Health Maternity Services Committee files, 1960–81; Department (Ministry) of Health maternity files, 1937–90.

Archives, Office of the Vice-Chancellor, University of Auckland (UOAA)
University of Auckland (College) Obstetrics and Gynaecology Advisory Committee files, 1949–; Postgraduate School (Department) of Obstetrics and Gynaecology, University of Auckland minutes, reports and correspondence, 1949–88.

University of Auckland Library, Special Collections (UOASC)
Auckland Division of the New Zealand Branch of the British Medical Association (NZBMA) minutes, 1950–70.
Douglas Robb Papers, c.1940–c.1970.
Herbert Green Papers, c.1940–c.1980.
Joan Donley Papers, c.1980–c.2000.

Auckland Museum Archives (AMA)
Transcripts of Committee of Inquiry into Maternity Services, 1937–38.
New Zealand Society for the Protection of Women and Children (NZSPWC) Auckland Branch minutes, 1936–39.
National Council of Women (NCW), Auckland Branch minutes, 1933–60.
Amy May Hutchinson 'Odd Memories at Eighty Odd and Life in 1900: Memories of a Social Worker', unpublished ms.
Dr Doris Clifton Gordon Papers, 1940–50.

Federation of New Zealand Parents' Centres Archives, Wellington (FNZPC)
Minutes, annual reports, newsletters and correspondence, 1951–c.1970.

Royal College of Obstetricians and Gynaecologists Archives, London (RCOG)
Annual reports, correspondence, New Zealand Regional Council minutes, 1947–71.

Hocken Library, Dunedin
Plunket Society Archives (PSA).

Private Collection (R. W. Jones)
New Zealand Obstetrical Society (NZOS) minutes, 1927–35; New Zealand Obstetrical and Gynaecological Society (NZOGS) minutes, 1935–1941.

Bibliography

INTERVIEWS

Neonatal Nursing Oral History Project, Alexander Turnbull Library.
National Women's Oral History Project 2002, interviews by Chanel Clark.
'The History of Women's Health with a special focus on National Women's Hospital' Project, interviews by Jenny Carlyon, 2004–6 (in author's possession).

UNPUBLISHED MANUSCRIPTS (in author's possession)

'Changing Trends, Attitudes, Structure and Design in Delivery Suite National Women's Hospital', 1962–88 (supplied to author by Glenda Stimpson).
Collison, Gabrielle, National Women's Hospital, Auckland, New Zealand, A Position Paper, July 1988.
Howie, Ross, 'Tangaroa and Beyond: The Newborn Service', Talk given to Auckland Medical History Society, 4 July 2002, and revised draft, 27 March 2004.
——, '"Historical Events at National Women's Hospital": Comments on the Booklet (Aug. 2004 version) Circulated at the Hospital's Farewell Function 24 Sep. 2004', 1 October 2004.
——, 'Newborn Services in Crisis, New Zealand 1980', 13 September 2010.
Liggins, G., 'A Brief Autobiography of Professor Sir Graham Liggins FRS', unpublished manuscript.
Robinson, Jeffrey, *National Women's Hospital Clinical Review*, April 1995, Review for Auckland Healthcare Services Ltd.
——, Review of Obstetric and Gynaecological Staffing at National Women's, September 1997 (review supplied to author by Professor Jeffrey Robinson).
Werry, John, transcript of speech at Dennis Bonham's funeral, 6 May 2005.

BOOKS AND ARTICLES

'A New Feature: Healthy Women: This Month: Childbirth', *Broadsheet*, December 1974, pp. 30–31.
Aickin, D. R., 'The Making of an Obstetrician', *New Zealand Medical Journal (NZMJ)*, vol. 81, 12 February 1975, pp. 92–95.
Albrechtsen, S., S. Rasmussen, S. Thoreson, L. M. Irgens and O. E. Iversen, 'Pregnancy Outcome in Women Before and After Cervical Conisation: Population Based Cohort Study', *British Medical Journal (BMJ)*, vol. 337, 2008, pp. 803–5.
Ansley, Bruce, 'Babies at Risk', *New Zealand Listener*, 5 April 1997, pp. 20–23.
——, 'Another Unfortunate Experiment?', *New Zealand Listener*, 14 August 1999, pp. 18–21.
Apgar, V., 'A Proposal for a New Method of Evaluation of the Newborn Infant', *Anesthesia and Analgesia Current Research*, vol. 32, 1953, pp. 260–7.
Arbyn, M., M. Kyrgiou, C. Simeons, A. O. Raifu, G. Koliopoulos, P. Martin-Hirsch, W. Prendiville and E. Paraskevaidis, 'Perinatal Mortality and Other Severe Adverse Pregnancy Outcomes Associated with Treatment of Cervical Intraepithelial Neoplasia: Meta-analysis', *BMJ*, vol. 337, 2008, pp. 798–802.
Armstrong, John, *Under One Roof: A History of Waikato Hospital*, Waikato Health Memorabilia Trust, Hamilton, 2009.
'Baby Boom: Who Can't Count? Why Can't the Maternity Services Cope?', *New Zealand Nursing Journal: Kai Tiaki (NZNJ)*, November 1990, pp. 17–19.
Bada, H. S., W. Hajiar, C. Chua and D. S. Sumner, 'Non-invasive Diagnosis of Neonatal Asphyxia and Intraventricular Haemorrhage by Doppler Ultrasound', *Journal of Pediatrics*, vol. 95, 1979, pp. 775–9.

Bibliography

Baird, M. A. H., 'Morbidity of Therapeutic Abortion in Auckland', *NZMJ*, vol. 83, 9 June 1976, pp. 395–9.
Baker, Jeffrey P., *The Machine in the Nursery: Incubator Technology and the Origins of Newborn Intensive Care*, Johns Hopkins University Press, Baltimore, 1996.
Bart, Pauline, 'Seizing the Means of Reproduction: An Illegal Feminist Abortion Collective – How and Why it Worked', in Helen Roberts (ed.), *Women, Health and Reproduction*, Routledge & Kegan Paul, London, 1981, pp. 109–28.
Begg, Neil C. and Rowland P. Wilson, 'Retrolental Fibroplasia: Report of a Case', *NZMJ*, vol. 52, February 1953, pp. 30–34.
Beinart, Jennifer, 'Obstetric Analgesia and the Control of Childbirth in Twentieth-Century Britain', in Jo Garcia, Robert Kilpatrick and Martin Richards (eds), *The Politics of Maternity Care: Services for Childbearing Women in Twentieth-century Britain*, Oxford University Press, Oxford, 1990, pp. 116–32.
Bell, Marie, *The Establishment of Parents' Centre: Successful Advocacy for Parents of Children under Three by the Parents' Centre Organisation in its First Decade 1952–1962*, Institute for Early Childhood Studies, Occasional Papers Series 18, Victoria University of Wellington, Wellington, 2006.
Bell, Terry and John Evans, 'Vasectomy, the "Snip and Tie" Operation is Booming', *Thursday*, 6 December 1973, pp. 21–22, 27.
Bevan-Brown, Maurice, *The Sources of Love and Fear, with Contributions by Members of the Christchurch Psychological Society*, A. H. & A. W. Reed, Wellington, 1950.
Bevis, D. C. A., 'Blood Pigments in Haemolytic Disease of the Newborn', *Journal of Obstetrics and Gynaecology of the British Empire*, vol. 63, 1956, pp. 68–75.
Blanchette, Glenn, 'The Changing Landscape of Maternity Services', in Robin Gauld (ed.), *Continuity and Chaos: Health Care Management and Delivery in New Zealand*, Otago University Press, Dunedin, 2003, pp. 137–49.
Bonham, Dennis G., 'The Evolution of Obstetrics and Gynaecology', *NZMJ*, vol. 63, November 1964, pp. 709–15.
——, 'Maternal and Child Health', in D. P. Kennedy (ed.), *Health in the 1970s: A Collection of Informed Opinions*, N. M. Peryer, Christchurch, 1970, pp. 22–32.
——, 'Leading Article: Caesarean Birth', *NZMJ*, vol. 96, 23 March 1983, pp. 205–6.
——, 'Leading Article: Advances in the Management of Infertility', *NZMJ*, 14 March 1984, pp. 146–7.
Bonham, D. G., D. J. Court, F. M. Graham, J. D. Hutton, G. C. Liggins, A. W. Liley, C. D. Mantell and E. B. Nye, 'Obstetric and Gynaecological Disorders: Advances in Treatment', *New Ethicals*, September 1980, pp. 69–79.
Bonita, Ruth, 'Contraceptive Research: For Whose Protection?', *Broadsheet*, vol. 76, January/February 1980, pp. 6–8.
Borst, Charlotte G., *Catching Babies: The Professionalization of Childbirth, 1870–1920*, Harvard University Press, Cambridge, Massachusetts, 1995.
Brahams, D., 'Medicine and the Law: In Vitro Fertilisation and Related Research: Why Parliament Must Legislate', *The Lancet*, vol. 2, 24 September 1983, pp. 726–9.
Brant, H. A., 'Childbirth with Preparation and Support in Labour: An Assessment', *NZMJ*, vol. 61, April 1962, pp. 211–19.
Brant, Herbert A. and Margaret Brant, *A Dictionary of Pregnancy, Childbirth and Contraception*, Mayflower, London, 1971.
British Medical Association (NZ Branch), *Report of the Committee of Inquiry into Maternity Hospital Staffing, 1946*, British Medical Association (NZ Branch), Wellington, 1947.
Brooks, Jocelyn, *Ill Conceived: Law and Abortion Practice in New Zealand*, Caveman Press, Dunedin, 1981.
Brown, Amy, 'The Maternity Technique, Enjoy Your Stay in Hospital', *Thursday*, 1 October 1970, pp. 62, 67.
Browne, Alan (ed.), *Masters, Midwives and Ladies-in-Waiting: The Rotunda Hospital*

1745–1995, A. & A. Farmar, Dublin, 1995.
Browne, Francis J., *Antenatal and Postnatal Care*, J. & A. Churchill, London, 1937.
Bryder, Linda, *Not Just Weighing Babies: Plunket in Auckland, 1908–1998*, Pyramid Press, Auckland, 1998.
——, 'Muriel Helen Deem', in Jane Thomson (ed.) *Southern People: A Dictionary of Otago Southland Biography*, Longacre Press in association with the Dunedin City Council, Dunedin, 1998, pp. 125–6.
——, *A Voice for Mothers: The Plunket Society and Infant Welfare 1907–2000*, Auckland University Press, Auckland, 2003.
——, 'Breastfeeding and Health Professionals in Britain, New Zealand and the United States, 1900–1970', *Medical History*, vol. 49, 2, 2005, pp. 179–96.
——, 'Debates about Cervical Screening: An Historical Overview', *Journal of Epidemiology and Community Health*, vol. 62, 2008, pp. 284–7.
——, *A History of the 'Unfortunate Experiment' at National Women's Hospital*, Auckland University Press, Auckland, 2009, reprinted as Linda Bryder, *Women's Bodies and Medical Science: An Inquiry into Cervical Cancer*, Palgrave Macmillan, London, 2010.
——, 'A Response to Criticisms of the History of the "Unfortunate Experiment" at National Women's Hospital', *NZMJ*, vol. 123, 1319, 30 July 2010, http://journal.nzma.org.nz/journal/123-1319/4240/.
——, 'Gordon, Doris Clifton – Biography', *Dictionary of New Zealand Biography. Te Ara – the Encyclopedia of New Zealand*, updated 1 September 2010, http://www.TeAra.govt.nz/en/biographies/4g14/1.
Bryder, L. and D. A. Dow (eds), *The History of Fetal Medicine with a Special Emphasis on Auckland, Witness Seminar at Old Government House, The University of Auckland, 19 February 2005*, The Australian and New Zealand Society of the History of Medicine, Auckland, 2006.
Bunkle, Phillida, 'Calling the Shots? The International Politics of Depo-Provera', in Rita Arditti, Renate Duelli Klein and Shelley Minden (eds), *Test-Tube Women: What Future for Motherhood?*, Pandora Press, London, 1984, pp. 165–87.
——, 'Dalkon Shield Disaster', *Broadsheet*, vol. 122, September 1984, p. 22.
——, *Second Opinion: The Politics of Women's Health in New Zealand*, Oxford University Press, Auckland, 1988.
Butler, Neville R. and Dennis G. Bonham, *Perinatal Mortality: The First Report of the 1958 British Perinatal Mortality Survey, under the Auspices of the National Birthday Trust Fund*, E. & S. Livingstone, Edinburgh, 1963.
Butler, Neville R. and Eva D. Alberman (eds), *Perinatal Problems: The Second Report of the 1958 British Perinatal Mortality Survey under the Auspices of the National Birthday Trust Fund*, E. & S. Livingstone, Edinburgh, 1969.
Carey, H. M. (ed.), *Modern Trends in Human Reproductive Physiology – 1*, Butterworths, London, 1963.
Carmalt Jones, D. W., *Annals of the University of Otago Medical School 1875–1939*, A. H. & A. W. Reed, Wellington, 1945.
Carrell, Robin, 'Essay Review: Trial by Media', *Notes and Records of the Royal Society*, 12 July 2012, p. 1, doi:10.1098/rsnr.2012.0028.
Cartwright, Ann, *The Dignity of Labour? A Study of Childbearing and Induction*, Tavistock, London, 1979.
Cartwright Report, *see* Committee of Inquiry into Allegations Concerning the Treatment of Cervical Cancer at National Women's Hospital and into Other Related Matters, *Report of the Committee of Inquiry into Allegations Concerning the Treatment of Cervical Cancer at National Women's Hospital and into Other Related Matters*, Government Printing Office, Auckland, 1988.
Casper, Monica J., *The Making of the Unborn Patient: A Social Anatomy of Fetal Surgery*, Rutgers University Press, New Brunswick, 1998.

Bibliography

Caton, Donald, *What a Blessing She Had Chloroform: The Medical and Social Response to the Pain of Childbirth from 1800 to the Present*, Yale University Press, New Haven, 1999.
Central Health Services Council, Standing Maternity and Midwifery Advisory Committee, *Human Relations in Obstetrics*, HMSO, London, 1961.
Chalmers, Iain, Murray Enkin and Marc J. N. C. Keirse (eds), *Effective Care in Pregnancy and Childbirth, vol. 1: Pregnancy & vol. 2: Childbirth*, Oxford University Press, Oxford, 1989.
Chamberlain, Geoffrey, *Special Delivery: The Life of the Celebrated Obstetrician William Nixon*, Royal College of Obstetricians and Gynaecologists, London, 2004.
Christie, D. A. and E. M. Tansey (eds), *Origins of Neonatal Intensive Care in the UK: A Witness Seminar held at the Wellcome Institute for the History of Medicine, London, 27 April 1999*, vol. 9, Wellcome Trust, London, 2001.
Clark, Anne, John C. Peek, Peter Forbes-Smith, Rodney C. Bycroft, Moya Shaw and Frederick M. Graham, 'Social and Reproductive Characteristics of the First 100 Couples Treated by in Vitro Fertilisation Programme at National Women's Hospital, Auckland', *NZMJ*, vol. 100, 24 June 1987, pp. 380–2.
Clark, F. L. and G. H. Green, *Obstetrical and Gynaecological Unit, Cornwall Hospital, Auckland, NZ, First Clinical Report, for the Year Ended 31st March 1949*, Auckland Hospital Board, Auckland, 1950.
Clark, Richard B., 'Epidural Anesthesia in Obstetrics: How Did Lumbar Epidural Technique Become the Prime Obstetric Anesthetic in the United States?', *American Society of Anesthesiologists Newsletter*, vol. 62, March 1998, http://www.asahq.org/Newsletters/1998/03_98/Epidural_0398.html.
Clarke, Alison, *Born to a Changing World: Childbirth in Nineteenth-century New Zealand*, Bridget Williams Books, Wellington, 2012.
Clarke, Rachel, 'National Homebirth Conference Report', *New Zealand College of Midwives Journal*, vol. 18, April 1998, p. 25.
Clarkson, J. E., 'Leading Article: Is Neonatal Intensive Care Effective?', *NZMJ*, vol. 96, 13 April 1983, pp. 242–3.
Clarkson, Sarah E., 'Viewpoint: On Being a Certifying Abortion Consultant: An Ethical Dilemma', *NZMJ*, vol. 91, 14 May 1980, pp. 346–7.
Clay, John, *R. D. Laing: A Divided Self*, Hodder & Stoughton, London, 1996.
Climie, C. R., 'Epidural Anaesthesia in Obstetrics', *NZMJ*, vol. 59, March 1960, pp. 127–30.
Cochrane, A. L., *Effectiveness and Efficiency: Random Reflections on Health Services*, Nuffield Hospitals Trust, London, 1972.
Collaborative Group on Antenatal Steroid Therapy, 'Effects of Antenatal Dexamethasone Administration in the Infant: Long-term Follow-up', *Journal of Pediatrics*, vol. 104, 1984, pp. 259–67.
Committee of Inquiry into Allegations Concerning the Treatment of Cervical Cancer at National Women's Hospital and into Other Related Matters, *Report of the Committee of Inquiry into Allegations Concerning the Treatment of Cervical Cancer at National Women's Hospital and into Other Related Matters*, Government Printing Office, Auckland, 1988 (Cartwright Report).
Coney, Sandra, 'Radicalising Childbirth', *Broadsheet*, March 1974, pp. 13–15.
——, 'Taking Childbirth Back', *Broadsheet*, May 1977, pp. 22–23, 25.
——, 'Alienated Labour – Foetal Monitoring', *Broadsheet*, May 1979, pp. 16–17, 38–39.
——, 'From Here to Maternity', *Broadsheet*, October 1984, pp. 4–6.
——, *The Unfortunate Experiment: The Full Story behind the Inquiry into Cervical Cancer Treatment*, Penguin, Auckland, 1988.
——, 'Fertility Action 1984–', in Anne Else (ed.), *Women Together: A History of Women's Organisations in New Zealand: Nga Ropu Wahine o te Motu*, Historical Branch, Department of Internal Affairs, Daphne Brasell Associates Press, Wellington, 1993, pp. 284–6.
——, 'Physiotherapy Technique Banned in Auckland', *The Lancet*, vol. 345, 25 February 1995, p. 510.

——, 'Cartwright Ten Years On: Access to Health Care the Over-Riding Issue', 1997, http://www.womens-health.org.nz/cartwright-ten-years-on.html.
——, 'New Zealand Inquires Further into Baby Deaths', *The Lancet*, vol. 354, 31 July 1999, p. 406.
Coney, Sandra and Phillida Bunkle, 'An Unfortunate Experiment at National Women's', *Metro*, June 1987, pp. 47–65.
Coombs, R. R. A., A. E. Mourant and R. R. Race, 'A New Test for the Detection of Weak and "Incomplete" Rh Agglutinins', *British Journal of Experimental Pathology*, vol. 26, 1945, pp. 255–66.
Cooter, Roger, 'The Ethical Body', in Roger Cooter and John Pickstone (eds), *Companion to Medicine in the Twentieth Century*, Routledge, London, 2002, pp. 451–69.
Coppleson, L. W. and B. W. Brown, 'Control of Carcinoma of Cervix: Role of the Mathematical Model', in Malcolm Coppleson (ed.), *Gynecologic Oncology: Fundamental Principles and Clinical Practice*, vol. 1, Churchill Livingstone, New York, 1981, pp. 390–7.
Coppleson, Malcolm, 'Colposcopy', in John Stallworthy and Gordon Bourne (eds), *Recent Advances in Obstetrics and Gynaecology*, Churchill Livingstone, Edinburgh, 12th edn, 1977, pp. 155–83.
Corbett, Jan, 'Second Thoughts on the Unfortunate Experiment at National Women's', *Metro*, July 1990, pp. 55–72.
Corkill, T. F., 'The Trend of Obstetric Practice in New Zealand', *NZMJ*, vol. 32, 1933, pp. 42–52.
——, 'Chloroform in Obstetrics', *NZMJ*, vol. 49, 1950, pp. 105–12.
Coulter, Shirley, '25th birthday of O & G: Postgraduate School's Beginnings', *University of Auckland News*, vol. 6, 7, September 1976, pp. 8–13.
Crowther, Vera, 'Maternity and the Working Woman', *Woman To-day*, October 1937, pp. 150–1, January 1938, p. 240.
Cull Report, *see* Ministry of Health, *Inquiry under S.47 of the Health and Disabilities Services Act 1993 into the Provision of Chest Physiotherapy Treatment Provided to Pre-term Babies at National Women's Hospital between April 1993 and December 1994*, Ministry of Health, Wellington, 1999 (chair Helen Cull).
Cumberlege, Geoffrey, *Maternity in Great Britain: A Survey of Social and Economic Aspects of Pregnancy and Childbirth Undertaken by a Joint Committee of the Royal College of Obstetricians and Gynaecologists and the Population Investigation Committee*, Oxford University Press, London, 1948.
Daly-Peoples, Linda, 'The Politics of Childbirth', *Broadsheet*, April 1977, pp. 14–21, 24.
Dalziel, Raewyn, *Focus on the Family: The Auckland Home and Family Society, 1893–1993*, The Home and Family Society, Auckland, 1993.
Dalziel, Stuart R., Natalie Walker, Varsha Parag, Colin Mantell, Harold H. Rea, Anthony Rodgers and Jane E. Harding, 'Cardiovascular Risk Factors after Antenatal Exposure to Betamethasone: 30-year Follow-up of a Randomised Controlled Trial', *The Lancet*, vol. 365, 9474, 28 May 2005, pp. 1856–62.
Dalziel, Stuart R., Varsha Parag, Anthony Rodgers and Jane E. Harding, 'Cardiovascular Risk Factors at Age 30 Following Pre-term Birth', *International Journal of Epidemiology*, vol. 36, 2007, pp. 907–15.
Daniels, K. R., 'The Practice of Artificial Insemination of Donor Sperm in New Zealand', *NZMJ*, vol. 98, 10 April 1985, pp. 235–9.
——, 'Demand for and Attitudes towards in Vitro Fertilisation: A Survey of Obstetricians and Gynaecologists', *NZMJ*, vol. 100, 11 March 1987, pp. 145–8.
Darlow, B. A., 'Viewpoint: How Small is Too Small – A Reappraisal', *NZMJ*, vol. 98, 24 July 1985, pp. 596–8.
Davis-Floyd, Robbie E., *Birth as an American Rite of Passage*, University of California Press, Berkeley, 2nd edn, 1992, 2003.

Bibliography

Dawes, G. S., 'Chairman's Closing Remarks', in G. E. W. Wolstenholme and Maeve O'Connor (eds), *Foetal Autonomy: A Ciba Foundation Symposium*, J. & A. Churchill, London, 1969, pp. 315–16.
Dawson, J. B., 'New Zealand Obstetrical Society Section: Doctor and Midwife, Colleagues or Rivals', *NZMJ*, vol. 32, 1933, pp. 20–23.
de Jong, Daphne, 'Birth Rights', *New Zealand Listener*, 18 June 1977, pp. 20–21.
de Lemos, R. A., D. W. Shermeta, J. H. Knelson, R. Kotas and M. E. Avery, 'Acceleration of Appearance of Pulmonary Surfactant in the Fetal Lamb by Administration of Corticosteroids', *American Review of Respiratory Disease*, vol. 102, 1970, pp. 459–61.
Department of Health, 'Maternal Mortality in New Zealand: Report of Special Committee set up by Board of Health to Consider and Report on the Question of the Deaths of Mothers in Connection with Childbirth', (Chairman, C. J. Parr), *AJHR*, 1921, H-31B, pp. 1–4.
——, *The Expectant Mother and Baby's First Month*, Government Printer, Wellington, 1935.
——, 'Report of the Committee of Inquiry into the Various Aspects of the Problem of Abortion in New Zealand', *AJHR*, 1937, H-31A, pp. 1–28.
——, 'Report of the Committee of Inquiry into Maternity Services', *AJHR*, 1938, H-31A, pp. 1–112.
Department of Justice, Law Reform Division, *New Birth Technologies: An Issues Paper on AID, IVF and Surrogate Motherhood*, Department of Justice, Wellington, March 1985.
Dick-Read, Grantly, *Revelation of Childbirth: The Principles and Practice of Natural Childbirth*, William Heinemann, London, 1943.
——, *Childbirth Without Fear: The Principles and Practice of Natural Childbirth*, Harper & Bros, New York, 1953, revised and enlarged.
Dobbie, Mary, 'A Wise and Lovable Woman . . . Rissa Scelly 1907–1983', *Parents Centre Bulletin*, vol. 98, 1984, p. 15.
——, *The Trouble with Women: The Story of Parents Centre New Zealand*, Cape Catley, Whatamongo Bay, 1990.
Donald, Ian, *Practical Obstetric Problems*, Lloyd-Luke, London, 1st edn, 1955.
——, *Practical Obstetric Problems*, Lloyd-Luke, London, 3rd edn, 1964.
Donald, I., 'On Launching a New Diagnostic Science', *American Journal of Obstetrics and Gynecology*, vol. 1, 1969, pp. 609–28.
Donald, I., J. MacVicar and T. G. Brown, 'Investigation of Abdominal Masses by Pulsed Ultrasound', *The Lancet*, vol. 1, issue 7032, 1958, pp. 1188–95.
Donley, Joan, 'Healthy Women', *Broadsheet*, October 1981, p. 40.
——, 'Having the Baby at Home', *Broadsheet*, September 1985, pp. 17, 47.
——, *Save the Midwife*, New Women's Press, Auckland, 1986.
——, *Herstory of N. Z. Homebirth Association*, New Zealand Homebirth Association, Auckland, 1992.
——, *Birthrites: Natural vs Unnatural Childbirth in New Zealand*, Full Court Press in association with New Zealand College of Midwives, Auckland, 1998.
Donnison, Jean, *Midwives and Medical Men: A History of the Struggle for the Control of Childbirth*, Historical Publications, London, 1988.
Dow, Derek A., 'Sir Douglas Robb', in Nicholas Tarling (ed.), *Auckland Minds and Matters*, University of Auckland, Auckland, 2003, pp. 128–46.
Dowbiggin, Ian, *The Sterilization Movement and Global Fertility in the Twentieth Century*, Oxford University Press, Oxford, 2008.
Dubow, Sara, *Ourselves Unborn: A History of the Fetus in Modern America*, Oxford University Press, Oxford, 2011.
Dunkley, P. A., 'Premature and Plural – Be Prepared', *NZNJ*, August 1967, pp. 8–12.
Dunn, H. P., 'Sequelae of Caesarean Section', *NZMJ*, vol. 59, April 1960, pp. 180–3.
——, 'Therapeutic Abortion in New Zealand', *NZMJ*, vol. 68, October 1968, pp. 253–8.
——, 'Natural Family Planning', *NZMJ*, vol. 82, 24 December 1975, pp. 407–8.
——, 'Come Back, Left-Lateral!', *NZMJ*, vol. 89, 14 March 1979, p. 180.

Bibliography

Dunn, Peter M., 'The Development of Newborn Care in the UK since 1930: American Academy of Pediatrics Thomas E. Cone, Jr. Lecture on Perinatal History', *Journal of Perinatology*, vol. 18, 6, 1, 1998, pp. 471–6.
Durand, R., 'Rooming-in – Results of an Inquiry', *NZMJ*, vol. 59, October 1960, pp. 457–8.
Ebbett, Eve, *Victoria's Daughter: New Zealand Women of the Thirties*, A. H. & A. W. Reed, Wellington, 1981.
'Editorial: The 1946 Committee of Inquiry into Maternity Hospital Staffing', *NZMJ*, vol. 46, April 1947, pp. 75–77.
'Editorial: Sterilisation as a Medical-Legal Problem', *NZMJ*, vol. 52, June 1953, pp. 153–6.
'Editorial: Intrauterine Transfusion', *BMJ*, 11 March 1967, pp. 583–4.
'Editorial: The Future of Obstetrics', *NZMJ*, vol. 73, March 1971, pp. 157–8.
'Editorial: Intrauterine Devices', *NZMJ*, vol. 86, 26 October 1977, pp. 387–8.
'Editorial: Mortality Rates With Oral Contraception', *NZMJ*, vol. 86, 14 December 1977, p. 525.
'Editorial: Abortion Again', *NZMJ*, vol. 88, 23 August 1978, pp. 150–1.
'Editorial: The Pattern of Abortion', *NZMJ*, vol. 93, 24 September 1980, pp. 237–8.
'Editorial: Adverse Pregnancy Outcomes after Treatment for Cervical Intraepithelial Neoplasia', *BMJ*, vol. 337, 2008, pp. 769–70.
'Editorial: Managing Low Grade and Borderline Cervical Abnormalities', *BMJ*, vol. 339, 28 July 2009, p. 3014, doi: http://dx.doi.org/10.1136/bmj.b3014.
Edwards, Martin, *Control and the Therapeutic Trial: Rhetoric and Experimentation in Britain, 1918–48*, Rodopi, Amsterdam, 2007.
Ehrenreich, Barbara and Deirdre English, *Witches, Midwives and Nurses: A History of Women Healers*, Glass Mountain Pamphlets, Oyster Bay, New York, 1973.
Erlam, Harry D., *A Notable Result: An Historical Essay on the Beginnings and the First Fifteen Years of the School of Medicine with a Chapter on the History of the Postgraduate School of Obstetrics and Gynaecology by G.H. Green*, University of Auckland, School of Medicine, Auckland, 1983.
Farquhar, Cynthia and Helen Roberts (eds), *Introduction to Obstetrics and Gynaecology*, University of Auckland, Auckland, 3rd edn, 2010.
Fenwicke, Rosy, *In Practice: The Lives of New Zealand Women Doctors in the 21st Century*, Random House, Auckland, 2004.
Field, Peggy Anne, 'Impressions of Women's Health in New Zealand', *Midwifery*, vol. 6, 1990, pp. 185–92.
Finer, N. and J. Boyd, 'Chest Physiotherapy in the Neonate: A Control Study', *Pediatrics*, vol. 61, 1978, pp. 282–5.
Flenady, V. J. and P. H. Gray, 'Chest Physiotherapy for Preventing Morbidity in Babies being Extubated from Mechanical Ventilation', *The Cochrane Library*, Oxford, Update Software, 2000: issue 4.
Forfar, John O., *Child Health in a Changing Society*, Oxford University Press, Oxford, 1988.
Foster, Peggy, *Women and the Health Care Industry: An Unhealthy Relationship?*, Open University Press, Buckingham, 1995.
Foundation Genesis, *Sir William Liley: A Tribute to the Father of Fetology*, Foundation Genesis, Strathfield, New South Wales, 1984.
France, J. T., 'Improving the Rhythm Method: An Outline of the Research into Ovulation at National Women's Hospital, Auckland', *Choice*, vol. 9, 2, May 1971, pp. 5–7.
Garcia, Jo, Robert Kilpatrick and Martin Richards (eds), *The Politics of Maternity Care: Services for Childbearing Women in Twentieth-century Britain*, Oxford University Press, Oxford, 1990.
Gattung, Theresa, 'When the Music Stops', *North & South*, April 2013, pp. 62–70.
Giesen, J. E., 'Practical Aspects in the Treatment of Sterility', *NZMJ*, vol. 50, August 1951, pp. 330–7.
Glasgow, Kathy, 'Maternity "shambles"', *New Zealand Health Review*, vol. 1, 1, Autumn 1998, pp. 9–10.

Bibliography

Gluckman, L. K., 'Some Unanticipated Complications of Therapeutic Abortion', *NZMJ*, vol. 74, August 1971, pp. 72–78.

Gluckman, Sir Peter and Tatjana Buklijas, 'Sir Graham Collingwood (Mont) Liggins 24 June 1926–24 August 2010', *Biographical Memoirs of Fellows of the Royal Society*, 2013, http://dx.doi.org/10.1098/rsbm.2012.0039.

Gordon, Doris, *Backblocks Baby-doctor: An Autobiography*, Faber & Faber, London, and Whitcombe & Tombs, Auckland, 1955.

——, *Doctor Down Under*, Faber & Faber, London, 1957.

Gordon, Linda, *The Moral Property of Women: A History of Birth Control Politics in America*, University of Illinois Press, Urbana, 2002.

Gornall, Jonathan, 'The Role of the Media in the Stoke CNEP Saga', *Journal of the Royal Society of Medicine*, vol. 103, 5, 2010, pp. 173–177, doi: 10.1258/jrsm.2010.10k011.

Graham, F. M., J. T. France and J. Clark, 'The Development of a Programme for in Vitro Fertilisation in New Zealand', *NZMJ*, vol. 98, March 1985, pp. 177–81.

Grant, Adrian, 'Monitoring the Fetus during Labour', in Iain Chalmers, Murray Enkin and Marc J. N. C. Keirse (eds), *Effective Care in Pregnancy and Childbirth, vol. 2: Childbirth*, Oxford University Press, Oxford, 1989, pp. 846–82.

Green, G. H., *Obstetrical and Gynaecological Unit, Cornwall Hospital, Auckland, NZ, Second Clinical Report, for the Year Ended 31st March 1950*, Auckland Hospital Board, Auckland, 1951.

——, 'Tubal Ligation', *NZMJ*, vol. 57, February 1958, pp. 470–7.

——, *Introduction to Obstetrics: A Theory and Practice for Obstetric Nurses*, N. M. Peryer, Christchurch, 1962.

——, 'Trends in Maternal Mortality', *NZMJ*, vol. 65, February 1966, pp. 80–86

——, 'Maori Maternal Mortality in New Zealand', *NZMJ*, vol. 66, May 1967, pp. 295–9.

——, 'The Foetus Began to Cry . . . Abortion' (Part 1), *NZNJ*, vol. 63, 7, 1970, pp. 11–12; (Part 2), *NZNJ*, vol. 63, 9, 1970, pp. 6–7; (Part 3), vol. 63, 9, 1970, pp. 11–12.

——, 'The Postgraduate School of Obstetrics and Gynaecology', in H. D. Erlam, *A Notable Result: An Historical Essay on the Beginnings and the First Fifteen Years of the School of Medicine*, University of Auckland, School of Medicine, Auckland, 1983, pp. 67–70.

——, 'William Liley and Fetal Transfusion: A Perspective in Fetal Medicine', *Fetal Therapy*, vol. 1, 1986, pp. 18–22.

Green, G. H., A. W. Liley and G. C. Liggins, 'The Place of Foetal Transfusion in Haemolytic Disease: A Report of 22 Transfusions in 16 Patients', *Australian and New Zealand Journal of Obstetrics and Gynaecology*, vol. 5, 1965, pp. 53–59.

Greenlees, Janet and Linda Bryder (eds), *Western Maternity and Medicine, 1880–1980*, Pickering Chatto UK, London, 2013.

Gregory, G. A., J. A. Kitterman, R. H. Phibbs, W. H. Tooley and W. K. Hamilton, 'Treatment of the Idiopathic Respiratory-distress Syndrome with Continuous Positive Airway Pressure', *New England Journal of Medicine*, vol. 284, 1971, pp. 1333–40.

Gregson, R. A. M. and Janet R. M. Irwin, 'Opinions on Abortion from Medical Practitioners', *NZMJ*, vol. 73, May 1971, pp. 267–73.

Grieve, B. W., 'Haemolytic Disease of the Newborn: Obstetric Aspects', *NZMJ*, vol. 52, June 1953, pp. 164–7.

Guilliland, Karen, 'Learning from Midwives', *NZNJ*, October 1996, p. 23.

——, 'National Director's Forum', *New Zealand College of Midwives National Newsletter*, vol. 7, December 1997, p. 8.

Guilliland, Karen and Sally Pairman, *The Midwifery Partnership: A Model for Practice*, Department of Nursing and Midwifery, Victoria University of Wellington, Wellington, 1995.

——, *Women's Business: The Story of the New Zealand College of Midwives 1986–2010*, New Zealand College of Midwives, Christchurch, 2010.

Gunn, A., P. D. Gluckman, J. S. Wyatt, M. Thoresen and A. D. Edwards, 'Selective Head

Cooling after Neonatal Encephalopathy', *The Lancet*, vol. 365, 2005, pp. 1619–20, doi:10.1016/S0140-6736(05)66505-1.

Gunn, A. J., P. D. Gluckman and T. R. Gunn, 'Selective Head Cooling in Newborn Infants following Perinatal Asphyxia: A Safety Study', *Pediatrics*, vol. 102, 4, 1998, pp. 885–992, doi:10.1542/peds.102.4.885.

Guy, Camille, '"I've Enjoyed My Life . . . Hard as it's Been at Times": Vera Jane Ellis Crowther', *Broadsheet*, September 1976, pp. 16–17, 25.

Hadley, Janet, 'The Case against Depo-Provera', in Sue O'Sullivan (ed.), *Women's Health: A Spare Rib Reader*, Pandora, London, 1987, pp. 170–4.

Hanson, Clare, *A Cultural History of Pregnancy: Pregnancy, Medicine and Culture, 1750–2000*, Palgrave Macmillan, New York, 2004.

Hanson, Elizabeth, *The Politics of Social Security: The 1938 Act and Some Later Developments*, Auckland University Press, Auckland, and Oxford University Press, Wellington, 1980.

Harding, J. E., F. K. I. Miles, D. M. O. Becroft, B. C. Allen and D. B. Knight, 'Chest Physiotherapy may be Associated with Brain Damage in Extremely Premature Infants', *Journal of Pediatrics*, vol. 132, 1998, pp. 440–4.

Harris, Aroha, *Measuring the Effectiveness of Health Services for Maori Consumers*, Ministry of Health, Wellington, 1994.

Harris, Aroha and Mary Jane Logan McCallum, '"Assaulting the Ears of Government": The Indian Homemakers' Clubs and the Maori Women's Welfare League in their Formative Years', in Carol Williams (ed.), *Indigenous Women and Work: From Labor to Activism*, University of Illinois Press, Urbana, 2012, pp. 226–39.

Hawgood, Barbara J., 'Physiologists: Professor Sir William Liley (1929–83): New Zealand Perinatal Physiologist', *Journal of Medical Biography*, vol. 13, 2, May 2005, pp. 82–88.

Hawksworth, W., 'The First Doris Gordon Memorial Oration: Progress of Obstetrics in the Last Twenty-five Years', *NZMJ*, vol. 62, January 1963, pp. 2–9.

Hay, Iain, *The Caring Commodity: The Provision of Health Care in New Zealand*, Oxford University Press, Oxford, 1989.

Heagney, Brenda (compiler), *Rubella: Essays in Honour of the Centenary of the Birth of Sir Norman McAlister Gregg 1892–1966*, The Royal Australasian College of Physicians, Sydney, 1992.

Health Benefits Review, *Choices for Health Care: Report of the Health Benefits Review*, Health Benefits Review, Wellington, 1986.

'Helen Brew: Closer to those Born at Home, a Star Talks', *Thursday*, 19 January 1976, pp. 30–31.

Hellman, Louis M., Gillian M. Duffus, Ian Donald and Bertil Sunden, 'Safety of Diagnostic Ultrasound in Obstetrics', *The Lancet*, vol. 1, 7657, 1970, pp. 1133–5.

Henaghan, Mark, *Health Professionals and Trust: The Cure for Healthcare Law and Policy*, Routledge, London, 2012.

Henderson, A. J., 'Childbirth – A Natural Function? A Report on One Hundred and Fifty Consecutive Cases of Relaxed Childbirth', *NZMJ*, vol. 53, February 1954, pp. 511–14.

Hercock, Fay, *Alice: The Making of a Woman Doctor, 1914–1974*, Auckland University Press, Auckland, 1999.

Hertzberg, Reuben, 'Michael Hugh Mulvihille Ryan', *Australian Journal of Ophthalmology*, vol. 10, 1982, pp. 3–4.

Hey, Edmund and Iain Chalmers, 'Mis-investigating Alleged Research Misconduct can Cause Widespread, Unpredictable Damage', *Journal of the Royal Society of Medicine*, vol. 103, 2010, pp. 132–7, doi: 10. 1258/jrsm.2010.09k045.

Hickey, R. F. J. and R. B. Dorofaeff, 'A Study of the Effects of Pain Relief in Labour', *NZMJ*, vol. 72, December 1970, pp. 377–82.

Holt, Betty, *Women in Council: A History of the National Council of Women of New Zealand*, National Council of Women, Wellington, 1980.

Hope-Robertson, W. J., 'Retrolental Fibroplasia', *NZMJ*, vol. 54, October 1955, pp. 531–40.
Howie, Ross, 'Prenatal Glucocorticoids in Preterm Birth: A Paediatric View of the History of the Original Studies by Ross Howie, 2 June 2004', in L. A. Reynolds and E. M. Tansey (eds), *Prenatal Corticosteroids for Reducing Morbidity and Mortality after Preterm Birth: The Transcript of a Witness Seminar held by the Wellcome Trust Centre for the History of Medicine at UCL, London, on 15 June 2004*, vol. 25, Wellcome Trust, London, 2005, appendix 2, pp. 89–95.
Howie, R. N. and G. C. Liggins, 'Clinical Trial of Antepartum Betamethasone Therapy for Prevention of Respiratory Distress in Pre-term Infants', in A. Anderson, R. W. Beard, J. M. Brudenell and P. M. Dunn (eds), *Preterm Labour: Proceedings of the Fifth Study Group of the Royal College of Obstetricians and Gynaecologists*, The College, London, 1978, pp. 281–9.
Hutchison, I. L. G., 'Neonatal Resuscitation Table', *NZMJ*, vol. 70, September 1969, pp. 175–8.
Jackson, Pauline, Betson Phillips, Elizabeth Prosser, H. O. Jones, V. R. Tindall, D. L. Crosby, I. D. Cooke, J. M. McGarry and R. W. Rees, 'A Male Sterilization Clinic', *BMJ*, vol. 4, 31 October 1970, pp. 295–7.
Jackson, Peter and J. Lew Lander, 'Female Sterilisation: A Five-year Follow-up in Auckland', *NZMJ*, vol. 91, 27 February 1980, pp. 140–3.
Jellett, Henry, *The Causes and Prevention of Maternal Mortality*, Churchill's Empire Series, J. & A. Churchill, London, 1929.
Jones, R. W., 'Performance of the Dalkon Shield Intrauterine Device', *NZMJ*, vol. 82, 13 August 1975, pp. 85–87.
Kedgley, Sue, *Mum's the Word: The Untold Story of Motherhood in New Zealand*, Random House, Auckland, 1996.
Keirse, Marc J. N. C., Murray Enkin and Judith Lumley, 'Social and Professional Support during Childbirth', in Iain Chalmers, Murray Enkin and Marc J. N. C. Keirse (eds), *Effective Care in Pregnancy and Childbirth, vol. 2: Childbirth*, Oxford University Press, Oxford, 1989, pp. 805–20.
Kinnock, Sandra and A. W. Liley, 'The Performance of an anti D Immunoprophylaxis Scheme', *NZMJ*, vol. 80, 23 October 1974, pp. 337–43.
Kitzinger, Jenny, 'Strategies of the Early Childbirth Movement: A Case-Study of the National Childbirth Trust', in Jo Garcia, Robert Kilpatrick and Martin Richards (eds), *The Politics of Maternity Care: Services for Childbearing Women in Twentieth-century Britain*, Oxford University Press, Oxford, 1990, pp. 92–115.
Kitzinger, Sheila, 'Childbirth and Society', in Iain Chalmers, Murray Enkin and Marc J. N. C. Keirse (eds), *Effective Care in Pregnancy and Childbirth, vol. 1: Pregnancy*, Oxford University Press, Oxford, 1989, pp. 99–109.
Klein, R., *The New Politics of the NHS: From Creation to Reinvention*, Radcliffe Publishing, Oxford, 2010.
Knight, D. B., D. J. Bevan, J. E. Harding, R. L. Teele, C. A. Kuschel, M. R. Battin and R. S. H. Rowley, 'Chest Physiotherapy and Porencephalic Lesions in Very Preterm Infants', *Journal of Paediatrics and Child Health*, vol. 37, 2001, pp. 554–8.
Koss, Leopold G., 'Dysplasia: A Real Concept or a Misnomer?', *Obstetrics and Gynecology: Journal of the American College of Obstetricians and Gynecologists*, vol. 51, 198, 1978, pp. 374–7.
Kyle, B. V. and T. J. Buckley, *The Obstetrical and Gynaecological Unit Cornwall Hospital, Green Lane West, Auckland, Third Clinical Report For the Year Ended 31st March 1951*, Auckland Hospital Board, Auckland, 1951.
Laing, Adrian Charles, *R. D. Laing: A Biography*, Chester Springs, Pennsylvania, and Peter Owen, London, 1994.
Larsson, Goran, *Conization for Preinvasive and Early Invasive Carcinoma of the Uterine Cervix*, Acta Obstetricia et Gynecologica Scandanavica, Supplement 114, Lund, 1983.

Bibliography

'Leading Article: Intrauterine Transfusion', *Scottish Medical Journal*, vol. 12, 1967, pp. 293–4.
'Leading Article: Legality of Sterilization', *BMJ*, vol. 1, 5698, 21 March 1970, pp. 704–5.
Lean, M. E. J., J. I. Mann, J. A. Hoek, R. M. Elliott and G. Schofield, 'Translational Research: From Evidence Based Medicine to Sustainable Solutions for Public Health Problems', *BMJ*, vol. 337, 27 September 2008, pp. 705–6.
Leap, Nicky and Billie Hunter, *The Midwife's Tale: An Oral History from Handywoman to Professional Midwife*, Scarlet Press, London, 1993.
Leavitt, Judith Walzer, *Brought to Bed: Childbearing in America, 1750 to 1950*, Oxford University Press, New York, 1986.
——, *Make Room for Daddy: The Journey from Waiting Room to Birthing Room*, University of North Carolina Press, Chapel Hill, 2009.
Lewis, Jane, *The Politics of Motherhood: Child and Maternal Welfare in England, 1900–1939*, Croom Helm, London, and McGill-Queen's University Press, Montreal, 1980.
——, '"Motherhood Issues" in the Late Nineteenth and Twentieth Centuries', in Katherine Arnup, Andrée Lévesque and Ruth Roach Pierson with the assistance of Margaret Brennan (eds), *Delivering Motherhood: Maternal Ideologies and Practices in the 19th and 20th Centuries*, Routledge, London, 1990, pp. 1–19.
——, 'Mothers and Maternity Policies in the Twentieth Century', in Jo Garcia, Robert Kilpatrick and Martin Richards (eds), *The Politics of Maternity Care: Services for Childbearing Women in Twentieth-century Britain*, Oxford University Press, Oxford, 1990, pp. 15–29.
Lewis, Milton J., 'Obstetrics: Education and Practice, 1870–1939, Part 2', *Australian and New Zealand Journal of Obstetrics and Gynaecology*, vol. 18, 1978, pp. 165–8.
Liggins, G. C., 'The George Addlington Syme Oration: Winds of Change', *Australia and New Zealand Journal of Surgery*, vol. 61, March 1991, pp. 169–72.
Liggins, Sir Graham, 'Geoffrey Sharman Dawes, CBE, 21 January 1918–6 May 1996', *Biographical Memoirs of Fellows of the Royal Society*, 44, November 1998, pp. 110–25.
Liggins, G. C. and R. N. Howie, 'A Controlled Trial of Antepartum Glucocorticoid Treatment for Prevention of the Respiratory Distress Syndrome in Premature Infants', *Pediatrics*, vol. 50, 4, 1972, pp. 515–25.
——, 'Prevention of Respiratory Distress Syndrome by Antepartum Corticosteroid Therapy', in Physiological Society, Barcroft Sub-committee, R. S. Comline, K. W. Cross, G. S. Dawes and P. W. Nathanielsz (eds), *Foetal and Neonatal Physiology, Proceedings of the Sir Joseph Barcroft Centenary Symposium, 1972*, Cambridge University Press, Cambridge, 1973, pp. 613–17.
Liley, A. W., 'Intrauterine Transfusion of Foetus in Haemolytic Disease', *BMJ*, vol. 2, 5365, 2 November 1963, pp. 1107–9.
——, 'A Case against Abortion', *Liberal Studies*, Whitcombe & Tombs, Auckland, 1971.
——, 'The Development of the Idea of Fetal Transfusion', *American Journal of Obstetrics and Gynecology*, vol. 3, 1971, pp. 302–4.
——, 'The Foetus as Personality', *Australian and New Zealand Journal of Psychiatry*, vol. 6, 1972, pp. 99–105.
——, 'The Foetus in Control of his Environment', in Thomas W. Hilgers and Denis J. Horan (eds), *Abortion and Social Justice*, Sheed & Ward, New York, 1972, pp. 27–36.
Litoff, Judy Barrrett, 'Midwives and History', in Rima D. Apple (ed.), *Women, Health, and Medicine in America: A Historical Handbook*, Garland, New York, 1990, pp. 443–58.
Loudon, Irvine, *Death in Childbirth: An International Study of Maternal Care and Maternal Mortality, 1800–1950*, Oxford University Press, Oxford, 1992.
——, 'Childbirth', in W. F. Bynum and Roy Porter (eds), *Companion Encyclopedia of the History of Medicine*, vol. 1, Routledge, London, 1993, pp. 1050–71.
Lovell-Smith, Margaret, 'Kent-Johnston, Agnes Gilmour', from the *Dictionary of New Zealand Biography. Te Ara – the Encyclopedia of New Zealand*, updated 30 October 2012, http://www.TeAra.govt.nz/en/biographies/5k8/kent-johnston-agnes-gilmour.

Lumley, Judith, 'Foetal Monitoring: A Look at the Evidence', *New Doctor (Journal of the Doctors' Reform Society of Australia)*, vol. 15, 1980, pp. 45–48.

Lumley, Judith and Jill Astbury, *Birth Rites, Birth Rights: Childbirth Alternatives for Australian Parents*, Nelson, Melbourne, 1980.

Macdonald, Margaret, 'Dr Pat Dunn and the Male Mastery of Birth', *Metro*, February 1991, pp. 130–2.

Maclaurin, J. C., 'Some Aspects of Neonatal Paediatrics', *Scottish Medical Journal*, vol. 14, 1969, pp. 321–8.

MacLean, A. B., D. R. Aickin and J. J. Evans, 'Artificial Insemination by Donor', *NZMJ*, vol. 97, 25 July 1984, pp. 484–6.

MacLean, Nancy, *The American Women's Movement, 1945–2000: A Brief History with Documents*, Bedford/St Martin's, Boston, 2009.

Manchester, Anne, 'Four Auckland Hospitals Become One: The New Auckland City Hospital the Largest Public Building in the Country, is Certainly Impressive, but Adapting to New Systems and a New Hospital Culture Continues to be Challenging for Nurses', *NZNJ*, October 2004, pp. 24–26.

Marks, Lara V., *Sexual Chemistry: A History of the Contraceptive Pill*, Yale University Press, New Haven, 2001.

Marland, Hilary, 'Childbirth and Maternity', in Roger Cooter and John Pickstone (eds), *Companion to Medicine in the Twentieth Century*, Routledge, London, 2003, pp. 559–74.

Marsh, Margaret and Wanda Ronner, *The Empty Cradle: Infertility in America from Colonial Times to the Present*, Johns Hopkins University Press, Baltimore, 1996.

——, *The Fertility Doctor: John Rock and the Reproductive Revolution*, Johns Hopkins University Press, Baltimore, 2008.

Martin, J. R., 'A Double Catheter Technique for Exchange Transfusion in the Newborn Infant', *NZMJ*, vol. 77, March 1973, pp. 167–9.

——, 'Phototherapy, Phenobarbitone and Physiological Jaundice in the Newborn Infant', *NZMJ*, vol. 79, 12 June 1974, pp. 1022–4.

Maternity Benefits Tribunal, *Report and Recommendations of the Maternity Benefits Tribunal*, Ministry of Health, Wellington, 1993.

'Maternity Services', *NZMJ*, vol. 83, 25 August 1976, pp. 158–9.

Maternity Services Committee, *Maternity Services in New Zealand: A Report by the Maternity Services Committee Board of Health*, Board of Health Report Series No. 26, Government Printer, Wellington, 1976.

——, *Obstetrics and the Winds of Change*, Board of Health, Wellington, 1979.

——, *Mother and Baby at Home: The Early Days*, Board of Health, Wellington, 1982.

——, *Special Care Services for the Newborn in New Zealand: A Report of the Maternity Services Committee*, Board of Health Report Series No. 29, Government Printer, Wellington, 1982.

McCalman, Janet, *Sex and Suffering: Women's Health and a Women's Hospital: The Royal Women's Hospital, Melbourne, 1856–1996*, Melbourne University Press, Carlton, Victoria, 1998.

McCauley, Sue, 'Everything You Wanted to Know about Sterilisation that Your Doctor Didn't Tell You', *Thursday*, 12 April 1973, pp. 20–21, 86.

McCredie, Margaret R. E., Katrina J. Sharples, Charlotte Paul, Judith Baranyai, Gabriele Medley, Ronald W. Jones and David C. G. Skegg, 'Natural History of Cervical Neoplasia and Risk of Invasive Cancer in Women with Cervical Intraepithelial Neoplasia 3: A Retrospective Cohort Study', *The Lancet Oncology*, vol. 9, 5, 2008, pp. 425–34.

McCulloch, Alison, *Fighting to Choose: The Abortion Rights Struggle in New Zealand*, Victoria University Press, Wellington, 2013.

McIndoe, W. A., M. R. McLean, R. W. Jones and P. R. Mullins, 'The Invasive Potential of Carcinoma in Situ of the Cervix', *Obstetrics and Gynecology: Journal of the American College of Obstetricians and Gynecologists*, vol. 64, 1984, pp. 451–8.

Bibliography

McKenzie, R, 'Laparoscopy', *NZMJ*, vol. 74, August 1971, pp. 87–91.

McKeown, Thomas, *The Role of Medicine: Dream, Mirage or Nemesis?*, Basil Blackwell, Oxford, 1979.

McKeown, Thomas and E. G. Knox, 'The Framework Required for Validation of Prescriptive Screening', in Thomas McKeown (ed.), *Screening in Medical Care: Reviewing the Evidence: A Collection of Essays with a Preface by Lord Cohen of Birkenhead*, Nuffield Provincial Hospitals Trust, Oxford University Press, London, 1968, pp. 159–73.

McLeod, Rosemary, 'The Importance of Being Sandra Coney', *North & South*, July 1988, pp. 54–67.

McLoughlin, David, 'The Politics of Childbirth: Midwives versus Doctors', *North & South*, August 1993, pp. 55–69.

Mein Smith, Philippa, *Maternity in Dispute: New Zealand, 1920–1939*, Historical Publications Branch, Department of Internal Affairs, Wellington, 1986.

——, 'Midwifery Re-innovation in New Zealand', in Jennifer Stanton (ed.), *Innovations in Health and Medicine: Diffusion and Resistance in the Twentieth Century*, Routledge, New York, 2002, pp. 169–87.

——, 'Hutchinson, Amy May', from the *Dictionary of New Zealand Biography. Te Ara – the Encyclopedia of New Zealand*, updated 30 October 2012, http://www.TeAra.govt.nz/en/biographies/4h40/hutchinson-amy-may.

Ministry of Health, *Inquiry under S.47 of the Health and Disabilities Services Act 1993 into the Provision of Chest Physiotherapy Treatment Provided to Pre-term Babies at National Women's Hospital between April 1993 and December 1994*, Ministry of Health, Wellington, 1999 (chair Helen Cull).

Mitchinson, Wendy, 'Agency, Diversity, and Constraints: Women and Their Physicians, Canada, 1850–1950', in The Feminist Health Care Ethics Research Network, co-ordinator Susan Sherwin, *The Politics of Women's Health: Exploring Agency and Autonomy*, Temple University Press, Philadelphia, 1998, pp. 122–49.

——, *Giving Birth in Canada, 1900–1950*, University of Toronto Press, Toronto, 2002.

Molloy, Maureen, 'Rights, Fact, Humans and Women: An Archaeology of the Royal Commission on Contraception, Sterilisation and Abortion in New Zealand', *Women's Studies Journal*, vol. 12, 1, August 1996, pp. 63–82.

Morris, N., 'Human Relations in Obstetric Practice', *The Lancet*, vol. 1, 23 April 1960, pp. 913–15.

Mortimer, Barbara, 'Introduction: The History of Nursing: Yesterday, Today and Tomorrow', in Barbara Mortimer and Susan McGann (eds), *New Directions in the History of Nursing: International Perspectives*, Routledge, London, 2005, pp. 1–21.

Moscucci, Ornella, *The Science of Woman: Gynaecology and Gender in England, 1800–1929*, Cambridge University Press, Cambridge, 1990.

'Mother Care', *Consumer*, no. 356, January/February 1997, pp. 4–7.

Mottram, Joan, 'State Control in Local Context: Public Health and Midwife Regulation in Manchester, 1900–1914', in Hilary Marland and Anne Marie Rafferty (eds), *Midwives, Society and Childbirth: Debates and Controversies in the Modern Period*, Routledge, London, 1997, pp. 134–52.

Murphy-Lawless, Jo, *Reading Birth and Death: A History of Obstetric Thinking*, Cork University Press, Cork, 1998.

National Institutes of Health, 'Consensus Statement: Effect of Corticosteroids for Fetal Maturation on Perinatal Outcomes, 28 February–2 March 1994', *Consensus*, vol. 12, 1994, pp. 1–24.

Neill, J. O. C., *Grace Neill. The Story of a Noble Woman, with a Contribution by Miss Flora J. Cameron*, N. M. Peryer, Christchurch, 1961.

Neilson, J. P., 'Doppler Ultrasound', *British Journal of Obstetrics and Gynaecology*, vol. 94, 1987, pp. 929–34.

Neilson, J. P. and C. R. Whitfield, 'Ultrasound in Obstetrics', *The Lancet*, 11 July 1981, p. 94.

Bibliography

Neilson, J. P. and Valerie D. Hood, 'Ultrasound in Obstetrics and Gynaecology: Recent Developments', *British Medical Bulletin*, vol. 36, 1980, pp. 249–55.

Neilson, Jim and Adrian Grant, 'Ultrasound in Pregnancy', in Iain Chalmers, Murray Enkin and Marc J. N. C. Keirse (eds), *Effective Care in Pregnancy and Childbirth, vol. 1: Pregnancy*, Oxford University Press, Oxford, 1989, pp. 419–39.

New Zealand Contraception and Health Study Group, 'New Zealand Contraception and Health Study: Design and Preliminary Report', *NZMJ*, vol. 99, 23 April 1986, pp. 283–6.

New Zealand Obstetrical and Gynaecological Society, Report of a Sub-Committee of the Wellington Division on Pain Relief in Obstetrics, *NZMJ*, vol. 50, December 1951, p. 616.

Nicol, Jennie, 'Abortion Services in New Zealand: A Report prepared for the Women, Children and Family Health Programme to Aid in Planning and Policy Formulation', Department of Health, Wellington, September 1987, http://www.moh.govt.nz/notebook/nbbooks.nsf/0/9C8646A92E9735404C2565D7000DD69E/$file/Abortion%20services.pdf.

Nicolson, Malcolm and John E. E. Fleming, *Imaging and Imagining the Fetus: The Development of Obstetric Ultrasound*, Johns Hopkins University Press, Baltimore, 2013.

Noble, Bernadette, 'Infertility and a New Miracle in Search for Motherhood', *Thursday*, 20 February 1969, pp. 5–6, 17.

Nolan, Melanie, *Breadwinning: New Zealand Women and the State*, Canterbury University Press, Christchurch, 2000.

Oakley, Ann, 'The Medicalized Trap of Motherhood', *New Society*, vol. 34, 18 December 1975, pp. 639–41.

——, *Women Confined: Towards a Sociology of Childbirth*, Schocken Books, New York, 1980.

——, *The Captured Womb: A History of the Medical Care of Pregnant Women*, Basil Blackwell, Oxford, 1984.

——, 'The History of Ultrasonography in Obstetrics', *BIRTH*, vol. 13, Special Supplement, December 1986, pp. 8–13.

'Obituary: Dennis Geoffrey Bonham', *NZMJ*, vol. 118, 1221, 26 August 2005, http://journal.nzma.org.nz.ezproxy.auckland.ac.nz/journal/118-1221/1639/.

'Obituary: Harvey McKay Carey', *Medical Journal of Australia*, vol. 152, 2 April 1990, p. 379.

'Obituary: V. Mary Crosse OBE, MD, MMSA, DObstRCOG, DPH', *BMJ*, vol. 2, 5859, 21 April 1973, p. 183.

'Obituary: Louis K. Diamond', *Transfusion*, vol. 42, October 2002, pp. 1381–2.

'Obituary: Irwin Bruce (Bill) Faris', *NZMJ*, vol. 123, 1319, 30 July 2010, http://journal.nzma.org.nz/journal/123-1319/4241/.

'Obituary: James Edmett Giesen', *NZMJ*, vol. 91, 14 May 1980, p. 357.

'Obituary: Bruce Walton Grieve', *NZMJ*, vol. 106, 9 December 1993, p. 532.

'Obituary: Tania Gunn', *University of Auckland News*, April 1999, p. 15.

'Obituary: William Hawskworth', *Journal of Obstetrics and Gynaecology of the British Commonwealth*, vol. 73, 1966, pp. 862–3.

'Obituary: Lady Celia Margaret Liggins, 1925–2003', *O & G Magazine: Royal Australian and New Zealand Society of Obstetricians and Gynaecologists*, vol. 5, 3, September 2003, p. 229.

'Obituary: Sir Graham Liggins', *The Economist*, 2 September 2010, http://www.economist.com/node/16941245.

'Obituary: Sir Graham Liggins 1926–2010', *New Zealand Listener*, 4 September 2010, p. 10.

'Obituary: Albert William Liley', *NZMJ*, vol. 96, 10 August 1983, pp. 631–2.

'Obituary: Sir Albert William Liley', www.rsnz.org/directory/yearbooks/ybook97/obitLiley.html.

'Obituary: William Woolf Mushin', *Anaesthesia*, vol. 48, 6, June 1993, pp. 461–2.

'Obituary: John Arthur Stallworthy', *NZMJ*, vol. 107, 26 January 1994, p. 23.

'Obituary: John Heywood Taylor', *NZMJ*, vol. 122, 1296, 5 June 2009, http://www.nzma.org.nz/journal/122-1296/xxxx/.

Bibliography

O'Connor, Mary Ellen, *Freed to Care, Proud to Nurse: 100 Years of the New Zealand Nurses Organisation*, New Zealand Nurses Organisation, Wellington, 2010.
Orr, Elizabeth, 'A Maternity Services Survey', *NZNJ*, vol. 55, 9, September 1962, pp. 6–7.
Overton, Graeme, 'The 1987 National Women's Hospital (NWH) "Unfortunate Experiment": Accusations of Unethical Experiments and Under-treatment, Resulting in Excess Deaths from Cervical Cancer. Facts and Fables', *NZMJ*, vol. 123, 1319, 30 July 2010, pp. 101–5, http://journal.nzma.org.nz/journal/123-1319/4244/.
Page, Dorothy, *The National Council of Women: A Centennial History*, Auckland University Press with Bridget Williams Books and National Council of Women, Wellington, 1996.
——, *Anatomy of a Medical School: A History of Medicine at the University of Otago 1875–2000*, University of Otago Press, Dunedin, 2008.
Pairman, Sally, 'Developing & Crafting A Vision: A Strategic Plan for Midwifery', *New Zealand College of Midwives Journal*, 18, April 1998, pp. 6–7.
Papps, Elaine and Mark Olssen, *Doctoring Childbirth and Regulating Midwifery in New Zealand: A Foucauldian Perspective*, Dunmore Press, Palmerston North, 1997.
Parboosingh, John, Marc J. N. C. Keirse and Murray Enkin, 'The Role of the Obstetric Specialist', in Iain Chalmers, Murray Enkin and Marc J. N. C. Keirse (eds), *Effective Care in Pregnancy and Childbirth, vol. 1: Childbirth*, Oxford University Press, Oxford, 1989, pp. 192–6.
Parker, Leigh, 'Scans . . . How Safe for Babies?', *New Zealand Woman's Weekly (NZWW)*, 9 October 1989, pp. 18–19.
Parker, R. B., 'Risk from the Aspiration of Vomit during Obstetric Anaesthesia', *BMJ*, vol. 2, 4879, 10 July 1954, pp. 65–69.
——, 'Maternal Death from Aspiration Asphyxia', *BMJ*, vol. 2, 4983, 7 July 1956, pp. 16–19.
Parkes, Charlotte, 'The Impact of the Medicalisation of New Zealand's Maternity Services on Women's Experience of Childbirth, 1904–1937', in Linda Bryder (ed.), *A Healthy Country: Essays on the Social History of Medicine in New Zealand*, Bridget Williams Books, Wellington, 1991, pp. 165–80.
Paterson, Kim, 'Birth . . . the Way You Want It', *NZWW*, 13 July 1987, pp. 56–57.
Peel, John (compiler), *The Lives of the Fellows of the Royal College of Obstetricians and Gynaecologists, 1929–1969*, RCOG, London, 1976.
——, *William Blair-Bell – Father and Founder*, RCOG, London, 1986.
Peretz, Elizabeth, 'A Maternity Service for England and Wales: Local Authority Maternity Care in the Inter-War Period in Oxfordshire and Tottenham', in Jo Garcia, Robert Kilpatrick and Martin Richards (eds), *The Politics of Maternity Care: Services for Childbearing Women in Twentieth-century Britain*, Oxford University Press, Oxford, 1990, pp. 30–46.
Perkins, Barbara Bridgman, *The Medical Delivery Business: Health Reform, Childbirth, and the Economic Order*, Rutgers University Press, New Brunswick, 2004.
Pool, D. I., *Te Iwi Maori: A New Zealand Population, Present and Projected*, Auckland University Press, Auckland, 1991.
'Position Paper: Issues Arising from in Vitro Fertilisation, Artificial Insemination by Donor and Related Problems in Biotechnology', *NZMJ*, vol. 98, 22 May 1985, pp. 396–8.
'Position Paper: Retinopathy of Prematurity: A Statement by the Committee on the Fetus and Newborn of the Paediatric Society of New Zealand', *NZMJ*, vol. 98, 12 June 1985, pp. 446–7.
Posner, Tina, 'What's in a Smear? Cervical Screening, Medical Signs and Metaphors', *Science as Culture*, vol. 2, 2, 11, 1991, pp. 167–87.
Raffle, Angela and Muir Gray, *Screening: Evidence and Practice*, Oxford University Press, Oxford, 2007.
Rakusen, Jill, 'Depo-Provera: The Extent of the Problem', in Helen Roberts (ed.), *Women, Health and Reproduction*, Routledge & Kegan Paul, London, 1981, pp. 75–108.

Rakusen, Jill, with help from Julia Segal and Sue Barlow, 'Depo-Provera – Third World Women Not Told this Contraceptive is on Trial', in Sue O'Sullivan (ed.), *Women's Health: A Spare Rib Reader*, Pandora, London, 1987, pp. 164–6.
Rankine, Jenny, 'More Anti-abortion Arson', *Broadsheet,* vol. 150, 1987, p. 9.
Ray, Pauline, 'Abortion: A Shift of Opinion', *Thursday*, 30 August 1973, pp. 33–35.
——, 'Whose Body is it? Whose Baby is it?', *New Zealand Listener*, 15 March 1980, pp. 20–22.
——, 'When Babies are Inconceivable', *New Zealand Listener*, 25 June 1983, pp. 20–21.
——, 'Midwives' Tales', *New Zealand Listener*, 5 November 1983, pp. 16–17.
Reagan, Leslie, *When Abortion was a Crime: Women, Medicine, and Law in the United States, 1867–1973*, University of California Press, Berkeley, 1997.
Redman, C. W. G., 'Geoffrey Sharman Dawes', Royal College of Physicians, *Lives of the Fellows*, http://munksroll.rc.london.ac.uk/Biography/Details/1197.
Reed, Richard K., *Birthing Fathers: The Transformation of Men in American Rites of Birth*, Rutgers University Press, New Brunswick, 2005.
Reid, Brett, 'From Here to Maternity – National Women's Takes a "Leap Forward"', *New Zealand General Practice*, 28 August 1990, p. 8.
Reiger, Kerreen M., 'The Politics of Midwifery in Australia: Tensions, Debates and Opportunities', *Annual Review of Health Social Sciences*, vol.10, 2000, pp. 53–64.
——, *Our Bodies, Our Babies: The Forgotten Women's Movement*, Melbourne University Press, Melbourne, 2001.
Reiss, H. E., 'Francis James Browne, 1879–1963: A Great Obstetrician and a Great Teacher', *Journal of Obstetrics and Gynaecology*, vol. 24, 6, September 2004, pp. 696–9.
'Report: Contraception, Sterilisation and Abortion in New Zealand', *NZMJ*, vol. 85, 25 May 1977, pp. 441–5.
Revington, Mark, 'Born Free', *New Zealand Listener*, 14 August 1999, pp. 18–21.
Reynolds, L. A. and E. M. Tansey (eds), *Prenatal Corticosteroids for Reducing Morbidity and Mortality after Preterm Birth: The Transcript of a Witness Seminar held by the Wellcome Trust Centre for the History of Medicine at UCL, London, on 15 June 2004*, vol. 25, Wellcome Trust, London, 2005.
Rich, Adrienne, *Of Woman Born: Motherhood as Experience and Institution*, Norton, New York, 1976.
Robb, George Douglas, *Medical Odyssey*, Collins, Auckland, 1967.
Roberton, N. R. C., 'Advances in Respiratory Distress Syndrome', *BMJ*, vol. 284, 27 March 1982, pp. 917–18.
Roberts, Helen (ed.), *Women, Health and Reproduction*, Routledge & Kegan Paul, London, 1981.
Robinson, Jean, 'Cervical Cancer: Doctors Hide the Truth', *Spare Rib*, vol. 154, 1985, reprinted in Sue O'Sullivan (ed.), *Women's Health: A Spare Rib Reader*, Pandora, London, 1987, pp. 49–51.
——, 'Shaken Baby Syndrome: Caused by Hospital Care', *AIMS Journal*, Spring 2003, vol. 15, 1, http://www.aims.org.uk/Journal/Vol15No1/ShakenBabySyndrome.htm.
Rodgers, J. A., "A good nurse . . . a good woman": Duty and Obedience in Early New Zealand Nursing', in Roger Openshaw and David McKenzie (eds), *Re-interpreting the Educational Past: Essays in the History of New Zealand Education*, New Zealand Council for Educational Research, Wellington, 1987, pp. 54–63.
Rogers, A. F. C. and Judith F. Lenthall, 'Characteristics of New Zealand Women Seeking Abortion in Melbourne, Australia', *NZMJ*, vol. 81, 26 March 1975, pp. 282–6.
Rosier, Pat, 'Broadcast: A Feminist Victory', *Broadsheet*, vol. 161, September 1988, pp. 6–7.
Rothman, David, *Strangers at the Bedside: A History of How Law and Bioethics Transformed Medical Decision Making*, Basic Books, New York, 1991.
Royal Commission of Inquiry into Contraception, Sterilisation, and Abortion in New Zealand, *Report of the Royal Commission of Inquiry into Contraception, Sterilisation, and Abortion in New Zealand*, Government Printer, Wellington, 1977 (chair Duncan McMullin).

Bibliography

Saffron, Lisa, 'Cervical Cancer – The Politics of Prevention', *Spare Rib*, vol. 129, April 1983, reprinted in Sue O'Sullivan (ed.), *Women's Health: A Spare Rib Reader*, Pandora, London, 1987, pp. 42–49.
Sandelowski, M., *Pain, Pleasure and American Childbirth: From the Twilight Sleep to the Read Method, 1914–1960*, Greenwood Press, Westport, Connecticut, 1984.
Sargison, Patricia A., *Notable Women in New Zealand Health: Te Hauora ki Aotearoa : O na Wahine Rongonui*, Longman Paul, Auckland, 1993.
Savage, Wendy, 'Family Planning in a Hospital Clinic', *NZMJ*, vol. 83, 28 April 1976, pp. 261–5.
——, *A Savage Enquiry: Who Controls Childbirth?*, Virago, London, 1986.
Scott-Vincent, Robyn, 'Infertility: New Hope . . . For Some', *NZWW*, 17 March 1986, pp. 53–55.
Shaw, Sir William Fletcher, 'Report on the Obstetrical and Gynaecological Services of NZ', Supplement to the *NZMJ*, vol. 47, June 1948, pp. 8, 568–70.
Shearer, Madeleine H., 'Maternity Patients' Movements in the United States 1820–1985', in Iain Chalmers, Murray Enkin and Marc J. N. C. Keirse (eds), *Effective Care in Pregnancy and Childbirth*, *vol. 1*, Oxford University Press, Oxford, 1989, pp. 110–30.
Sinclair, Keith, *A History of the University of Auckland, 1883–1983*, Auckland University Press and Oxford University Press, Auckland,1983.
——, *A History of New Zealand*, Penguin, Auckland, revised edn, 2000.
Smith, D. M. and H. M. Carey, 'Continuous Integration of the Fetal Heart Rate', *NZMJ*, vol. 55, February 1956, pp. 309–12.
Smyth, Helen, *Rocking the Cradle: Contraception, Sex and Politics in New Zealand*, Steele Roberts, Wellington, 2000.
Sparrow, Margaret, *Abortion Then and Now: New Zealand Abortion Stories from 1940 to 1980*, Victoria University Press, Wellington, 2010.
Stace, Hilary, 'Fraser, Janet', from the *Dictionary of New Zealand Biography. Te Ara – the Encyclopedia of New Zealand*, updated 30 October 2012, http://www.TeAra.govt.nz/en/biographies/4f21/fraser-janet.
Stewart, C. R., K. R. Daniels and J. D. H. Boulnois, 'The Development of a Psychosocial Approach to Artificial Insemination by Donor Sperm', *NZMJ*, vol. 95, 8 December 1982, pp. 853–6.
Stewart, Sarah, 'Midwifery in New Zealand: A Cause for Celebration', *MIDIRS [Midwives' Information and Resource Service] Midwifery Digest*, vol. 11, 3, September 2001, pp. 319–22.
Stirling, Pamela, 'Hard Labour', *New Zealand Listener*, 12 March 1990, pp. 10–15.
Stojanovic, Jane, '"Leaving your dignity at the door": Maternity in Wellington 1950–1970', *New Zealand College of Midwives (Inc.) Journal*, vol. 31, October 2004, pp. 12–18.
——, 'Midwifery in New Zealand, 1904–1971', *Birthspirit Midwifery Journal*, vol. 5, February 2010, pp. 53–60.
Strid, Judi, 'Midwifery in Revolt', *Broadsheet*, November 1987, pp. 14–17.
Tansey, E. M. and D. A. Christie (eds), *Looking at the Unborn: Historical Aspects of Obstetric Ultrasound*, Wellcome Witnesses to Twentieth Century Medicine, March 1998, vol. 5, The Wellcome Trust, London, 2000.
Temkin, Elizabeth, 'Rooming-in: Redesigning Hospitals and Motherhood in Cold War America', *Bulletin of the History of Medicine*, vol. 76, 2, 2002, pp. 271–98.
Tennant, Margaret, 'Grace Neill in the Department of Asylums and Hospitals', *New Zealand Journal of History*, vol. 12, 1, April 1978, pp. 3–16.
Tew, Marjorie, *Safer Childbirth?: A Critical History of Maternity Care*, Free Association Books, London, 2nd edn, 1998.
'The Abortion Doctors: A Nationwide Survey of Certifying Consultants under the CS & A Act', *Broadsheet*, vol. 68, April 1979, pp. 20–23.
Thomas, G. T., 'Laparoscopy in Southland', *NZMJ*, vol. 91, 9 January 1980, pp. 10–12.

Bibliography

Thomas, Mary (ed.), *Post-war Mothers: Childbirth Letters to Grantly Dick-Read, 1946–1956*, University of Rochester Press, Rochester, 1997.
Tone, A., *Devises and Desires: A History of Contraceptives in America*, Hill & Wang, New York, 2001.
Topham-Kindley, Liane, 'Never Say Die: GPOs Meet for CME Talks', *New Zealand Doctor*, 6 October 2004, p. 9.
Tudehope, D. I. and C. Bagley, 'Techniques of Physiotherapy in Intubated Babies with Respiratory Distress Syndrome', *Australian Paediatric Journal*, vol. 16, 1980, pp. 226–8.
Urquhart-Hay, D., 'Voluntary Sterilisation in the Male', *NZMJ*, vol. 71, April 1970, pp. 230–2.
van der Krogt, Christopher, 'Barrer, Nina Agatha Rosamond – Biography', *Dictionary of New Zealand Biography. Te Ara – the Encyclopedia of New Zealand*, updated 1 September 2010, http://www.TeAra.govt.nz/en/biographies/4b6/1.
Wakely, Gerald, *For the Women of New Zealand: The Story of the National Women's Hospital: The Background, the Idea, the Chair, the Building*, Auckland Hospital Board, Auckland, 1963.
Walker, A. H. C., 'Liquor Amnii Studies in the Prediction of Haemolytic Disease of the Newborn', *BMJ*, vol. 2, 17 August 1957, pp. 376–8.
Walker, Arnold L., A. J. Wrigley, A. D. Marston, Katherine M. Hirst and W. J. Martin, *Report on Confidential Enquiries into Maternal Deaths in England and Wales 1952–1954*, Reports on Public Health and Medical Subjects, No. 97, HMSO, London, 1957.
Walker, Sir Arnold L., A. J. Wrigley, G. S. Organe, Marjorie Kuck and M. A. Heasman, *Confidential Maternal Mortality Report for 1961–63*, No. 115, HMSO, London, 1966.
Wall, Carroll, 'The Glamorous Gynaecologists: An Anarchy of the Heart', *Metro*, June 1984, pp. 32–50.
Warnock, Mary (chair), *Report of the Committee of Inquiry into Human Fertilisation and Embryology*, HMSO, London, 1984.
Wassner, Adelheid, *Labour of Love: Childbirth at Dunedin Hospital 1862–1972*, The Author, Dunedin, 1999.
Weisz, George, *Divide and Conquer: A Comparative History of Medical Specialization*, Oxford University Press, Oxford, 2006.
Wheeler, Jenny, 'Home or Hospital Birth? The Case for Both . . .', *NZWW*, 30 October 1978, pp. 28–30.
White, Heather J., S. C. Hawes and D. Heginbotham, *Report of the Abortion Supervisory Committee for the Year Ended 31 March 1986*, Abortion Supervisory Committee, Wellington, 1986.
Wichtel, Diana, 'Delivering with Style', *New Zealand Listener*, 21 September 1985, pp. 14–15, 34.
Wiles, Anton, 'Maternity – A Drastic Cut in Options for Women', *New Zealand Medical Association Newsletter*, 14 November 1997, pp. 3–4.
Williams, A. N. and R. Sunderland, 'Controversy: Neonatal Shaken Baby Syndrome: An Aetiological View from Down Under', *Archives of Disease in Childhood: Fetal and Neonatal Edition*, vol. 87, 2002, F29–F30.
Williams, A. Susan, *Women and Childbirth in the Twentieth Century: A History of the National Birthday Trust Fund 1928–93*, Sutton Publishing, Stroud, 1997.
Williams, Lynda, 'Dreaming the Impossible Dream: The Fate of Patient Advocacy', in Sandra Coney (ed.), *Unfinished Business: What Happened to the Cartwright Inquiry*, Women's Health Action, Auckland, 1993, pp. 88–102.
Williamson, N. W., 'Viewpoint: Abortion: A Legal View', *NZMJ*, vol. 72, October 1970, pp. 257–61.
Willocks, J. and A. A. Calder, 'The Glasgow Royal Maternity Hospital 1834–1984: 150 Years of Service in a Changing Obstetric World', *Scottish Medical Journal*, vol. 30, 1985, pp. 247–54.
Wolf, Jacqueline H., *Deliver Me From Pain: Anesthesia and Birth in America*, Johns Hopkins University Press, Baltimore, 2009.

Bibliography

Wolstenholme, G. E. W. and Maeve O'Connor (eds), *Foetal Autonomy: A Ciba Foundation Symposium*, J. & A. Churchill, London, 1969.
Wood, Pamela, 'Guest Editorial', *New Zealand College of Midwives (Inc.) Journal*, vol. 31, October 2004, pp. 4–6.
Woodford, F. Peter, *The Ciba Foundation: An Analytical History 1949–1974*, Associated Scientific Publishers, Amsterdam, 1974.
World Health Organization International Agency for Research on Cancer, *IARC Handbooks on Cancer Prevention, vol. 10, Cervix Cancer Screening*, IARC Press, Lyon, 2005.
Wright, Teresa, 'The Stoke CNEP Saga – How it Damaged All Involved', *Journal of the Royal Society of Medicine*, vol. 103, 7, 2010, pp. 277-82, doi: 10.1258/jrsm.2010.10k012.
Young, Gail, 'A Woman in Medicine: Reflections from the Inside', in Helen Roberts (ed.), *Women, Health and Reproduction*, Routledge & Kegan Paul, London, 1981, pp. 144–62.
'Your Choices in Childbirth', *Consumer*, no. 324, March 1994, pp. 6–9.
Zallen, D. T., D. A. Christie and E. M. Tansey (eds), *The Rhesus Factor and Disease Prevention: The Transcript of a Witness Seminar held by the Wellcome Trust Centre for the History of Medicine at UCL, London, on 3 June 2003*, vol. 22, Wellcome Trust, London, 2004.

THESES

Abel, Sally, 'Midwifery and Maternity Services in Transition: An Examination of Change following the Nurses Amendment Act 1990', PhD thesis, University of Auckland, 1997.
Barnett, Richard, 'Obstetric Anaesthesia and Analgesia in England and Wales 1945–1975', PhD thesis, University College London, 2007.
Bourke, Gabrielle, 'Illuminating the Dark Hour: Auckland's St Helens Hospital, 1906–1990', MA thesis, University of Auckland, 2006.
Brown, Hayley Marina, '"A Woman's Right to Choose": Second Wave Feminist Advocacy of Abortion Law Reform in New Zealand and New South Wales from the 1970s', MA thesis, University of Canterbury, 2004.
Daellenbach, Rea, 'The Paradox of Success and the Challenge of Change: Home Birth Associations of Aotearoa/ New Zealand', PhD thesis, University of Canterbury, 1999.
Gooder, Claire, 'A History of Sex Education in New Zealand, 1939–1985', PhD thesis, University of Auckland, 2010.
Grehan, Madonna May, 'Professional Aspirations and Consumer Expectations: Nurses, Midwives and Women's Health', PhD thesis, University of Melbourne, 2009.
Jeffery, Christina A., 'Whanautanga: The Experiences of Maori Women who Gave Birth at National Women's Hospital 1958–2004', MA thesis, University of Auckland, 2005.
Jenkins, Helen and Jocelyn Tracey, 'Comparison of Te Puke Maternity Hospital and National Women's Hospital, Community Health Project 1977/28', Medical School, University of Auckland.
Jowitt, Deborah, 'The H-Bug Epidemic: The Impact of Antibiotic-resistant Staphylococcal Infection on New Zealand Society and Health 1955–1963', MSc (Midwifery) thesis, AUT, 2004.
Wilson, Jennifer C., 'Hypertension of Pregnancy: A Study of Foetal Mortality and Maternal Prognosis in Pre-eclampsia and Essential Hypertension of Pregnancy Carried Out at National Women's Hospital, Auckland', Preventive Medicine dissertation, University of Otago, 1956.

INDEX

Abel, Sally, 207, 208, 235
abortion, 3, 7, 19, 113, 115, 140, 143, 144, 148, 151, 152–60, 160–5, 166
Abortion Act 1967 (UK), 157, 160
Abortion Law Reform Association of New Zealand, 154–5
Abortion Supervisory Committee, 161, 162, 165
Accident Compensation Corporation, 132–3, 229, 291n133; ACC Medical Misadventure Advisory Committee, 229
Adams, Jan, 229
Adams, Mrs, 34
Adamson, Karliss, 100
adrenocorticotrophin (ACHT), 121–2
Agricultural Research Council, Unit of Reproductive Physiology and Biochemistry (UK), 121
Aickin, Donald, 170
Aitken, (Sir) Robert, 40
Allan, Fred, 95
alternative birthing centres, 183–4
American College of Obstetricians and Gynecologists, 124, 126
American Society for the Study of Sterility, 107
amniocentesis, 96–7, 98, 115, 132, 133, 156
anaesthesia in childbirth, 13, 15–16, 17, 19, 54–5, 56–60, 61, 62, 63, 80, 101, 110, 121, 170, 171, 180, 206, 226, 234. *See also* pain relief, twilight sleep
Anaesthetic Appeal Fund (UK), 17
antenatal blood transfusion. *See* intrauterine blood transfusion
antenatal education, 61, 62, 66, 79, 177, 178–9, 188. *See also* Parents' Centre
Apgar scale, 66, 101
Apgar, Virginia, 101
artificial insemination: by donor, 111–12; by husband, 111
Asia-Oceania Congress on Perinatology, 198
Association of Radical Midwives (UK), 193
Auckland Area Health Board, 210, 214
Auckland Central Crown Health Enterprise, 223
Auckland City Hospital, 224, 232

Auckland District Health Board, 224, 231–2
Auckland Hospital Board, 22, 26, 34, 36, 39, 46, 68, 74, 76, 111, 113, 163, 170, 171, 174, 175, 176
Auckland Hospital, 22, 150, 231; Department of Critical Care, 137
Auckland Infertility Society, 114
Auckland Maternity Services Consumer Council, 216
Auckland Medical Aid Centre, 159
Auckland Medical Research Foundation, 119
Auckland University College *see* University of Auckland
Auckland Women's Health Council, 204, 216
Australian College of Midwives, 207
Averill, Isabel, 34
Averill, Leslie, 31
Avery, Mary E., 122, 268n36

Baird, (Sir) Dugald, 40
Baird, M. A. H. ('Tony'), 130, 159, 164, 197–8, 199, 218, 220
Baker, Jeffrey, 138
Baldwin, Mrs Stanley, 17
Barnes, Elsie, 149
Barrer, Nina, 33, 43, 250n43
Barrowclough, Ian, 168, 279n5
Bart, Pauline, 240
Bassett, Michael, 147, 201, 203, 204
Batcheler, Lynda, 148, 187, 188, 205
Beard, Richard, 198
Becroft, David, 271n102
Begg, Daisy, 36
Begg, Neil, 156
Bell, Robert, 38
Belsham, Sue, 164, 211, 213
Bethany Hospital, 22, 23, 63, 170
Bevan-Brown, Maurice, 61, 62
Bevis, Douglas, 96–7
bidets, 83
Billings, Margaret, 78
birth control. *See* contraception, family planning
birth, hospitalisation of, 4, 6, 7, 13–14, 15, 54, 62, 82, 85, 189, 195, 196, 197, 217, 237, 238, 246n32

Index

Birthcare, 224
Blanchette, Glenn, 222
Bloodworth, Rhoda, 34
Bonham, Dennis, 2, 6, 7, 46, 100, 104–7, 111, 112, 113–14, 116, 117, 118, 119, 120, 127, 130, 137, 138, 142–5, 149, 150–1, 155–6, 159, 160, 163–4, 164–5, 166, 167, 168, 169–70, 172, 173, 174, 176–7, 179, 180, 183, 187–8, 190, 191, 193, 196, 198–9, 200, 203, 204–6, 225, 226, 232, 239, 264n7, 279n12, 282n124
Bonham, Nancie, 106, 187
Bonita, Ruth, 146
Bonney, Victor, 30–1
Bourne, Aleck, 152
Boyd, Vivienne, 162
Brant, Herbert A. ('Bert'), 66–7
Brant, Margaret, 66–7
breastfeeding, 55, 73, 74, 75, 78, 79, 173, 174, 178, 195
Brew, Helen, 61–2, 83–4, 195
Brew, Quentin, 62
Bridgman, Geoffrey, 197
British College of Obstetricians and Gynaecologists. *See* Royal College of Obstetricians and Gynaecologists
British Medical Association, New Zealand Branch, 32, 34, 67, 80, 83, 143, 144, 204. *See also* New Zealand Medical Association
British Perinatal Mortality Survey, 169
Broadsheet, 7, 146, 147, 163–4, 191–2, 193, 194, 196, 197, 203, 239
Brown, James B., 108–9
Brown, Louise, 112
Brown, Miss G., 78
Brown, Tom, 128
Browne, Alan, 93, 101, 128–9, 133
Browne, Francis J., 60
Budd, Sandra, 213, 216, 223–4
Bunkle, Phillida, 145, 146, 147, 158, 192, 201, 204, 209
Burgess, Sian, 198–9
Bush, Alice, 67, 90
Buzzard, Sir Farquhar, 30

caesarean section, 24–5, 54, 64–6, 106, 170, 171, 180–1, 219
Calverley, Jill, 196
Calvert, Nora, 183–4
Cameron, Flora, 81, 83
Campaign Against Depo-Provera, 146
Campbell, Kate, 93
carcinoma *in situ*, 51, 106, 201–3

Cardiovascular Research Institute, University of California Medical Center, 118–19, 121
Carey, Harvey M., 6, 43, 45, 46, 47–8, 50, 51–3, 54, 57, 59, 60, 61, 62–3, 65, 66–7, 67–9, 72, 73, 74, 76, 79, 80, 81, 82–3, 93, 96, 100, 101, 106, 143, 239, 240–1. *See also* Pinkerton, Grace
Carey, Mark W., 47
Carlyon, Jenny, 234
Cartwright Inquiry/Report, 2, 3, 7, 146, 191, 201–2, 203–5, 206–7, 209, 210, 211, 212, 214, 215, 216, 220, 224, 225, 227, 228, 231, 240, 242
Cartwright, Ann, 174
Cartwright, Silvia, 2, 4, 201, 202, 203–4, 214
Casper, Monica, 99, 100, 156, 158
Cassey, Mrs, 21
Caton, Donald, 16
Caygill, David, 204
Central Health Services Council, Standing Maternity and Midwifery Advisory Committee (UK), 172
cervical cancer, 2, 51, 106, 201, 202, 204
Chalmers, Sir Iain, 124, 125
Chamberlain, Geoffrey, 78, 169
Chapman, Sylvia, 11
chest physiotherapy, 120, 228–30
Ciba Foundation Symposium 1968, 121–2, 127
Clark, Frederick, 46, 59
Clark, Helen, 200, 206–8, 221, 227
Clark, Patricia, 197
Clarke, Alison, 14, 16
Clarke, (Sir) Cyril, 134
Clarkson, John, 139
Clarkson, Pat, 188
Clarkson, Sarah, 162–3
Clentworth, Howard, 221
Clifton, Jan, 199
Climie, Richard ('Dick'), 57, 58, 59–60, 63, 101
clomiphine citrate, 110, 265n42
Coalition for Maternity Action, 199
Cochrane Centre (UK), 124
Cochrane Collaboration, 239; Coordinator in Menstrual Disorders, 226
Cocker, William H., 38, 39, 48
Cole, Christine, 85
Cole, David, 111, 225
Collison, Gabrielle, 164, 186, 211
Colombo Plan, 50
Columbia-Presbyterian Medical Center (US), 97

315

Combined Auckland Housewives' Associations, 83
Committee of Inquiry into Maternity Services 1937, 11, 13, 15, 19, 21, 22, 23–4, 25
Coney, Sandra, 146, 147, 148, 158, 187, 191, 192, 193, 196, 201, 203, 204, 209, 215–16, 221, 229, 283n10
consumer representatives, 2, 6, 8, 9, 62, 70, 78, 79, 83–4, 87, 136, 166, 173, 174, 183, 193, 199, 207, 211, 215–16, 224, 235, 236, 239, 242
continuous positive airways pressure, 119–20, 135
contraception, 3, 7, 69, 143. See also family planning
Contraception, Sterilisation, and Abortion Act 1977, 151, 161, 162, 163, 164
Contraceptive Choice Committee, 148
contraceptive pill, 145–6, 148, 151, 165; Roman Catholic pill, 69
cooling cap, 230–1
Coombs, Robin, 102; Coombs test, 102
Cooper, Deryn, 194, 197, 199
Coppleson, Malcolm, 202
Corbett, Jan, 204
Corkill, Brian, 160
Corkill, Thomas, 12–13, 57, 80
Cornwall Hospital. See National Women's Hospital
corticosteroids, 6–7, 120–6, 239
Coulter, Robert, 57
Council for the Single Mother and her Child, 191
Court, Denys, 217
Craven, Joseph, 22
Crick, Anthony, 64
Crimes Act: 1908, 152; 1961, 152, 206; Crimes Amendment Act 1977, 161
Crosse, Mary, 93
Crowley, John, 144
Crowley, Patricia, 124
Crowther, Vera, 18, 60–1, 193–4, 283n18
Crozier, Margaret, 197
Cull Report, 227, 229, 230, 242
Cull, Helen, 229

Daellenbach, Rea, 194–5
Dalkon Shield, 3, 147
Daly-Peoples, Linda, 197–8
Darlow, Brian, 139–40, 272n145
Dawes, Geoffrey, 121, 125, 126, 127, 128
Dawson, (Sir) Bernard, 12, 13, 29, 30, 35, 37, 48
Deem, Helen, 27, 28, 36, 88, 90

Delargey, Cardinal, 144
Depo-Provera, 145–7
Devonport Housewives' Union, 21
diagnostic ultrasound. See ultrasound
Diamond, Louis K., 95
Diasonograph, 129
Dickens, Val, 182, 188
Dick-Read, Grantly, 60–1, 62, 66, 74, 80, 82, 85, 93, 177, 182, 241, 255n87
direct-entry midwifery programmes, 199, 208, 238. See also midwives, training of
Dixon, Louisa, 74
Dobbie, Mary, 63, 68, 69, 74, 79, 81, 82, 83, 173
Dodd, Joan, 86
Doe v Bolton (US), 155
domiciliary confinement. See home birth
domiciliary midwives, 190, 193–4, 198–9, 200–1, 238. See also independent midwives
Donald, Ian, 47, 48, 64, 128, 129, 131, 157
Donley, Joan, 4–5, 7, 21, 169–70, 172, 184, 190, 193–4, 198, 199, 200, 204, 206–7, 209, 216, 237–8
Donnison, Jean, 54
Doppler ultrasound, 132
Doris Gordon Memorial Oration, 41
Dowbiggin, Ian, 149
Dower, John, 137, 138
Down's syndrome, 133, 140, 156–7
Du Chateau, Carroll. See Wall, Carroll
Dunkley, Penelope, 136, 197
Dunn, Hugh P. ('Pat'), 65–6, 112, 115, 144–5, 154, 175, 179–80, 281n80
Dunn, Peter, 94, 101, 119

East, Paul, 114
Eccles, John, 51
Edwards, Robert, 112, 115
Ehrenreich, Barbara, 3
Eickhoff, Louise, 178–9
Elliott, Bob, 138
Ellis, Joy, 114
Ellis-Crowther. See Crowther, Vera
English Population Investigation Committee (UK), 20
English, Deirdre, 3
Epsom Day Hospital, 160, 163–5
European Society of Perinatal Medicine, 125
exchange transfusion, 94, 95–6, 99, 102, 133, 134, 135–6

Falconer, Phoebe, 4
family planning, 55, 67, 82, 143–5, 148, 149, 150, 155, 205, 215. See also contraception

Index

Faris, Irwin B. ('Bill'), 42, 43, 129, 136, 158, 164, 170–1, 174
Farmer, Keitha, 188
Farquhar, Cynthia ('Cindy'), 205, 226, 232
fatherhood classes, 178
Federation of New Zealand Parents' Centres. *See* Parents' Centre
feminism, 3, 4, 5, 7, 18, 28, 60, 131, 133, 142, 145–6, 160, 162, 166, 174, 179, 181, 189, 190–209 *passim*, 216–17, 218, 235, 236, 238, 239–40. 242. *See also* women's health movement, women's liberation movement
Feminist Club, Sydney, 28
Feminists for Life, 174
Fenwick, George, 93
Fenwicke, Rosy, 186
Ferguson, William, 223
Fergusson, Lady Alice, 36
Fergusson, Sir Bernard, 104
Fertility Action, 131, 146–7, 204, 215
Fertility Associates, 111, 114
fertility services, 6, 103–16
fetal medicine, 6, 99, 100, 117, 224, 226, 241. *See also* maternal fetal medicine
Fisher, Geoffrey J. St C. ('Geoff'), 37–8, 39
Fisher, Isobel, 78
Fisher, Richard, 111, 112, 114, 115
Fleming, John, 132
forceps deliveries, 27, 54, 56, 59, 63–4, 219
Ford, Mrs, 55
Foucault, Michel, 235
France, John, 144, 226, 227, 282n124
Fraser, Florence, 129–30, 188
Fraser, Janet, 13, 19
Fraser, Peter, 13, 18, 22, 25
Freda, Vincent, 100

Garcia, Jo, 239
Gardiner, Cedric, 57–8
Gemzell, Carl, 108
Giesen, J. E. ('Ed'), 41, 108
'Glamorous Gynaecologists', 103, 209, 239
Gluckman, (Sir) Peter, 227, 230–1
Gluckman, Laurie, 153–4
Godber, Sir George, 167
Gordon, Doris, 5, 16–17, 21, 23, 26–30, 32–4, 35–7, 40–1, 43–4, 44–5
Gordon, Linda, 156
Gordon, William ('Bill'), 27
Graham, Frederick M. ('Freddie'), 112, 114, 115, 117
Graham, John, 227
Green, George Herbert ('Herb'), 38, 42, 46, 50–1, 51–2, 53, 59, 64, 81–2, 83, 91, 95, 96, 97–8, 106–7, 143, 146, 153, 155, 158, 159–60, 164, 167, 174, 176, 188, 190, 191, 201–3, 205, 280n51
Green Lane Clinical Centre, 232
Green Lane Hospital, 121, 164, 195, 215, 224, 232, 233
Gregory, George, 119
Grierson, John, 46
Grieve, Bruce, 53, 95, 96, 97, 102, 162, 177
Grieve, Ronald J. K. ('Ron'), 197
Grigor, R. Renton, 90, 95
Guilliland, Karen, 172, 205, 206, 216–17, 218, 220, 221, 222
Gunn, Alastair, 230
Gunn, Tania, 228, 230–1
gynaecology teaching associates, 215

Hamberger, Lars, 128
Hamilton, Rebecca, 112, 266n58
Hammersmith Hospital, London, 2, 47–8; Intensive Care Unit for Neonates, 90
Hanson, Clare, 128
Harbutt, Jefcoate, 39, 57
Harbutt, Kate, 183
Harding, Jane, 118, 226–7
Hare, Joyce, 77, 102
Harris, Aroha, 224
Hawksworth, William, 41, 45, 48, 251n91
H-bug, 73, 74, 104
Health Alternatives for Women Inc., 216
Health and Disability Commissioner, 221
Health and Disability Services Act 1996, 222
Health Benefits Review 1986, 206–7
Health, Minister of, 13, 18, 20, 23, 25, 29, 36, 37, 41, 55, 81, 84, 114, 147, 167, 168, 198, 201, 204, 206, 207
Henderson, Albert, 171
Henry, Gary, 223, 229–30
Hercus, Ann, 147, 200
Hercus, Charles, 23–4, 31
Hercus, Macky, 90
Hess, Julian, 89–90, 92
Hogan, Mrs, 55
Hogg, Vanya, 196
Holland, Eardley, 38
home birth, 5, 7, 13, 21, 62, 79, 84, 166, 167, 170, 184, 193–9, 200–1, 208, 209, 213, 217, 220, 224, 236, 238, 244n9
home-birth associations, 194–5. 197. *See also* New Zealand Home Birth Association
home-birth midwives. *See* domiciliary midwives

317

Index

Honeyman, Leslie, 113
Hood, John, 226, 227
Hope-Robertson, Walter, 93
Hospital Boards Employee Regulations 1947, 72
Hospitals Act 1957, 67
Hospitals and Charitable Institutions Amendment Act 1947, 40
Howie, Ross, 91, 92, 96, 101, 118–19, 120, 123, 125, 134, 135, 137–8, 139, 188, 205, 239
Human Assisted Reproduction Technology Act 2004, 112
human pituitary gonadotrophin, 108–10, 265n42
Humanae Vitae, 144
Hunter, Sir Thomas, 35, 37
Hutchinson, Amy, 13, 17, 22, 25, 34, 35
Hutchison, Ian, 183
Hutton, John, 176, 217
Hyman, Kay, 232

Ibbertson, Kaye, 109, 265n38
in vitro fertilisation, 107, 110, 112–16
incubators, 92, 109, 136
independent midwives, 7 208, 209, 213, 217–21, 222, 224. See also domiciliary midwives
infant mortality, 10, 33, 47, 58–9, 62, 64, 95, 196
infant welfare, 27, 88–9
Inquiry into Cervical Cancer at National Women's Hospital. *See* Cartwright Report
International Childbirth Conference 1973 (US), 192
International Childbirth Education Association, 195
intrauterine blood transfusion, 1, 98, 100, 104, 117, 129, 133–5
intrauterine device (IUD), 145, 147–8
Ironside, Wallace, 79

Jackson, Peter, 151–2
Jamieson, Murray, 132
Jeffcoate, Norman, 49
Jeffery, Christina, 75, 185, 214
Jellett, Henry, 11, 12, 24–5, 28, 64
Jenkin, Norma, 44–5
Jockel, Charles, 197
Jones, Ronald W. ('Ron'), 147, 151, 155–6

Kane, Amy, 34, 35
Karitane hospitals, 89–90, 93, 104
Kedgley, Sue, 172, 209

Kenrick, Selwyn, 24
Kent-Johnston, Agnes, 13, 19–20, 24
Kilpatrick, Robert, 239
King, (Sir) Frederic Truby, 88–9
King, James, 219
King, Nicky, 213
Kirk, Miss, 34
Kirk, Norman, 161
Kitzinger, Sheila, 181, 241
Knight, David, 138, 140–1, 173, 273n150
Knights, Lilian, 39
Kyle, Bernard ('Bernie'), 43, 63, 64, 179

La Leche League, 5, 174
Laing, R. D., 195, 241
Landsteiner, Karl, 94
Lawson quintuplets, 107, 109
Leavitt, Judith W., 3, 14, 15, 16, 85, 180, 181, 184
Leech, Valerie, 173
Lejeune, Jerome, 157
Levine, Philip, 95
Levy, Louis, 31, 34–5, 35
Lewis, Cecil, 38–9
Lewis, Jane, 14, 15
Liddell, Hilary, 148, 187, 205, 232
Liggins Institute. *See* University of Auckland
Liggins, Cecelia ('Celia'), 164, 188
Liggins, (Sir) Graham ('Mont'), 7, 52, 92, 107, 109, 119, 120–3, 124, 125, 126–8, 141, 145–6, 156, 160, 182, 183, 188, 203, 205, 226, 227, 232, 238–9
Liley, (Sir) William ('Bill'), 6, 7, 51–2, 65, 69, 75, 96–100, 102, 104, 106–7, 117, 120, 133–4, 141, 156–8, 161, 164, 178, 182, 227, 238, 241, 276n99
Liley, Margaret, 75, 77, 156, 179, 188
Limtrakarn, Jiree, 50
Loudon, Irvine, 16
Ludbrook, Samuel, 90
Lumley, Judith, 132

Macfarlane, Alastair, 39, 78
Macfarlane, Barbara, 194
MacGregor, Duncan, 10
Macintosh, (Sir) Robert, 30
Mackay, Joan, 169, 170, 173, 174, 193
Mackintosh, Andrew, 178, 197, 198, 199
Maclean, Hester, 13
MacLean, Norman, 115, 163
Malcolm, Aussie, 198
Mantell, Colin, 113, 164, 185, 196, 200, 204–5, 225, 226

Maori and maternity, 51, 82, 184–6, 195, 224
Maori Women's Welfare League, 186
Marsh, Margaret, 107, 110
Martin, John, 134
Mater Misericordiae Maternity Unit, 170
maternal fetal medicine, 219, 224, 226, 241. *See also* fetal medicine
Maternal Mortality Research Act 1968, 106, 167–8
maternal mortality, 12, 15, 28, 65, 106, 166, 167–8, 173, 196, 206; in Maori, 51
Maternity Action (Tauranga), 216
Maternity Action Alliance, 205
maternity benefit, 21, 25, 193, 216, 218, 222; in Canada, 247n67
Maternity Benefits Tribunal 1992, 216, 218
maternity nurses, training of, 24, 33, 40, 51, 55, 71–2, 73, 77, 80–1, 86, 170, 257n8
Maternity Patients' Bill of Rights, 174–5
Matheson, Clare, 206
Matthews, Jack D., 53, 72, 78, 90–2, 93, 94, 96, 101–2, 118, 119, 133, 135, 136, 138, 195–6
McAleer, Dorothy, 77, 104
McArthur, Barton, 123–4, 139
McCalman, Janet, 70, 72, 74, 77, 107, 109
McCowan, Lesley, 132, 148, 187, 205
McGeorge, Victor, 197
McGuire, Mrs, 13
McIndoe, William A. ('Bill'), 163, 201
McIntosh, Agnes, 34, 35
McKay, Don, 84
McKeown, Thomas, 202
McKinnon, Emily Siedeberg, 15
McLaren, Hugh, 155
McLeod, Grant Liley, 99
McMillan, David, 9
McMullin, Duncan W., 161
mechanisms of labour, 121–2, 126–7
Medical Council of New Zealand, 24, 205, 229; Central Ethical Committee, 160
Medical Practitioners Disciplinary Committee, 220
Medical Research Council of New Zealand, 51, 100, 121, 126, 134, 145, 146, 230; National Hormone Committee, 110; report on neonatal and infant health 1973, 138; Standing Committee on Therapeutic Trials, 146
Mein Smith, Philippa, 207–8
Metro, 103, 112, 116, 117, 158, 201, 203, 209, 239

Middlemore Hospital, 171, 172, 226, 279n30
Midwives Act, England and Wales 1901, 244n7
Midwives Registration Act 1904, 10
midwives, training of, 10–11, 23–4, 28, 33, 40, 71, 86, 170, 208, 212, 238. *See also* direct-entry midwifery programmes
Millar, Margaret, 73, 76
Miller, Mrs L. F., 171
Minnitt, R. J., 18
Mitchinson, Wendy, 5, 14
Moir, J. Chassar, 29
Molesworth, Nellie, 19
Moncrieff, Alan, 88, 90
Moody, Allan, 34
Morris, Norman, 172
Morton, William T. G., 15
Muldoon, Robert, 170, 279n22
Munn, Stephen, 140
Murphy-Lawless, Jo, 3
Murray, Nigel, 223
Murray, Verna, 136, 178, 182, 197, 238
Mushin, William, 59

Nash, (Sir) Walter, 79
Nash, Diana, 208, 217
National Birthday Trust Fund (UK), 17–18, 169
National Consumer Council, 84
National Council of Women, 14, 17, 18, 22, 23, 25, 28, 32, 33–4, 37, 41, 45, 47, 55, 78, 81, 82, 83, 84, 87, 162, 235; Maternity Services Sub-committee, 36
National Institutes of Health (US), 124, 132
National Organisation of Women, 174
National Twilight Sleep Association (US), 16
National Women's Health, 232
NATIONAL WOMEN'S HOSPITAL: Care and Respect of Public Patients at National Women's Hospital Sub-committee, 176; Child Development Unit, 139; clinical director of maternal fetal medicine, 226; clinical director of newborn services, 138; clinical reports, 46, 51, 54, 59, 63, 64, 91, 92, 219, 220; clinical services general manager, 232; Clinico-Pathological Discussions of all Stillbirths and Neonatal Deaths, 53, 94; Cornwall Hospital, 39, 46, 90, 185; Cornwall Suite, 224; Department of X-raying and Ultrasound Scans, 130; endocrine laboratory, 108; Ethical Committee, 188; Family Planning Clinic, 143; Fertility Plus, 115; fundraising,

35–6, 37; general manager, 164, 211, 213, 218, 223, 229; hospital logo, 243–4n22; Hospital Medical Committee, 53, 56–7, 65, 68, 73, 74, 75, 80, 85, 90, 91, 94, 96, 101, 102, 108, 122, 123, 129, 130, 136, 143, 150, 152, 153, 154, 155–6, 174, 176, 177, 180, 182, 183–4, 188; Infertility Clinic, 107, 110; Infertility Research Trust, 114; IVF Unit, 114; Lactation Department, 78; Maori health manager, 224; male charge midwife, 188; male maternity nurse, 71, 257n7, 259n77; manager of maternity and neonatal services, 211, 216, 220, 223, 224; maternity access rights co-ordinator, 224; medical social worker, 76; medical superintendent, 52, 68, 69, 159; medical superintendent (first female), 186; medical superintendent post disestablished, 211; miscarriage support programme, 131; Neonatal Intensive Care Unit, 133, 135, 137, 227–8; neonatal tutor specialist, 135; Nursing Advisory Committee, 177; official opening 1964, 1, 103–4; Paediatric Department, 90, 96, 101–2, 133; Parents' Hospital Committee, 63; patient advocate, 131, 214–15; pink room, 184, 186, 236; Postgraduate School of Obstetrics and Gynaecology, 2, 5, 26–45 *passim*, 50, 51–2, 56, 69, 97, 100, 106, 113, 119, 166, 173, 190, 209, 225–6, 236; Premature Baby Unit, 133; private beds in, 41, 48, 49; Project 95, 223; purpose-built hospital, 1, 49, 60, 75, 102, 103, 232; radium treatment facilities, 104; recurrent miscarriage clinic, 187; relocation (2004), 8, 224, 232; resident paediatric officer, 51; Rh Sub-committee, 96, 125; Special Care Babies Unit, 227–8; Termination Committee, 152, 153; Women's Health Information Centre, 216; 'Whanau Room', 184–6

natural childbirth, 6, 60–3, 74, 173, 181, 193, 196, 240–1

Natural Childbirth Association. *See* Parents' Centre

Natural Family Planning Association, 144

Neal, Sue, 146

Neill, Grace, 23

neonatal intensive nursing care course, 136

neonatal paediatrics, 75, 93, 100–102, 118, 119, 137, 181, 228

neonatology, 75, 89, 90–1, 101, 226–7

New Zealand Board of Health, 15, 84; Maternity Services Committee, 83–4, 106, 144, 151, 166, 200; Women's Health Committee, 200

New Zealand Board of Physiotherapists, 229

New Zealand College of Midwives, 206, 207, 213, 216, 221; *Journal*, 237, 238

New Zealand Department of Health, 11, 16–17, 22, 23, 32, 34, 35, 67, 68, 83, 113, 154, 168, 235; consultant in maternity, 166, 169; consultant obstetrician, 11, 28; director of maternal and child welfare, 169; director of maternal welfare, 83; director of nursing, 13, 81; director-general of health, 23, 75, 83, 148, 229; medical statistician, 57; nursing regulations, 72; 'safe maternity campaign', 27

New Zealand Diploma in Obstetrics, 49–50

New Zealand Doctors for Life, 115, 163

New Zealand Family Planning Association, 55, 67, 143–4, 145, 151, 166, 215

New Zealand Federation of University Women, 75–6, 77, 78, 84, 87

New Zealand Home Birth Association, 5, 197, 199, 224

New Zealand Labour Party, women's branches, 19, 25

New Zealand Medical Association, 204. *See also* British Medical Association, New Zealand Branch

New Zealand Medical Women's Association, 67

New Zealand Nurses Association, 197, 207; Midwives Section, 5, 205; Midwives and Obstetric Nurses Special Interest Section, 207

New Zealand Obstetrical and Gynaecological Society, 9, 11–12, 20, 21, 26, 27, 28–9, 31, 32, 34, 35, 36, 39, 54, 57, 83, 122, 146; renamed Royal New Zealand College of Obstetricians and Gynaecologists, 289n65

New Zealand Obstetrical Society. *See* New Zealand Obstetrical and Gynaecological Society

New Zealand Perinatal Society, 106, 117, 125

New Zealand Registered Nurses Association, Obstetrical Branch, 20

New Zealand Society for the Protection of Women and Children, 15, 18, 19, 20, 22, 23, 25, 34, 235

New Zealand Women's Health Network, 200

Nicolson, Malcolm, 132

Nightingale, Anne, 22, 72, 211, 212, 214, 220, 223

Nilsson, Lennart, 128

Index

Nixon, William, 46, 78, 105, 143, 169, 172, 173
North, Derek, 205, 209
Nordmeyer, Arnold, 36, 37, 55–6
North Shore Hospital, 171, 172
Northcroft, Hilda, 34, 35
Nurses Act 1971, 193, 206
Nurses Amendment Act 1990, 7, 206–8, 217, 218, 219, 221, 236
Nurses and Midwives Registration Act 1925, 71
Nurses and Midwives Registration Board, 67, 70, 71, 73–4, 80, 81–3, 136, 257n2
Nurses Registration Act 1901, 10
Nursing Council of New Zealand, 136, 221, 229, 257n2

Oakley, Ann, 4, 130–1, 169, 209, 243n12, 283n10
Oamaru Mothers' Group, 82, 84
Obstetrical Endowment Appeal, 28–9, 35–6, 43
Obstetrics and Gynaecology Endowment Fund, 225
Obstetrics and the Winds of Change 1979, 166, 175, 183
obstetrics, establishment of chairs: Auckland, 37–8, 39–40; Otago, 31; Melbourne, 28; New South Wales, 69; Sydney, 28
Odent, Michel, 181
Olssen, Mark, 4, 237
Oxford Database of Perinatal Trials (UK), 124

Paediatric Society of New Zealand, 90, 139
Paget, Tom, 11, 12, 13, 19, 23, 27, 32
pain relief, 12, 15–20, 27, 29, 55–6, 57, 60–1, 63, 86, 191, 236, 240. *See also* anaesthesia, twilight sleep
Pairman, Sally, 206, 216, 218
panning and swabbing, 72–3, 79
Papps, Elaine, 4, 237
Parents' Centre, 5, 6, 61, 62–3, 66, 67–8, 69, 74, 78–81, 82, 83–5, 87, 142, 166, 173, 174, 195, 198, 208, 216, 222, 235, 236, 239; Educational Advisory Council, 80, 259n74; first Dominion conference, 61, 62, 78–9
Parker, R. B., 58
Patients' Rights Advocacy Waikato Inc., 216
Pattison, Neil, 134–5, 223–4
Pattrick, Anne, 89
Peek, John, 112, 114
Peel, Sir John, 105, 264n7
Pelvin, Bronwen, 208

perinatal medicine, 3, 6, 96, 103, 117–41 *passim*
perinatal mortality, 97, 106, 118, 133, 166, 169, 198
Phillips, Leo, 74, 94, 96
phototherapy, 134
Pickup, Dennis, 223
Pincus, Gregory, 145
Pinkerton, Grace, 47, 67, 252n4. *See also* Carey, Harvey M.
Pitt, Albert, 10
Plunket Society, 5, 27, 36, 62, 89, 139, 158, 228; Plunket nurses, 72, 186; director of nursing, 89; medical adviser, 88; mothers' clubs, 82
Plunkett, Tom, 37–8, 39, 55, 58, 61, 90, 91
Port, Elizabeth ('Betty'), 48
Posner, Tina, 202
Postgraduate School of Obstetrics and Gynaecology. *See* National Women's Hospital
prematurity, 6, 51, 58–9, 63, 75, 78, 88–94, 96–7, 102, 104, 118–20, 122, 123, 125, 126, 133, 134, 135, 137, 138–9, 140, 228, 230, 241
Pot, Marjet, 224
Public Health and Disability Act 2000, 290n80
Purdue, Connie, 174, 183

Queen Mother's Maternity Hospital, Glasgow, 129

Read, Charles, 40
Reagan, Leslie, 152, 154
rectal examination, 81, 260n82
Reid, Stanley, 183
Reports on Confidential Enquiries into Maternal Deaths (UK), 57, 59, 65
respiratory distress syndrome (RDS), 6, 99, 102, 118–20, 122, 123, 126, 135
retrolental fibroplasia, 92–3, 119, 139
Rhesus haemolytic disease, 94–100, 102, 106, 133–4, 135
Richards, Martin, 239
Riley, Frederick, 29
Robb, (Sir) Douglas, 1, 36, 37, 40, 44, 104, 117, 238
Roberts, Helen, 148, 215, 240
Robins, A. H., 147. *See also* Dalkon Shield
Robinson, Jeffrey, 210, 224
Robinson Review (1995), 211, 215, 217, 217, 223, 231
Rock, John, 107

321

Rodeck, Charles, 100
Roe v Wade (US), 157
Roke, Christine, 148
Ronner, Wanda, 107, 110
rooming-in, 74–6, 79, 84, 86, 173, 174, 258–9n40
Ross, Dame Hilda, 79
Ross, Sir James Paterson, 53
Rothman, David, 140
Rotunda Hospital, Dublin, 11, 93, 101, 128–9, 133
Rowley, Simon, 140, 181
Rowling, Wallace E. ('Bill'), 161
Royal College of General Practitioners, maternity spokesperson, 223
Royal College of Obstetricians and Gynaecologists, 30, 32, 35, 38, 39, 44, 49, 83, 124, 132; New Zealand council of, 160; president of, 30, 32, 38, 40, 105, 203
Royal New Zealand Plunket Society. *See* Plunket Society
Royal Women's Hospital, Melbourne, 27, 60, 70, 72, 74, 77, 78, 93, 107, 109, 112, 223, 231
Ruakura Agricultural Research Station, 120
Rutter, Frank, 113, 171
Ryan, Hugh, 93

Salvation Army, 22, 23, 63, 170
Sargison, Patricia, 194
Savage, Wendy, 204–5
Save the Midwife Association, 5, 199
Sayers, Susan ('Sue'), 135–6
Sayes, Edwin, 50
Scelly, Rissa, 76
Scoggins, Bruce, 231
Scott, Sir John, 69, 105, 146, 205
Seaman, Barbara, 145
Seddon, Richard (obstetrician), 109, 143, 148, 200
Seddon, Richard (politician), 10, 14, 23
sex education, 142–3
Sex Hygiene and Birth Regulation Society. *See* New Zealand Family Planning Association
Shaw, Percy, 37
Shaw, William Fletcher, 29, 30, 32, 36, 38
Shieff, Bernard, 110
Short, Roger, 121
Simpson, James Young, 15, 29
Sinclair, Sir Keith, 106
Sisters Overseas Service, 162
Smail, Sheryl, 218
Smith, Mrs David, 34

Smyth, Gerald Spence, 42, 43, 49, 71, 78
Smyth, Helen, 143
Social Security Act 1938, 20, 21, 49
Society for the Promotion of Health of Women and Children. *See* Plunket Society
Society for the Protection of the Unborn Child, 7, 154, 155, 156, 157–8, 161, 162
Soljak, Miriam, 174
Sorrento Maternity Hospital, Birmingham (UK), 93, 118
Special Care Services for the Newborn in New Zealand report, 1982, 139
Spence, Matthew ('Matt'), 137
SPUC. *See* Society for the Protection of the Unborn Child
St Helens hospitals, 10, 11, 14, 15, 16, 17, 18, 19, 20, 22–3, 24, 28, 31, 32, 33, 40, 71, 76, 83, 86, 137, 170, 171, 188, 194, 197, 211, 238, 244n9, 245n27
Stacey, Gwen, 84, 261n105
Stallworthy, (Sir) John, 29–30, 36, 40–1, 43, 45, 99, 108, 264n7
Stallworthy, Arthur, 29
Status of Children Act 1987, 112
Stent, Robyn, 221
Steptoe, Patrick, 112, 115
sterilisation, 7, 64, 110, 143, 148–52, 174
Stewart, Alice, 128
Stewart, John, 53
Stewart, Mrs, 21
Stimpson, Glenda, 182
Stojanovic, Jane, 237
Stone, Peter, 219, 224, 226, 227
Strang, Leonard, 122
Strid, Judi, 193, 209, 216, 239
Sullivan, John, 94
surfactant, 122
Sutherland, Allan, 220

Tarnier, Stephane, 92
Taylor, Howard C., 97
Taylor, John, 143, 151, 153, 163, 164
termination of pregnancy. *See* abortion
test tube babies, 112–13. *See also in vitro* fertilisation
Tew, Marjorie, 4
Thailand, training of doctors from, 50
Thomas, Mary, 54
Thomson, Heather, 162
Tizard, Bob, 168
Townsend, Lance, 62
toxaemia, 48, 53, 91
Treaty of Waitangi Act 1975, 185

Tretheway, Moira, 99
tubal ligation, 148–9, 151–2, 274n43
Turbott, Harold, 83
Turner, Gillian, 2, 205, 218, 225–6
twilight sleep, 16–17, 35
Twydle, Barry, 188

ultrasound, diagnostic, 6, 47, 114, 128–33, 135, 270n76
unborn child, 6, 7, 99–100, 102, 115, 126–8, 140, 156, 157, 158, 161, 163, 226, 241. *See also* Society for the Protection of the Unborn Child
Unemployed Workers' Union, Women's Auxiliary, 21
'Unfortunate Experiment', 2, 201–6, 209
United Women's Convention, 200
University College Hospital, London, 46, 66, 77–8, 100, 105, 122, 143
University of Auckland: Auckland University College, 37–8, 39, 43; dean of medicine, 38, 111, 205, 209, 225; Department of Obstetrics and Gynaecology, 204, 225–6, 227; Liggins Institute, 126, 227; post-graduate professor of obstetrics and gynaecology, 46, 47, 169, 225, 232; professor of maternal fetal medicine, 226, 241; professor of neonatology, 226–7; professor of obstetric and gynaecological endocrinology, 126; Research Centre in Reproductive Medicine, 226; research professor in perinatal physiology, 100, 117; Ryburn Committee, 209; School of Medicine, 36, 37, 38, 106, 187, 191, 209, 225; Women's Liberation Group, 154
University of California Davis, 120–1
Upjohn Company, 145, 146, 147
Urquhart-Hay, Donald, 150

vasectomy, 149–51
Veale, Arthur, 156
ventilators, 118, 119–20, 135, 272n137

Waikato Women's Hospital, 137
Wairoa Hospital, 82–3
Waitakere Hospital, 172, 194
Walker, A. H. C., 96
Wall, Carroll, 103, 113, 117, 209
Wallace, Augusta, 162
Waller, Harold, 78
Walsh, Ngaire, 144

Warnock, Mary, 115
Warren, Alexander, 150
Warren, Algar, 68, 102, 109, 136, 159–60, 178
Watt, James, 79–80
Watt, Michael, 23
Wealthall, Stephen, 135
Welch, Robert, 120
Welfare of Women and Children, Minister for, 79
Wellington Women's Hospital, 217
Wells, Horace, 15
Werry, John, 154, 159, 187
West Auckland Women's HealthWatch, 131
Weston, Philip, 229
Wheeler, Jenny, 196
whenua, 99, 185, 263n63
White, Heather, 162
White, Mrs Charles, 34
Whiteman, Carolynn, 224
Whither Obstetrics? 1982, 198
Wiener, Alexander, 94
Williams, Lynda, 131, 215, 217
Wilson, Alexander, 34
Wilson, Jennifer, 148, 188, 282n127
Windeyer, J. C., 28
Wolf, Jacqueline, 63
Women's Affairs, Ministry of, 147, 200, 203
Women's Electoral Lobby (Waikato) Inc., 216
women's health movement, 7, 130, 166, 191. *See also* feminism
Women's Health Special Interest Group, 216
women's liberation movement, 142, 146, 160. *See also* feminism
Women's National Abortion Action Campaign, 161
Wood, Elizabeth, 181
Wood, Pamela, 237
Wood, W. L., 22
Woolf, Virginia, 17
Woolnough, James, 159
World Health Organization, 93, 200; Advisory Panel on Maternal and Child Health, 106; Advisory Panel on Perinatal Mortality, 106; Human Reproduction Program, 123
Wright, Lawrence, 83
Wright, Liam, 49, 162, 164, 183

Young, Carolyn, 194
Young, Diony, 195
Young, Gail, 240